Progress in Drug Research

Founded by Ernst Jucker

Series Editors

Prof. Dr. Paul L. Herrling
Novartis International AG
CH-4002 Basel
Switzerland

Alex Matter, M.D., Director
Novartis Institute for Tropical Diseases
10 Biopolis Road, #05-01 Chromos
Singapore 138670
Singapore

Progress in Drug Research

Imaging in Drug Discovery and Early Clinical Trials

Vol. 62

Edited by
Markus Rudin

Birkhäuser Verlag
Basel · Boston · Berlin

Editor:

Prof. Dr. Markus Rudin
Institute for Biomedical Engineering
University of Zürich/ETH Zürich
Moussonstr. 18
CH – 8092 Zürich
Switzerland

ISBN-10: 3-7643-7157-9   Birkhäuser Verlag, Basel – Boston – Berlin
ISBN-13: 978-3-7643-7157-9

© 2005 Birkhäuser Verlag, P.O. Box 133, CH-4010 Basel, Switzerland
Part of Springer Science+Business Media
Printed on acid-free paper produced from chlorine-free pulp. TCF ∞
Cover design and layout: Micha Lotrovsky, CH-4106 Therwil, Switzerland
Printed in Germany

ISBN-10:7643-7157-9   e-ISBN: 3-7643-7426-8
ISBN-13: 978-3-7643-7157-9

9 8 7 6 5 4 3 2 1   www.birkhauser.ch

Contents

Contents

Foreword

Imaging techniques are undergoing a tremendous development. The clinically established methods such as X-ray computerized tomography (CT), magnetic resonance imaging (MRI), ultrasound imaging, and nuclear imaging provide structural and functional data of ever increasing quality. Today, the speed of data acquisition allows making efficient use of the measurement time; the collection of multiple complementary datasets during a single imaging session enhances the reliability of the diagnostic/prognostic information. Improved image processing tools enable three-dimensional visualization of imaging data as well as the derivation of biomedical relevant information from the primary imaging data. In the recent years, target-specific, so-called molecular imaging approaches have been developed at a rapid pace. Information such as target expression, target function, pathway activities (e.g., protein-protein interactions), or cell migration can meanwhile be studied in the intact organism with reasonable spatial and temporal resolution. While most of these methods are currently confined to animal studies, they will be translated in a not too distant future also to the clinical arena. The value of these techniques, which allow visualizing the underlying molecular mechanism associated with disease, as a basic research tool and, most importantly, for diagnostics will be enormous. In addition, the use of multiplexed imaging methods will enable the comprehensive characterization of a therapeutic intervention, visualizing and measuring the biodistribution of both the drug and the drug target, the drug-target interaction, the activation of signal transduction pathways, and ultimately the morphological and physiological consequences of these molecular events.

It is obvious that aside from the already established relevance in medical diagnostics, imaging techniques will play a major role in the development of novel therapies. As non-invasive modalities they are readily translatable from a preclinical to a clinical setting. There is considerable hope that imaging methods, in conjunction with other bio-analytical techniques, will provide early information of drug efficacy, much earlier than conventional pharmacological readouts. Drug development resources could then be focused on the most promising development candidates, for which pilot clinical trials using imaging readouts have demonstrated proof of the therapeutic concept. This potentially would save considerable resources and might expedite translational and clinical studies, from which ultimately the patient would profit. Non-invasive imaging enhances the diagnostic accuracy, enabling medical personnel to select and tailor the therapy strategy in an optimal way; monitoring the patient's therapy response will allow optimizing the treatment regimen.

The objective of this volume is to illustrate the role of non-invasive imaging for modern drug discovery and development. There is considerable expectation by many different stakeholders that investments in imaging technology will add value to the process of developing a novel drug: for biomedical researches imaging should enhance the basic understanding of the disease process, for the drug development it should yield unambiguous information that facilitates proper decision making allowing to focus resources, for management it should expedite the development process and thus reduce costs, for marketing it should provide compelling visual evidence of drug efficiency that would convince prescribers to choose this drug, for the regulators validated imaging data might replace softer endpoints that are currently used for many indications. Most importantly, patients would profit from better monitoring and better medicine.

The layout of the book follows the drug discovery process, from the target selection/validation (molecular imaging) to the clinical drug evaluation and ultimately to the approval by regulatory authorities. Chapter 1 by Paul L Herrling gives an overview of the drug discovery process from the selection of a potential drug target to the handover to the clinical development. The layout of the volume essentially follows this process. In Chapter 2, Tobias Schäffter discusses the basic principles of the individual non-invasive imaging techniques that are used as clinical diagnostic tools.

The information provided by modern imaging techniques extends far beyond the structural-anatomical readouts obtained from the first X-ray studies. Today, information on molecular and cellular events, physiological and metabolic processes can be gathered in the intact organism, which complements structural information. Molecular and cellular imaging approaches translate many assays developed for molecular and cell biological studies into paradigms suited for in vivo visualization. These aspects are discussed in Chapters 3 by David Sosnovik and Ralph Weissleder focusing on MRI and optical (fluorescence) imaging techniques, and in Chapter 4 by Olivier Gheysens and Sam Gambhir with special emphasis on nuclear and optical (bioluminescence) methods. Molecular imaging approaches will impact drug discovery at all phases: from the visualization of the target expression and target function, to the molecular proof-of-therapeutic mechanism at a molecular level in the intact organism – ultimately in the patient.

The use of genetically modified organisms, and in particular mice, for testing biological hypotheses or as models of human diseases has become indispensable in modern biomedical research. This demands tools for rapid and efficient characterization of such animals with the intention to link molecular, physiological, metabolic or structural peculiarities to genetic modifications (phenotyping). Transgene insertion is a random process, correspondingly large numbers of mice have to be analyzed to identify the desired phenotypes. Non-invasive methods play an important role in this task; these aspects are addressed by R. Mark Henkelman et al. in Chapter 5.

Following target identification and validation and the screening of large compound libraries, potential drug candidates have to be optimized with regard to efficacy, pharmacokinetic properties, and safety. This lead optimization phase involves the qualitative and quantitative evaluation of drug effects in models of human disease, as discussed by Markus Rudin et al. in Chapter 6. Mark Tengowski and John Kotyk illustrate the role of imaging, and in particular MRI for the evaluation of potential safety issues and toxicological effects.

A prerequisite for clinical drug evaluation is knowledge of the drug's pharmacokinetic (PK) properties. *In vivo* PK studies are based on positron-emission tomography (PET) using radiolabeled drug molecules. Aspects of tracer synthesis, PET experiments, and the extraction of quantitative information from PET data are topic of Chapter 8 by Mats Bergström and Bengt Langström. Clinical drug evaluations, in particular when targeting chronic diseases require large patient populations, are time consuming and therefore expensive. To optimize the chances for success, pilot studies aiming to demonstrate proof of the pharmacological concept would be of outmost importance. Such studies depend on the availability of biomarkers that are indicative of treatment outcome. Biomarkers would also be of value for stratifying patient groups, a higher homogeneity of the population, increasing the relevance of the study. In Chapter 9 Janet Miller and Greg Sörensen discuss the potential of imaging biomarkers for diagnosis and prognosis of human stroke as well as for the evaluation of therapeutic interventions. In particular, the concept of using the patient as its own control is highly attractive. Finally, Chapter 10 is devoted to the use of imaging readouts for clinical drug trials. David Lester puts special emphasis on regulatory aspects, discussing efforts by the regulatory authorities regarding the use of innovative methodologies such as imaging in drug approval process.

Zürich, May 2005   Markus Rudin

Progress in Drug Research, Vol. 62
(Markus Rudin, Ed.)
© 2005 Birkhäuser Verlag, Basel (Switzerland)

The drug discovery process

By Paul L. Herrling

Novartis International AG
Corporate Research
CH-4002 Basel, Switzerland
<paul.herrling@novartis.com>

1   Introduction

In recent years drug discovery science has evolved into a distinct branch of science. It is highly multidisciplinary including among others, the disciplines of chemistry, multiple branches of biology (from molecular to behavioral biology), biophysics, computer sciences, mathematics and engineering. It distinguishes itself from academic biomedical sciences by having as its goal and measure of success a pharmacological therapy, while the focus of the academic environment is the generation of new knowledge. Scientists in a drug discovery environment must, therefore, be able to work in multidisciplinary teams, often not of their choosing, and must be able to communicate their specialist knowledge to scientists in other disciplines. They must equally be able to understand the contributions of other specialists towards their common goal. Drug discovery scientists adapt their scientific activities to the requirements of the project to which they contribute, and are often required to abandon one of their own ideas to contribute to somebody else's. This is distinctly different from the academic environment where scientists typically follow their own ideas and their interests, generated usually by the results of their previous research or occasional scientific 'hot topics'.

However, the interaction between academic and drug discovery sciences is essential. The life sciences (including chemistry) are absolutely central to drug discovery because they are needed to improve the knowledge about disease processes to enable progress in pharmacological (and biological) therapies. The life sciences are currently in an exponential phase of knowledge generation, which occurs primarily in the academic environment; therefore, drug discovery scientists need to have very close and frequent interactions with their colleagues in academia.

The tremendous progress in biomedical knowledge and technology in the last 10 years necessitated a complete redesign of the drug discovery process. Some of the key factors mandating change were: (1) an exponential increase in the number of therapeutic targets (a therapeutic target is the precise molecular entity in the human body that interacts with a therapeutic compound to achieve a biological effect in the context of disease), and (2) the discovery of very high levels of complexity in terms of interactions among genes (gene networks) and their products, as exemplified by the combinatorial interaction of proteins in signaling pathways. In 1996, all existing therapeutic agents interacted with an estimated 500 drug targets [1], but the sequencing of the human genome revealed about 25000–30000 protein-coding genes [2, 3]. If one takes into account splicing and post-translational modifications, it can be estimated that there must be more than 100000 functionally different proteins assuming 25000 protein-coding genes [4], and a conservative average of five splice variants per protein. It is estimated that 57% of the human protein-coding genes display alternative splicing, and that they contain an average of 9 (8.94) exons [5], this would result in about 125000 proteins. This number does not take into account post-translational modifications such as proteolytic processing of larger proteins into smaller active ones or RNA editing [6, 7]. Some estimates indicate that only 5000–10000 of these proteins might be useful drug targets (or 'drugable') [8]. However, this was based on an estimate of 'disease' genes, and there might be many more proteins involved in disease processes than the number of 'disease' genes. Whatever the correct number is, it is orders of magnitudes larger than the past number of available targets, necessitating a high throughput strategy to validate and screen them.

This chapter summarizes some of the key steps in the drug discovery process, and describes some of the main activities at the different stages of the process. It aims at helping to understand the contributions of imaging described in the following chapters in the context of the whole drug discovery process.

2 The drug discovery (and development) phases: overview

The drug discovery community distinguishes four main discovery phases and four clinical phases (Fig. 1)

2.1 The D0 phase

Before the drug discovery process can begin, the strategic selection of therapeutic areas of interest to the company must be made, as no company will address all areas of medicine.

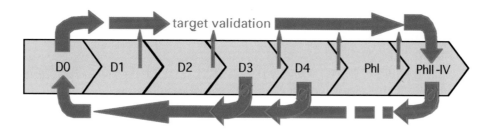

Figure 1.
The phases of drug discovery and development. D0: Basic sciences, target selection. D1: Assay devel-opment for high-throughput screening *in vitro*. D2: High-throughput screening of public and pro-prietary compound libraries, ligand finding (hits). D3: Lead optimization by medicinal chemistry, *in vitro* and *in vivo* models, initial pharmacokinetics and safety. D4: Preparation for human studies: bio-markers, extensive pharmacokinetics, safety, metabolism in animals, formulation, chemical up-scal-ing. PhI: Proof of concept/mechanism in human, tolerance. PhII: Dose finding. PhIII: Efficacy, regis-tration studies. PhIV: Post-marketing studies.

2.1.1 Choice of therapeutic areas and indication

Discovery research departments need to understand their company prior-ities, which are usually defined by a group of internal and external dis-covery scientists, clinical and development scientists, as well as commer-cial experts from marketing. Key criteria to select the areas for research include:
- expected added medical benefit at the time of introduction in comparison to existing therapy and therapies expected to be in place at that time, i.e., medical need
- existence of a viable scientific hypothesis
- number of patients and expected commercial return
- synergy potential (i.e., will working in this area/indication also contribute to other fields addressed by the company?)
- company skills and history.

2.1.2 Choice of therapeutic target

Once the therapeutic areas are chosen, the drug discovery process begins by selecting the appropriate therapeutic target. Therapeutic targets are the

exact molecular site in the human body at which a proposed therapy is aimed to beneficially modify the course of a disease or even prevent it. They include:
- Cell membrane receptors and ion channels
- Intra- or extracellular enzymes
- Proteins of signaling pathways
- Nuclear receptors
- Genes or gene regulatory processes.

Except for the last target class all others are exclusively proteins. The choice of a particular target depends on the level of scientific knowledge concerning its involvement in the disease process to be addressed. Some targets are clinically validated, i.e., it has been demonstrated in patients that affecting this particular target is of therapeutic benefit. Yet, the most innovative targets have a much lesser degree of validation, such as a genetic linkage with disease, pure speculation based on approximate knowledge about the disease process, or some evidence from gene inactivation experiments. Transgenic animals expressing human disease mutations have become an invaluable tool for intermediary validation [9, 10].

Once a protein has been chosen as a target, it is important to begin efforts to determine its three-dimensional structure so that a structure-based medicinal chemistry effort can be begun as soon as possible and in parallel to high throughput screening.

2.2 The D1 phase

Following target selection, the target protein must be obtained in sufficient quantities and in pure form to allow the design of appropriate high-throughput screening assays [11]. The protein is usually produced by recombinant methods either in bacterial, insect or human cell line systems. It is then included in the appropriate assay for high-throughput screening of large compound libraries to allow measurement of its interaction with a therapeutic tool. At this point, the nature of the therapeutic tool to be developed is selected based on the target characteristics. Therapeutic tools are usually one of the following.

2.2.1 Low molecular weight compounds, synthetics

Synthetic low molecular weight (MW) compounds (usually MW <500) mimic nature's use of small molecules, such as hormones and neurotransmitters, to modulate biological processes. Their main advantages are:
- potential access to all compartments of the human body
- potentially low cost of manufacturing (exceptions are molecules requiring many and complex synthetic steps)
- amenable to a large number of synthetic variations to improve their "drugability", i.e., solubility, membrane permeability, specificity for the target, reduced side effects.

One of the main drawbacks is that, due to their small size, they may have difficulty to interfere with large surface protein-protein interactions.

2.2.2 Low molecular weight molecules, natural products

Such compounds are isolated from natural sources, often as secondary metabolites of organisms that use them in biological functions, e.g., toxins or antibiotics for defensive purposes. Their MW ranges from 100 to about 1000. Their main advantages are:
- they are the result of millions if not billions of years of combinatorial chemistry and selection, so that the probability that they will display biological activity is very high
- they can reach most compartments of the human body
- they can be synthetically modified for drugability.

These are counterbalanced by a principal disadvantage, i.e. natural compounds are, in general, of highly complex structure, including many chiral centers and are difficult to synthesize by methods of synthetic chemistry; often, they can only be obtained by biological processes such as fermentation.

2.2.3 Proteins: antibodies and growth factors

Therapeutic antibodies can be made to interfere with specific molecular

processes and endogenous growth factors to sustain/rectify disease-related deficiencies. Their main advantages are:
- they can be mined from the human genome
- several efficient methods are available to make fully human antibodies
- very high specificity and affinity can be achieved;

on the other hand:
- they can usually only reach extracellular/cell surface targets (in particular antibodies)
- their synthesis, purification and refolding for activity can be expensive and difficult
- in nature, growth factors are very tightly controlled, both spatially and in time and in concentration, so that therapeutic systemic application can cause unwanted side effects.

2.2.4 Gene therapy

A conceptually very elegant method to substitute deficient gene functions found in many diseases such as cystic fibrosis, hemophilia, Gaucher's disease, ADA deficiency etc. [12] is gene therapy, where an engineered vector, often of viral origin, is used to convey an intact functional gene to deficient cells to restore their function. The main advantage of the approach is the direct causal reversal of disease generating malfunction.

However, this has to be balanced against the disadvantages (today) of:
- an often insufficient expression of the repair gene to achieve a therapeutic effect
- insufficient or absent regulation of the foreign gene causing unwanted effects
- imperfect genome integration control (retroviral vectors) can lead to onco-genicity [13]
- insufficient tissue specificity.

2.2.5 Organ transplantation, including xeno-transplantation

The repair of deficient organs can be achieved by transplanting organs from a compatible donor. Due to the development of immunosuppressive regimes, human to human allo-transplantation today has become a routine procedure [14]. Its main advantage is that it is life saving.

However, today:
- there is an insufficient number of donor compared to medical need
- the immunosuppressive regimes are still imperfect, and have partly life-threatening side-effects.

To address the donor organ shortage, the strategy of transplanting organs from animals that have been genetically modified to inhibit the hyper-acute rejection usually observed in interspecies transplantation has been explored using pigs as donors (xeno-transplantation) [15].

Xeno-transplantation would offer the advantage of:
- 'unlimited' organ supply
- potential replacement of many damaged organs.

At present, the main disadvantage of the approach are:
- rejection mechanisms can not be sufficiently controlled to allow a sufficiently long-lasting donor organ survival in the host
- incompatible physiology between donor and recipient remains a prohibitive problem
- perceived safety concerns about reactivation of endogenous retroviruses [16].

2.2.6 Cell therapies: tissues as well as adult and embryonic stem cells derived

Blood transfusion is the oldest life-saving cell therapy. Newer versions of cell therapy aim at repairing damaged specialized tissue in the host by taking advantage of stem cells occurring in the human body that have the potential to regenerate specific cell types (adult stem cells) or all cell types (embryonic stem cells) [17]. Cell/stem cell therapy offers as main advantages:
- potential repair of many tissues
- no rejection is to be expected if autologous stem cell transplantation is performed.

Main disadvantages (today):
- to date, the ability to multiply of adult stem cells in sufficient quantities without differentiation has had only limited success
- because of their origin there is ethical concern to use human embryonic stem cells [17].

The scientific exploration of the potential of both embryonic and adult stem cells is at its very beginning, in particular the potential to repair complex organs.

2.2.7 Artificial organs

In some cases fully artificial organs can be considered to replace damaged ones [18]. Main advantages of using artificial organs are:
- their potentially unlimited supply
- the possibility to replace tissue/organ function without the drawbacks of biological transplantation and cell therapy methods.

Today, the approach is facing several hurdles:
- only a very limited number of functions can be artificially replaced, such as locomotory functions, cardiovascular pumping and acoustic deficiencies
- the size of artificial organs is technologically highly challenging and often prohibitive.

2.3 The D2 phase: ligand screening

During the D2 phase, the search for ligands for the selected target is performed. Ligands are obtained from a number of sources:
- diverse proprietary libraries, typically around 1 million compounds for a large pharmaceutical company. Compound handling is highly automated to allow for efficient screening operations.
- commercially available compound collections
- tailored combinatorial chemistry libraries [19]
- natural compound libraries from microorganisms or plants that can be preselected based on traditional medicinal knowledge [20]

- proteins and antibodies from genome mining [21].

Ligands that interact with the target are called 'hits' and are usually validated by repeating experiments and recording full dose-response curves. These original hits are then also selected for drugability (solubility, membrane permeability, *in vitro* genotoxicity, selectivity, etc.) before moving into the next phase. The compounds thus selected are then called 'leads', on which the medicinal chemists and pharmacologist perform optimization work.

2.4   The D3 phase: lead optimization

During the D3 phase, the low MW leads obtained in D2 are modified and subjected to structure-activity evaluation to optimize their solubility, potency, selectivity, metabolic properties, as well as their side effect profile both in *in vitro* and in whole animal models. An example of such a lead optimization is shown in Figure 2 and Table 1.

The most promising compounds are then evaluated in at least two relevant animal species to obtain an indication of the species specificity of the target modulation. Longer term studies in intact animals are performed to evaluate the effect of repeated applications, including the occurrence of potential tachyphyllaxis (the attenuation of pharmacological effects after repeated applications). One of the most important aspects of this phase is to obtain data allowing judgment of the potential medical benefit for the patient, as compared to existing therapies or therapies believed to be available at the time of introduction. This is often done in extensive comparative studies with the competing therapeutic agents. The only relevant competitive advantages are advantages that bring a significant medical benefit compared to previous therapy in the patient's perception. A different molecule or mechanism of action as such is not sufficient unless it will plausibly translate into such a medical advantage for the patient.

The patenting of the new therapeutic principle occurs at the latest during the D3 phase. The optimized compound progresses to the next phase, but leads of different chemical structures are kept for potential backups in case the first candidate moving forward fails. However, backups are best selected when the nature of the limiting factors of the first candidate become apparent.

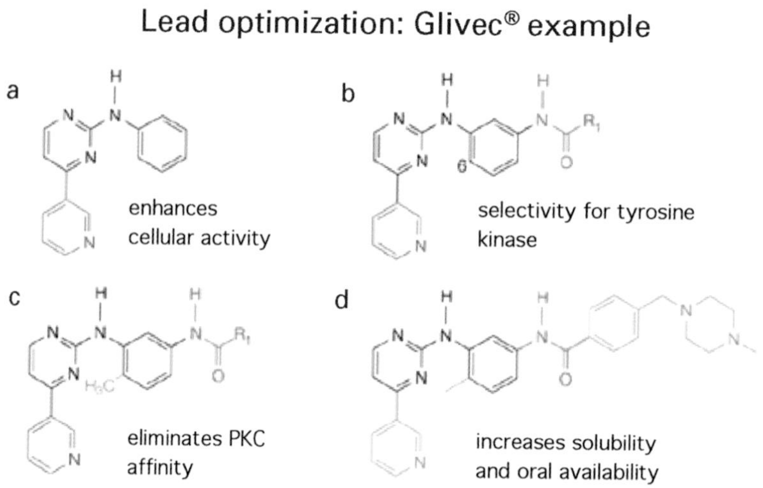

Lead optimization: Glivec® example

a

enhances
cellular activity

b

selectivity for tyrosine
kinase

c

eliminates PKC
affinity

d

increases solubility
and oral availability

Figure 2.
Lead optimization: the Glivec® example. Glivec® is a new and revolutionary mechanism-directed therapy for chronic amyotrophic leukemia (CML). The addition of the colored substituents to the original lead structure allowed different desired properties of the compound to be improved as indicated.
(from [22], reproduced with permission).

2.5   The D4 phase

This phase is the final preparation for the clinical evaluation of a potential
drug candidate. It involves extensive pharmacokinetic, metabolic and safety
studies in whole animals in at least two species. During D4, chemical up-scal-
ing is carried out, from milligram to kilogram quantities, and an appropriate
formulation for compound administration is developed. The clinical research
strategy is defined, in recent times with a strong emphasis on biomarkers,
that should indicate already during the early clinical testing phase whether
the scientific therapy concept is likely to be achieved with the selected therapeutic approach (proof-of-concept studies).

Throughout the process, methods that provide temporo-spatial information on the distribution of potential drug targets, the drug candidate, the
drug-target interaction and consequences thereof are of high relevance.
Among such techniques, methods such as imaging, which provide non-invasive readouts, are highly attractive as they frequently allow a one-to-one

Table 1.
Selectivity of Glivec® against a panel of kinases. The optimized compound was selected for maximal selectivity towards the Abl kinase (red) but a residual affinity to the platlet-derived growth factor (PDGF, green) and c-kit receptors(blue) remained, which turned out to confer therapeutic benefit for cancers other than CML (from [22]).

Kinases	IC_{50} [μM]
v-Abl	0.1–0.3
p210$^{bcr-abl}$	0.25
p190$^{bcr-abl}$	0.25
TEL-Abl	0.35
TEL-Arg	0.5
PDGF receptor	0.1
TEL-PDGF receptor	0.15
c-Kit (stem cell factor receptor)	0.1
Flt-3	>10
c-Fms and v-Fms	>10
KDR	>10
EGF receptor	>100
c-erbB2	>100
Insulin receptor	>100
IGF-I receptor	>100
v-Src	>10
Jak-2	>100

translation from preclinical to clinical drug evaluation. The remainder of this book addresses the many parts of the drug discovery process, where imaging techniques can make major contributions.

References

1   Drews J (2000) Drug discovery: a historical perspective. *Science* 287: 1960–1964
2   International Human genome sequencing Consortium (2001) Initial sequencing and analysis of the human genome. *Nature* 409: 860–921
3   Venter JC, Adams MD, Myers EW, Li PW, Mural RJ, Sutton GG, Smith HO, Yandell M, Evans CA, Holt RA et al (2001) The sequence of the human genome. *Science* 291: 1304–1351
4   Orchard S, Hermjakob H, Apweiler R (2005) Annotating the human proteome. *Mol Cell Proteomics* 4: 435–440
5   Modrek B, Lee CJ (2003) Alternative splicing in the human, mouse and rat genomes is

associated with an increased frequency of exon creation and.or loss. *Nat Genet* 34: 177–180

6 Eisenberg E, Nemzer S, Kinar Y, Sorek R, Rechavi G, Levanon EY (2005) Is abundant A-to-I RNA editing primate specific? *Trends Genet* 21: 77–81

7 Sommer B, Kohler M, Seeburg PH (1991) RNA editing in brain controls a determinant of ion flow in glutamate gated channels. *Cell* 67: 11–19

8 Drews J (2000) Drug discovery: a historical perspective. *Science* 287: 1960–1964

9 Stuerchler-Pierrat C, Abramwoski D, Duke M, Wiederhold KH, Mistl C, Rothacher C, Ledermann B, Buerki K, Frey P, Paganetti PA et al (1997) Two amyloid precursor protein transgenic mouse models with Alzheimer disease-like pathology. *Proc Natl Acad Sci USA* 94: 13287–13292

10 Stuerchler-Pierrat C, Sommer B (1999) Transgenic animals in Alzheimer disease research. *Rev Neurosci* 10: 15–24

11 Bleicher KH, Boehm H-J, Mueller K, Alanine AJ (2003) Hit and lead generation: beyond high-throughput screening. *Nat Rev Drug Discov* 2: 369–378

12 Victor A. McKusick et al: OMIM™ Database – Online Mendelian Inheritance in Man™: *http://www.ncbi.nlm.nih.gov/entrez/query.fcgi?db=OMIM* (Accessed May 2005)

13 Fischer A, Hacein-Bey-Abina S, Cavazzana-Calvo M (2004) Gene therapy of children with X-linked severe combined immune deficiency: efficiency and complications. *Medicine/Sciences* 20: 115–117

14 Borel JF (1994) Cyclosporine. In: MM Dale, JC Foreman, T-P Fan (eds): *Textbook of Immunopharmacology*, 3rd edition. Blackwell Scientific Publications, Oxford, Chapter 29

15 Fishman J, Sachs D, Shaikh R (eds) (1998) Xenotransplantation: Scientific Frontiers and Public Policy. Proceedings of a conference. New York, New York, USA. May 18–20, 1998. *Ann NY Acad Sci* 862: 1-251

16 Van der Laan LJW, Lockey C, Griffeth BC, Frasier F, Wilson CA, Onions CW, Hering BJ, Long Z, Otto E, Torbett BE, Salomon DR (2000) Infection by porcine endogenous retrovirus after islet transplantation in SCID mice. *Nature* 407: 90–94

17 Aldhous P (2000) Stem cells: panacea, or Pandora's box? *Nature* 408: 897–898

18 Pescovitz D (2004) Parts for vital organs. *Scientific American*, Special Edition Vol. 14/3: 78–83 (www.sciam.com)

19 Furka A (1995) History of combinatorial chemistry. *Drug Discovery Research* 36: 1–12

20 Yan X, Zhou J, Xie G (1999) *Traditional Chinese Medicines*. MPG Books, Ashgate, Aldershot UK

21 Ostendorn R, Frisch C, Urban M (2004) Generation, engineering and production of human antibodies using HuCAL®. In: G Subramanian (ed): *Antibodies*, Volume 2: Novel technologies and therapeutic use; Kluwer Academic/Plenum Publishers, New York, 13–52

22 Capdeville R, Buchdunger E, Zimmermann J, Matter A (2002) Glivec: CGP057148 (STI571, imatinib), a rationally developed, targeted anticancer drug. *Nat Rev Drug Discov* 1: 493–502

Progress in Drug Research, Vol. 62
(Markus Rudin, Ed.)
© 2005 Birkhäuser Verlag, Basel (Switzerland)

Imaging modalities: principles and information content

By Tobias Schaeffter

Philips Research Hamburg
Roentgenstr. 24–26
D-22335 Hamburg, Germany
<Tobias.Schaeffter@philips.com>

Glossary of abbreviations

ADC, apparent diffusion coefficient; CCD, charged coupled device; CT, computed tomography; CNR, contrast-to-noise ratio; FIR, far infrared; GI, gastrointestinal; HU, Hounsfield units; IR, infrared; LOR, line-of-response; MRI, magnetic resonance imaging; MTC, magnetization transfer contrast; NIR, near infrared; NMR, nuclear magnetic resonance; PMT, photomultiplier tubes; PET, positron emission tomography; rf, Radiofrequency; Sv, Sievert; SNR, signal-to-noise ratio; SPECT, single-photon emission computed tomography; SPIO, superparamagnetic iron oxide; NaI(Tl), sodium iodide single crystal doted with thallium; T, Tesla; USPIO, ultra-small superparamagnetic iron oxide; UV, ultraviolet; VIS, visible.

1 Historical introduction: From X-rays to optical tomography

In 1895, W. Röntgen discovered a new type of rays, which he named "X" for unknown. Röntgen found out that these X-rays could pass through the soft tissue of humans, but not bones and metal objects. One of Röntgen's first experiments late in 1895 was a film of the hand of his wife. On 28 December 1895 Röntgen gave his preliminary report "Über eine neue Art von Strahlen" and already several months later X-rays were used in clinical medicine. In 1896, C. Müller began building X-ray tubes in a small factory in Hamburg, Germany, for use at a nearby hospital. His factory became the basis for today's most advanced X-ray tube factory worldwide. In 1901, Röntgen was awarded with the first Nobel Prize in physics, but he declined to seek patents or proprietary claims on the X-rays. Over the next few decades, X-rays grew into a widely used diagnostic tool in medical practice. Since bones show up clearly as white objects against a darker background, Röntgen's rays proved particularly suited for examining fractures and breaks, but they could also spot diseases of the respiratory system such as tuberculosis, and a variety of other tissue abnormalities. All X-ray images based upon projection imaging until the 1970s, when G. Hounsfield and A. Cormack developed the basis for three-dimensional X-ray imaging, i.e. computed tomography (CT) In 1979, this work was awarded the Nobel Prize in Medicine.

Shortly after the discovery of X-rays, another form of penetrating rays was discovered. In 1896, H. Becquerel discovered natural radioactivity during his work on fluorescence crystals. One of the minerals was a uranium compound and Becquerel found that this compound had exposed photographic plates although stored in a box. Becquerel concluded that the uranium compound gave off a type of radiation that could penetrate heavy paper and expose photographic film. Bequerel's discovery was, unlike that of the X-rays, more or less unnoticed by scientific community. In 1898, Marie and Pierre Curie discovered two other radioactive elements, which they named "polonium" and "radium". Both elements were more radioactive than uranium and allowed radiographic castings for industrial applications, whereas the first use of radionuclides in medicine was for treatment, i.e. radiation therapy. In 1903, Bequerel and the Curies received the Nobel Prize in Physics. In 1913, G. de Hevesy invented the "tracer principle", which states that radioactive isotopes can be used to trace materials even as they undergo chemical change. This work was awarded the Nobel Prize in Chemistry in 1943. Although H. Blumgart tested the tracer principle in humans in 1926 to determine the circulation time of blood, it took another 20 years until radionuclides were used for medical imaging. In 1950s, B. Cassen and H. Anger developed instruments for the detection of γ-rays. This allowed the development of single-photon emission computed tomography (SPECT) by D. Kuhl and others as well as Positron Emission Tomography (PET) by M Phelps during 1970s.

The hazards of radiation from nuclides and X-ray exposure were clearly known by the early 1900s. In fact many pioneers of the new techniques suffered for their efforts, for instance Madame Curie died in 1934 from pernicious anemia, presumable due to an overexposure to radiation. The first radiation-free imaging technique in medicine was ultrasound. The development of modern ultrasonics started about 1917, when P. Langevin developed a device he named "hydrophone" for underwater detection and navigation. In 1928, S. Sokolov proposed an ultrasound transmission technique for flaw detection in metals. This technique was tested for preliminary brain imaging by the K. Dussik in 1942. The development of diagnostic ultrasound instrumentation was strongly influenced by radar techniques developed during World War II. In particular, D. Howry and J. Wild showed that tissue interfaces could be detected in ultrasound echoes in the late 1940s. However, it took another 20 years until ultrasound became a clinical tool.

Another medical imaging modality that avoids ionizing radiation is magnetic resonance imaging (MRI). This technique is based on the nuclear magnetic resonance (NMR) effect that was discovered in 1946 independently by two groups at Stanford and at Harvard University. For this discovery, F. Bloch and E. Purcell were awarded with the Nobel Prize for Physics in 1952. It could be shown that the frequency of the NMR effect depends on the strength of the magnetic field and the chemical environment of the nuclei. With this discovery NMR spectroscopy was born and soon became an important analytical method in the study of the composition of chemical compounds. Fundamental developments in NMR spectroscopy resulted in two Nobel Prizes in Chemistry: R.R. Ernst in 1991 and K. Wüthrich in 2002. In the early 70s, R. Damadian demonstrated that NMR relaxation times of tumor samples, measured in vitro, differed significantly from values of normal tissue. This discovery built the basis for using NMR as a tool for medical diagnosis. In 1973, P. Lauterbur published the first MRI experiment. In the following years tremendous developments have improved MRI to make the technique applicable for daily clinical practice. In particular, the early work of P. Mansfield showed how extremely fast imaging could be achievable. In 2003, the work of P. Lauterbur and P. Mansfield was awarded the Nobel Prize in Medicine.

Nowadays, the 'big four' imaging modalities, i.e. X-ray (CT), nuclear imaging, ultrasound and MRI continue to dominate the medical imaging practice in many variants and combinations. However, other interesting techniques are appearing. For instance, new types of optical techniques are on their way into clinical practice. Although P. Bozzini developed the first endoscope in 1806, it took until the mid of the last century until this technique was widely used in medicine. Apart from surface imaging, other techniques allow three-dimensional optical imaging. In 1929, Cutler developed a technique called transillumination, where light was shined on one side of a human breast and the absorption behavior on the other side was examined. During the last decade, diffuse optical tomography was developed. Especially, B. Chance at University of Pennsylvania made significant contributions in instrumentation, optical contrast agents and reconstruction algorithms. Although the application of diffuse optical tomography in medicine is still under investigation, this technique has the potential to make a major contribution in preclinical imaging in animals.

2 Main principles in biomedical imaging

Images of the human body can be derived from the interaction of energy with human tissue. In biomedical imaging, the energy is applied as acoustic or electromagnetic waves. Depending on the energy of the waves, which can be

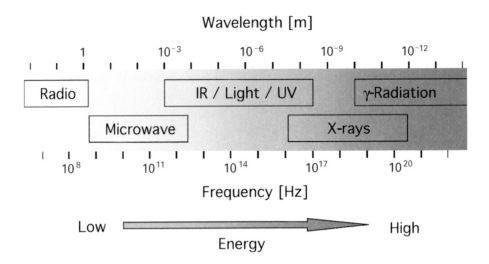

Figure 1
Energy spectrum of electromagnetic waves ranging from low energy of radio waves to high energy for γ-radiation.

expressed in terms of the wavelength, different types of interaction with bio-logical tissue are induced. A broad energy spectrum of electromagnetic waves (Fig. 1) ranging from radio waves to X-ray radiation is used for investigation of tissue. Imaging methods involving high energy use ionizing radiation, i.e., the applied energy is sufficient to ionize atoms and molecules. This is, for instance, the case for X-ray based and nuclear imaging techniques, which bear the potential of causing radiation damage. MRI and optical imaging, on the other hand, use non-ionizing radiation, while ultrasound is based on pressure waves, and correspondingly are considered safe.

Imaging methods that use either non-ionizing radiation or ionizing radi-ation interact with tissue at the molecular or atomic level, involving a vari-ety of interaction mechanisms such as absorption, reflection, scattering and transmission. During absorption, a fraction of the total energy of the wave is transferred to the tissue's molecules or atoms; hence, the intensity of a wave is reduced upon passage through tissue. In particular, strong absorption of energy occurs at resonance, i.e., when the frequency of the incident wave matches with the resonance frequency of a certain property of tissue. For instance, strong absorption of light can be observed, if the frequency of the light matches with electronic transitions, as well as with rotation and vibration modes of molecules. In addition, electromagnetic energy is absorbed, if there is a match between the frequency of the electromagnetic wave with the electron or nuclear spin resonance. Often, the absorption of energy by molecules in tissue results in the emission of energy as a secondary process. Reflection occurs at tissue interfaces, where the direction of the wave is altered in a defined way, i.e., the angle of the incoming wave is the same as of the reflected wave. The direction of a wave is also changed in scattering. In elastic scattering the direction of the wave is changed but the energy stays the same, whereas in inelastic scattering energy loss occurs. In addition to amplitude changes, the phase relation of a wave can also be altered, which happens in incoherent scattering. Ideally, transmission occurs if none of the described interactions occurs (i.e., the direction, the amplitude and phase of the wave is not modified). Usually absorption and scattering processes will alter both amplitude and phase of the wave upon passage through tissue; these changes are lumped into an overall attenuation factor.

In general, the interactions described determine the image contrast in the different imaging techniques. Which type of the interactions is prominent depends on the energy of the wave and properties of the tissue. In the following, different modalities are characterized by describing the type and amount of energy applied. Furthermore, the interactions and factors, which influence the image contrast, are discussed.

3   X-ray imaging

X-ray imaging is a transmission-based technique, in which X-rays pass from a source through the patient and are detected on the opposite side of the patient (Fig. 2). This portion of the radiation is directly measured by the detector and is called primary radiation. The contrast in X-ray images arises from the different attenuation of X-rays in different tissues. The amount of absorption depends on the tissue composition, e.g., dense bone matter absorbs more X-rays than soft tissues, such as muscle, fat and blood. Another important factor for the overall image quality of X-ray imaging is the X-ray source, which defines the energy spectrum and the resolution of the X-ray beam. In planar X-ray, the line integral of the location-dependent attenuation is measured, and the resulting intensities are displayed as a two-dimensional image. However, such a projection image makes it difficult to interpret

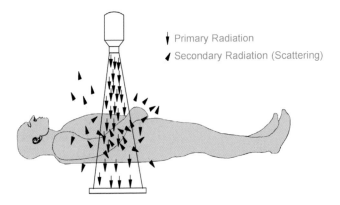

Primary Radiation

Secondary Radiation (Scattering)

Figure 2.
Principle of X-ray imaging.

overlapping layers of soft tissue and bone structures. To resolve three-dimensional structures, X-ray CT is used, which generates cross-sectional, two-dimensional images of the body. Due to the high spatial resolution of X-ray and CT images, these techniques are widely used to depict the anatomy and structural information.

3.1 Contrast mechanisms

The contrast in X-ray imaging depends on the interaction of X-rays with tissue (Fig. 3). A small number of the initial X-rays pass through the body without any interaction. Some fraction of the radiation is absorbed within the body and does not reach the detector on the other side. Energy absorption occurs via the photoelectric interaction of the X-rays with tightly bound electrons from the inner shell. These electrons are emitted with a kinetic energy that is equal to difference of the initial energy of X-ray and the binding energy of the electron. After emission of an electron the resulting hole is filled up with an electron from an outer shell that leads to the emission of radiation. This radiation has a low energy and is thus often absorbed in the vicinity. The amount of photoelectric interaction depends on the atomic number of the tissue elements and the X-ray energy, i.e., the amount of absorption becomes smaller with increasing X-ray energy. However, as soon as the energy of the radiation is above the binding energy of the innermost electrons (K-

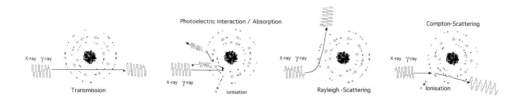

Figure 3.
Interaction principles of X-rays. In transmission, no interaction with the atoms of the tissue occurs. In absorption, the photoelectric interaction with the electrons of the atoms result in transfer of energy from the X-ray to the atoms of the tissue. In scattering, the direction of the X-ray is changed either without (Rayleigh) or with loss of energy (Compton).

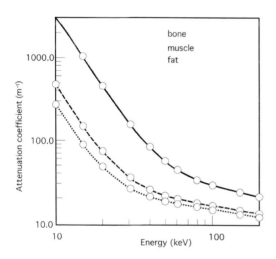

Figure 4.
Attenuation coefficients as function of the X-ray energy.

shell), the amount of photoelectric interaction increases significantly. This phenomenon is called K-edge, and is in the order of 4 KeV for calcium (bone). For energies above this value the probability of photoelectric interaction decreases further. Figure 4 shows the mass absorption coefficients for different tissues. It is clear that soft tissue contrast (e.g., between muscle and fat) can only be achieved at lower energies.

Apart from transmission and absorption, another fraction of the incident radiation is scattered. Scattering is also called secondary radiation and degrades the image contrast. Two main mechanisms contribute to scattering: Compton and Rayleigh scattering. Compton scattering is based on the interaction of X-rays with loosely bound electrons in the outer shell of atoms. A fraction of the energy of the X-radiation is transferred to such electrons. The X-ray radiation changes its direction and looses a small amount of energy. Rayleigh, also called coherent, scattering represents a non-ionizing interaction between the X-rays and tissue, where X-ray energy is converted into harmonic motions of the electrons in atoms of the tissue. The atoms then reradiate the energy with the same wavelength but in a different direction. The amount of Rayleigh scattering depends on the atomic number of the atoms in tissue and the initial energy of the X-ray, whereas Compton scattering is independent from atomic number and depends only weakly on the energy of the initial radiation. For X-rays in the diagnostic range Compton scattering is the dominant mechanism and Rayleigh scattering is negligible. Usually, scattering is an undesired process in X-ray imaging, which degrades the image contrast and thus quality.

3.2 Instrumentation

An X-ray system consists of two main components: the X-ray source and a detection unit to measure non-absorbed X-rays. The X-rays are produced in an X-ray tube, which comprises a cathode and an anode. The cathode is usually made of a tungsten wire, which is heated up to about 2000 °C by an electric current to produce free electrons. A high electric voltage (20–150 kV) between the anode and cathode accelerates these free electrons towards the anode. The anode is usually also made of tungsten, which has a high atomic number and a high melting point. The latter is important since most of energy produced in the X-ray tube is converted into heat. To distribute the heat over a large surface area, the anode is often made as a rotating disk. The frequency of modern rotating anodes is in the order of 200 Hz. Electrons hitting the surface of the anode cause the generation of two different types of radiation: Bremsstrahlung and characteristic radiation. Bremsstrahlung is caused by electrons that pass close to a nucleus of the anode's material. During this process the electrons are losing some of their kinetic energy, which is emitted as X-ray radiation. Each electron has a number of such interactions until their total kinetic energy is converted into X-rays. Therefore, X-rays with a wide range of energies are produced. X-rays with maximal energy are produced in a situation, when the complete kinetic energy of an electron is converted at once, i.e., the maximal energy of X-rays depends on the applied accelerating voltage. The energy spectrum of the Bremsstrahlung is characterized by a linear behavior, the intensity of the Bremsstrahlung decreasing with increasing energy. The spectrum contains also sharp peaks, due to characteristic radiation. These peaks are caused by photoelectric interaction of the X-rays with electrons of the inner shell of the atoms of the anode material.

An important design factor of an X-ray tube is the focal spot size of the X-ray beam. This spot size is determined by two factors: the cross-section of the electron beam and the angle of the anode to the electron beam. The focal spot size ranges from 0.3 to 1.2 mm. Often X-ray tubes contain two cathodes of different sizes to change the focal spot size of the electron beam and thus the focal spot size of the X-ray beam. In addition, a collimator is applied between the X-ray tube and the object to restrict the dimensions of the X-ray beam to the field of view required for imaging.

In X-ray imaging, the primary radiation should be detected to form an image. However, in practice, a large contribution of the detected X-rays has been scattered. This secondary radiation contains no spatial information and is often randomly distributed over the image. In order to reduce the contribution from scattered X-rays, an anti-scatter grid is placed in front of the detector. Such a grid consists of lead septa, which are aligned in the direction of the primary radiation. Therefore, X-rays with large deviation from this direction, due to scattering are absorbed in the septa, whereas X-rays with a direction parallel to the septa are registered by the detectors.

There is a number of different X-ray detectors. The simplest type is a film, which is usually used in combination with an intensifying screen. The intensifying screen converts X-rays into light photons, to which film is sensitive. Dark areas on the developed films correspond to tissue with a low X-ray attenuation (i.e., strong transmission), whereas bright areas correspond to highly attenuating tissue. Although X-ray films are still being used, modern systems are based on digital X-ray detection systems. In these detectors, X-rays are converted into an electrical signal that can be digitized. Three basic detector types can be differentiated: ionization chambers, scintillation detectors, and direct converters.

Ionization chambers are filled with gas, usually xenon, under high pressure to ensure high number of interactions between the gas and the X-ray radiation. X-rays transmitted through the chamber ionize the gas, i.e., produce electron–ion pairs. Charged electrodes attract these ions and electrons, thereby producing an electrical current that is proportional to the number of X-rays. The advantages of ionization chambers in contrast to a scintillation detector are the relatively low prize and fast temporal response. A disadvantage is that multi-row detectors are difficult to manufacture.

Scintillation detectors consist of a scintillation material and an array of photodiodes. The former converts the X-ray radiation into visible light, which then is converted into an electrical signal. Usually, thallium-doped cesium iodide or cadmium tungstate crystals are used as scintillation material. In flat panel detectors the crystals are formed as thin rods (10-μm diameter), which are aligned parallel to each other and are connected to thin film transistor switches. The advantage of these rods is that light produced by the X-rays is kept inside the rods with only limited cross-talk between the elements. Commercial available flat-panel detectors have a dimension of 43×43 cm with 3000×3000 elements with a pixel dimension of about 150 μm. The frame rate of these detectors is limited to about 100 Hz.

Direct converters are made from semiconductor material that converts radiation directly to an electrical signal. Se, GaAs, CdZnTe and other high-density solid-state materials are good candidates for the detection of X-rays at the typical energies (1–100 keV), but are also applicable when using higher energy radiation (up to 511 keV). While CdZnTe detector modules offer good energy resolution and potentially sub-millimeter intrinsic spatial resolution, a significant number of material-related difficulties and limitations are yet to be overcome. In particular, the charge collection and transport properties of CdZnTe are poor due to high rate of recombination and trapping of generated charge carriers (especially for holes). In addition, CdZnTe is rather expensive and difficult to manufacture in large volumes. Therefore, direct detectors are still in a research phase.

3.3 Planar X-ray

Planar X-ray imaging has a number of applications, like bone scans, chest X-ray, mammography or angiography. Each application has special demands concerning spatial resolution, the signal-to-noise ratio (SNR) and the contrast-to-noise ratio (CNR). Ideally, all these parameters should have a high value, but usually trade-offs have to be made. The spatial resolution of an X-ray image is affected by a number of factors, the most relevant ones being the focal spot size of the X-ray tube and the position of the object with respect to the X-ray tube and the detector. The fact that the X-ray source has a finite size results in blurring. For a given focal spot size, the spatial resolution can be improved if the distance between the object and the detector is increased at a given distance between the object and the focal spot. In general, the object should be placed as close as possible to the source while keeping the detector at a large distance.

The SNR depends on the properties of the X-ray beam. The signal of each pixel depends on the number of high-energy X-rays, since these have a high probability to reach the detector. Therefore, the higher the accelerating voltage, the greater is number of high-energy X-rays produced, resulting in a higher SNR. The noise in an X-ray image is mainly influenced by the statistical variance in the X-ray beam for a given area which can be reduced by using a higher X-ray tube current and/or a longer exposure time. However, this also results in a higher X-ray dose (see below).

Even if an image has a very high SNR, there is little information in the image, if the contrast between different tissues is low, i.e., for diagnostic applications CNR is more relevant than SNR. Since the CNR is defined in terms of signal differences, all factors that influence the SNR, affect also the CNR. In contrast to the SNR, the CNR can often be improved using low energy X-rays. In this case, Compton scattering is reduced and the photoelectric interaction is the dominant effect. However, the beam energy must be sufficient to penetrate through the object with a given attenuation.

3.4   X-ray CT

X-ray CT allows the reconstruction of three-dimensional images. For this, an X-ray tube is rapidly rotated 360° around the patient and a number of projections are obtained from different angles. The development of CT began with Hounsfield's experiment, which is also called "first generation" of CT (Fig. 5). In this setup a translation-rotation approach is used, i.e., a single line-integral for each translational position is obtained and the procedure is

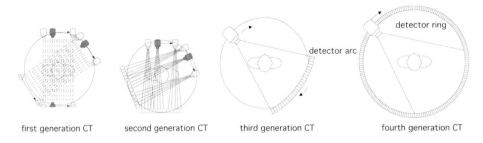

first generation CT   second generation CT   third generation CT   fourth generation CT

Figure 5.
Principles of X-ray CT.

repeated for different angles. This approach, however, results in rather long scan times (several minutes). To speed up the acquisition, a 'fan-beam' geometry was applied in the second and third generation of CT scanners. In the latter, a rotating fan beam source–detector pair are is used. An extension of this principle is the forth generation CT, in which a complete detector ring is used with only the tube rotating. Most of the modern CT scanners are third generation instruments using a number (16–64) of detector rows. These scanners are also called multi-slice CTs, because a number of slices can be recorded simultaneously. In addition, the use of a two-dimensional detector can be used in combination with a cone-beam X-ray geometry to obtain a true three-dimensional dataset. Further reduction of the scan time can be achieved by faster rotation times. Therefore the improvement of the mechanical design of the gantry, which carries the X-ray tube and the detector, is essential. Currently, the rotation times of the gantry are ranging between 0.3 and 1 s.

The CT image is commonly reconstructed by applying a filtered back projection algorithm. Since this reconstruction technique assumes that the line integrals correspond to parallel X-ray trajectories, the use of fan-beam geometry requiring a modification of the original algorithm, which takes the beam angulation into account. Recently, more advanced iterative reconstruction techniques were developed. These techniques use an estimate of the image, which is changed iteratively with respect to the measured data. The process is repeated until the error (e.g., mean squared error) is below a certain threshold. After reconstruction each pixel contains the averaged attenuation values within the corresponding voxel. This number is compared to the attenuation value of water and displayed on a scale of Hounsfield units (HU),

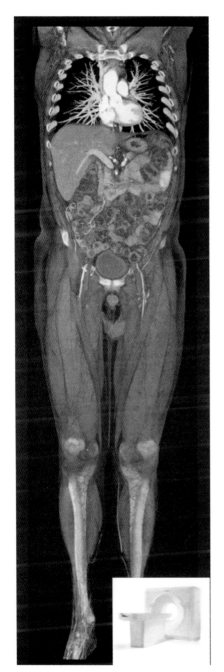

Figure 6.
Whole-body image obtained with 40-slice CT scanner.

which assigns an attenuation value (HU) of zero to water. The attenuation value ranges between –1000 and 3000 HU for medical applications with attenuation values for soft tissue in the range between 40 and 100 HU. The contrast also depends on the energy of the X-rays, which leads to the undesired process in CT called "beam-hardening". Since an X-ray beam contains a spectrum of energies and the lower energies are attenuated in soft tissue, the average energy of the X-ray beam increases during its passage through the tissue. Therefore the energy spectrum of the beam and, hence, the contrast changes for different path length of the beam through tissue. Usually, this effect is accounted for during the image reconstruction.

The spatial resolution in X-ray CT depends on the focal spot of the X-ray tube, the size of the detector elements and the position and size of the object. The spatial resolution of clinical CT scanner is less than 0.5 mm in the center of the CT scanner. Figure 6 shows the result of a whole-body acquisition. The spatial resolution of small bore animal (rodents) scanners is much higher and can be less than 50 µm. A detailed description of CT can be found in [1].

3.5   X-ray contrast agents

X-ray contrast agents are chemicals that are introduced into the body to increase the image contrast. X-ray contrast agents contain substances with a high atomic number (high electron number) that increase the attenuation value in regions, where they accumulate. Barium sulfate is a typical X-ray agent for imaging the gastrointestinal (GI) tract and the colon. Alternatively air is used for GI imaging due to its very low beam attenuation. Iodine-based X-ray contrast agents are widely used for angiographic studies and cancer imaging. The extent of the beam attenuation depends on the iodine load of the agent.

3.6   Safety and biological effects

Both absorption and Compton scattering lead to the emission of electrons (i.e., ionization), which can cause cell damage and/or genetic mutations that might lead to malignant tissue transformation. In general, whether cell death or mutations occur depend on the dose of the radiation. At lower dose there is a certain probability for tissue damage, while high radiation doses inevitably and reproducibly cause cell death. The absorbed dose is defined as energy of the radiation per unit mass of tissue and is given in units of grays (1 Gy = 1 J/kg). The radiation dose, however, is a physical definition and gives only little indication about the biological effect of radiation on different types of tissue. Therefore, the effective dose equivalent was introduced, which is defined as the weighted sum over the dose delivered to different organs. The weighting factors describe the different sensitivities of organs to radiation with respect to cancer. For example gonads and breast have a larger sensitivity to radiation than thyroids and skin. In addition, the delivered dose for each organ is weighted by a quality factor that describes the effect of different types of radiation. The quality factor is 1 for X-rays and γ-radiation, whereas larger values are used for other radiation types applied in radiation therapy (e.g., 20 for α-radiation). The dose equivalent is given in units of Sievert (1 Sv). It differs for different clinical exams, e.g., the equivalent dose of a chest X-ray is about 0.03 mSv, for abdominal X-ray about 1 mSv and for abdominal CT about 10 mSv.

4   Nuclear imaging

In contrast to X-ray and other imaging modalities, nuclear imaging does not provide morphology information, but images physiological processes due to injected radionuclides.

Nuclear imaging is based upon the detection of γ-rays that are emitted due to the radioactive decay of such radionuclides. Radioactivity occurs for isotopes with a high number of protons and neutrons (i.e., for heavy atoms). There are different types of radioactive decays, α-, β-, and γ-decay, which result in the emission of α- (4He nucleus), β- (electron or positron), and γ-particles. Another additional decay mechanism is based on the capture of an orbital electron by the nucleus with the subsequent emission of γ-photons. In nuclear imaging only γ-rays are used, whereas α- and β-particles are used in radiotherapy. No radionuclide decays completely with the emission of γ-rays only: For instance, γ-radiation results from the interaction of tissue electrons with a β^+-particle or from the decay of an intermediate species (metastable isotopes) that was formed by the decay of a different nuclide (mother nuclide). Important properties of radionuclides are the activity and half-life time. The activity describes the number of decays per second and is given in units of Bequerel (Bq). Occasionally, activity values are still given in Curies (Ci) defined as 1 Ci = 3.7×10^{10} Bq. The half-life time is the point in time when half of the nuclides have decayed. For nuclear imaging, a radionuclide should have a half-life that is short enough to limit the radiation to the organism, but long enough to allow detection.

For imaging, small amounts (typically nanograms) of radionuclides are injected into the body. These nuclides are usually incorporated into a biological active molecule also called radiopharmaceutical. The distribution of the radionuclide strongly depends on the pharmacokinetic and binding properties of the radiopharmaceutical. Therefore, the development and synthesis of radiopharmaceuticals is of key importance in nuclear imaging to obtain meaningful physiological, metabolic and molecular information.

Nuclear imaging is applied to study physiological and metabolic processes such as tissue perfusion and glucose utilization. In addition, novel radio-pharmaceuticals have been developed that provide information on apoptosis, angiogenesis, cell proliferation, cell migration and immunological events. Radioactive labeling of antibodies, peptides and low-molecular weight ligands allows imaging of cell receptors. Recently, a concept of reporter probes were developed in nuclear imaging to visualize gene expression *in vivo* [2, 3].

Two principal nuclear imaging techniques can be differentiated due to the use of different radionuclides: Single photon emitters decay under the emission of γ-rays with energies between 100 and 360 keV. Positron emitters decay under the emission of positrons that result in a pair of high-energy γ-rays (511 keV) after annihilation with an electron. The corresponding three-dimensional imaging techniques are single photon emission computed tomography (SPECT) and positron emission tomography (PET). Both nuclear imaging techniques have a rather poor spatial resolution and often a low SNR. The CNR, on the other hand, can be rather high when compared to other imaging techniques, provided the radiopharmaceutical is accumulating in a certain region only. In this case, there is no or little signal from the background, i.e., from tissue, to which the radiopharmaceutical has not been distributed.

An advantage of nuclear imaging techniques is that the tracer uptake rate can be quantified more or less directly from the imaging data. A widely used semi-quantitative parameter is the standard uptake value (SUV), which is defined as the ratio of the tissue activity divided by the injected dose. Unfortunately, there is a large variability of this parameter depending on the time point when the activity in tissue is measured. In addition, a high uptake of a targeted tracer can also be caused by other factors than just the concentration of the molecular targets, for instance by high perfusion values. To account for such factors, parametric maps have been introduced that provide more relevant information on the ligand-target interaction. These maps reflecting tracer kinetics are derived from dynamic scan data and are based on pharmacokinetic models, which describe the transport mechanisms of the tracer [4]. The models assume a number of tissue compartments (e.g., plasma, extracellular and intracellular space), which are volumes with homogeneous contrast agent concentrations $c_n(t)$. The exchange between these compartments is describe by rate constants $k_1, k_2, ..., k_n$. The rate constants are usually determined on the assumption of a first order process, i.e., the temporal change of the concentrations $dc_n(t)/dt$ is proportional to the differences in concentration between the compartments, which can be described by first order differential equations. The rate constants are obtained from regression analysis (curve fitting), comparing the time-activity data with the results obtained from multi-compartment modeling. The time-activity data of the tracer in the blood plasma (arterial input function) are also required as independent data for the regression analysis. They are usually measured from blood samples, which are taken at different points in time. Curve fitting is carried out either in certain regions-of-interest or on a pixel-by-pixel basis. A practical method that uses a graphical solution (also called Patlak-plot) is based on a three-compartment model, which assumes unidirectional transport of the tracer into the third compartment (intracellular space) [5].

4.1   Contrast mechanisms

The contrast in nuclear imaging is determined by the differences in the distribution of the radiopharmaceuticals. The contrast strongly depends on the pharmcokinetic properties and the target affinity of the radiopharmaceutical: the higher ratio between specific and unspecific binding of the radiopharmaceutical, the greater the CNR. While contrast is largely given by the local activity of the radiopharmaceutical, other factors will influence the appearance of the image as well. Emitted γ-rays interact with the tissue on an atomic level similarly to the interaction of X-rays. Scattering and photoelectric interactions result in a degradation of image quality. Since the emitted γ-rays have a high energy, the scattering process is predominantly influenced by the Compton scattering. Compton scattering translates into a reduction of the CNR, while photoelectric interactions result in an attenuation of the γ-rays. The attenuation depends on their energy, i.e., the higher the energy of γ-rays, the lower the attenuation in tissue and thus a higher SNR. Effects of γ-ray attenuation and Compton scattering depend on the path length of the photons through tissue, and are, therefore, more pronounced for radiation sources located from regions deep in the body. Usually, accurate quantification account for this effect using a location-dependent attenuation correction. A detailed description can be found in [6].

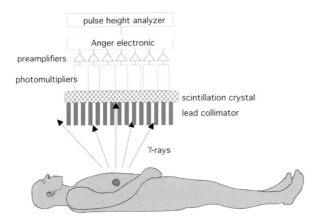

Figure 7.
Principle of γ-ray detection. A γ-camera consists of a lead collimator, a scintillation crystal and photo-multipliers. The position and the energy of the detected γ-rays are determined by a Anger-electronic and a pulse-height analyzer.

4.2   Single-photon emission computed tomography

Figure 7 shows the basic principles and instrumentation of SPECT. The radio-pharmaceutical injected is assumed to have accumulated in a specific region of the body. During the decay of the radionuclides γ-rays are emitted in all directions. Some of the γ-photons are attenuated and scattered in the body due to photoelectric interaction and the Compton effect. The γ-rays that leave the body can be detected by a γ-camera. Similar to X-ray imaging, two imaging modes can be distinguished. In planar scintigraphy the two-dimensional distribution of the activity distribution is measured, where the intensity in each pixel represents the total number of emitted γ-rays that have passed the collimator stage (see below). Hence, planar scintigraphy yields projection images with no depth information. In contrast to X-ray imaging, the attenuation of g-rays degrades planar scintigraphy images and affects the quantification of the concentration of radiopharmaceuticals. Three-dimensional imaging can be performed, by rotating the γ-camera around the body. Due to its similarity to X-Ray CT this approach is called single-photon emission CT (SPECT). Usually one or several γ-cameras are rotated around the patient (Fig. 8). The camera acquires a number of planar images from different view angles in a "stop-and-go" mode. Typically 32 to 128 views are acquired and

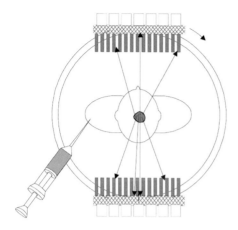

Figure 8.
Principle of SPECT. Injected radiopharmaceuticals decay under the emission of γ-rays. A single or multiple γ-cameras that are rotated around the body to detect the γ-rays.

a filtered back-projection algorithm is then applied to reconstruct a three-dimensional image of the activity distribution within the body. Usually, images with a numerical resolution of $64 \times 64 \times 64$ and $128 \times 128 \times 128$ are reconstructed. To improve the image quality in SPECT, tissue attenuation has to be corrected. The location-dependent tissue attenuation can be determined from the Hounsfield values derived from a CT scan acquired prior to the SPECT experiment. Alternatively, an approximation of an attenuation correction can be applied using a 360° rotation SPECT scan. In such a scan the differences in the signal amplitude from views obtained in upper half and the lower half can be determined, and the signal amplitudes can be corrected to the mean value.

4.2.1 Instrumentation

The basic design of a γ-camera was described by Anger in 1953 [7]. It consists of three components (Fig. 7): the collimator, the scintillation crystal and a number of photomultiplier tubes (PMT). Spatial information is encoded by geometrical collimation. The collimator selects only those γ-rays that have a trajectory at an angle of $90° \pm \alpha$ to the detector plane, the cone angle α being

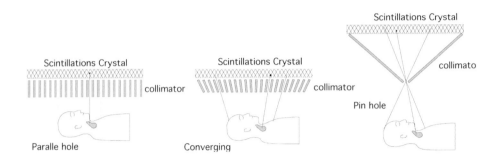

Figure 9.
Different types of collimators for single photon detection.

defined by the diameter and length of the collimator; γ-rays with other incident angles are blocked. The collimator is generally a lead structure with a honeycomb array of holes. The holes are either drilled in a piece of lead or formed by lead foils, where the lead walls (septa) are designed to prevent penetration of γ-ray from one hole to the other. The parallel hole collimator is the most widely used collimator. Apart from parallel-hole collimator, there are also other types of collimators that can be used to magnify or reduce the size of an object on the image. For instance, a diverging collimator is used to image structures that are larger than the size of the γ-camera. On the other hand, a converging collimator is used to image small structures (Fig. 9). A pinhole collimator is an extreme form as of a converging collimator to magnify small objects placed very close to the pinhole [8]. The principal disadvantage of geometrical collimation is low efficiency; only a small fraction of the γ-rays is detected (a cone with an small angle α out of a sphere), as most of the γ-photons are either absorbed by the collimator or never reach the camera. Typically about 1 of 10000 of emitted γ-rays is transmitted through the collimator, resulting in dramatic reduction of the SNR.

The γ-rays that passed through the collimator are converted into a detectable signal. Usually, the detector device consists of a sodium iodide single crystal doted with thallium NaI(Tl). When a γ-ray hits this scintillation crystal, it loses energy through photoelectric and Compton interactions with the crystal. The photoelectric interaction results in the emission of light, the intensity of which is proportional to the energy of the γ-rays. Overall, approximately 15% of the absorbed energy is converted into visible light. The light emitted in the scintillation crystal is converted to detectable electronic signals by a PMT. This conversion is linear and the amplitude of the output signal is therefore be proportional to the absorbed energy of the radiation. In the photo-cathode of the PMT, the incoming light stimulates electron emission. The electrons are accelerated by a potential to an electrode, called a dynode, which has a properly selected surface to give a multiplying effect. Tubes with 10–14 dynodes are available, and the number of electrons is multiplied in the dynode chain of the pulse. Typically, the electrical signal is amplified by more than a factor of 10^6. For detection of the light, a number of PMTs are closely coupled to the scintillation crystals to convert the light signal into an electrical signal. In a SPECT system, about 100 PMTs are used, which are distributed on a hexagonal grid. This geometry ensures that the distance from the center of each PMT to its neighbor is the same. The PMT nearest to the scintillation event converts the most light. The position of the scintillation point is determined from the relative signal outputs of the PMT using an Anger position network. This network produces four outputs, from which the position of the light source can be determined. In addition, the sum of the signals is proportional of the energy of the absorbed γ-rays, which can be used to differentiate between non-scattered with from scattered γ-rays. This is done by a pulse-height analyzer, which selects energies within a certain window. The selection process can improve image quality, because scattered γ-rays have lost their geometrical information and, thus, contribute to a high background noise. Furthermore, windows at different energies can also be used to differentiate between γ-rays at different energies that are emitted from different radionuclides. Hence, multi-energy windows allow for simultaneous imaging of multiple tracers. Currently, new types of γ-cameras are under development, which are based on solid-state detectors. Such devices, e.g., a cadmium zinc telluride (CdZnTe)-based semiconductor, allow a direct conversion of γ-rays into an electrical signal. In contrast to a combination of a scintillation crystal and photomultipliers, such devices can measure more events and have a better energy resolution. However, high production costs of such materials have prevented a widespread application so far.

The spatial resolution of SPECT is mainly determined by the γ-camera. The resolution of the scintillator-photomultiplier combination is in the order of 3 mm and depends on thickness of the scintillation crystal and the diameter of the photomultiplier. However, the practical resolution of γ-cameras is less than this value and is mainly limited by the collimator. The spatial resolu-

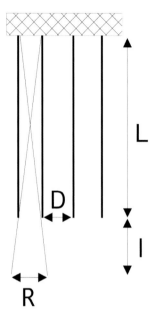

Figure 10.
Design of a collimator. The distance D and the length l of the septa as well as the distance l from the source determine the achievable resolution R of the collimator.

tion (R) of a collimator depends on its geometry, i.e., length (L) and the distance of the lead strips (D), and its distance (l) to γ-ray source (Fig. 10). The overall spatial resolution of clinical SPECT ranges between less than 1 cm to about 2 cm, depending on the collimator type and its distance from the γ-ray source. In general, the collimator should be placed as close to the γ-ray source as possible. Figure 11 shows a modern SPECT system that can move γ-cameras on an optimal trajectory around the patient. Dedicated animal scanners have much higher spatial resolution, i.e., below 3 mm; most of them are based on pinhole collimation.

4.2.2 SPECT agents

Nuclear imaging can be considered as pure molecular imaging techniques, since they can directly detect the molecules, in which the radionuclides have been incorporated. These compounds are called radiopharmaceuticals or

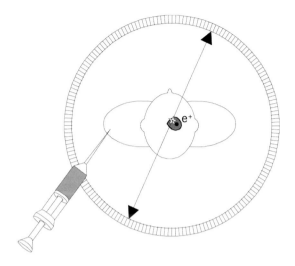

Figure 11.
Principle of PET. A radiopharmaceutical is injected into the body that decays under the emission of a positron. After traveling a short distance the positron captures an electron, resulting in the emission of two antiparallel γ-rays. Since those γ-rays are measured in coincidence no collimator is required.

Table 1.
Properties of important radionuclides used in single emission tomography (SPECT)

Radionuclide	Half-life time	Energy of γ-rays (keV)
^{99m}Tc	6.02 h	140
^{111}In	2.8 days	171, 245
^{123}I	13 h	27, 159
^{131}I	8 days	284, 364, 637

radiotracers. Typical radionuclides for SPECT imaging are ^{99m}Tc, ^{111}In, ^{123}I, ^{201}Tl, and ^{67}Ga. The half-life times and energies of the emitted γ-ray are summarized in Table 1. Radionuclides for SPECT are either produced in a nuclear reactor or in a radionuclide generator. Typical products from nuclear reactors are ^{201}Tl or ^{111}In and molybdenum, where the isotope is produced with neutron activation. On-site molybdenum generators are used to produce ^{99m}Tc, which a product of the radioactive decay. Uptake and biodistribution of the radiopharmaceuticals is governed by their pharmacokinetic properties. Targeting a radiopharmaceuticals to a disease-specific marker or process might lead to its accumulation in certain pathological tissue and thus constitute an early diagnostic indicator. The main advantages of SPECT agents are their relatively long half-life times and a relatively simple chemistry that allow the synthesis of targeted SPECT ligands on-site. Major applications of SPECT imaging are assessment of cardiac function, measurement of blood perfusion in various organs (e.g., heart, brain or lung), detection of tumors and measurement of the renal function. Furthermore, new SPECT agents are approved and under development that allow the detection of specific biological processes, like metabolism, apoptosis and hypoxia.

4.3 Positron emission tomography

A different and more sophisticated nuclear imaging technique is positron emission imaging. The radiopharmaceuticals used in this technique decay under the emission of positrons. A positron is the antimatter of an electron, i.e., it has the same mass as an electron but a positive charge. The kinetic energy of emitted positrons depends on the radionuclide. The emitted positron travels a short distance (0.3–2 mm) within matter (tissue) until it is captured by an electron. The two particles annihilate and the mass of both particles is transformed into energy, i.e. into the generation of two γ-rays with an energy of 511 keV. Due to the conservation of the positron's momentum, the γ-rays are statistically emitted at angles of $180 \pm 0.5°$. These γ-rays can be detected by a detector system enclosing the object (Fig. 11). An important advantage of positron emission imaging is that no geometrical collimation is required. Collimation occurs electronically, i.e., by coincidence detection: γ-rays belonging to the same annihilation event will reach the detector system almost simultaneously, i.e., within a narrow coincidence time window, which is of the order of 10 ns. The source of the γ-emission lies on a line connecting the two responsive detector elements, the so-called line-of-response (LOR). In contrast to SPECT, PET requires two parallel detectors or a complete detector ring. After acquisition the data are usually corrected for attenuation effects, and for accidental and multiple coincidences. Both errors in the coincidence detection can occur, if γ-ray pairs are emitted simultaneously in the body causing ambiguities in defining the LOR. Accidental coincidences represent events that are determined from a wrong LOR connecting detection events originating from different annihilation processes. Multiple coincidences describe the combination of true coincidences with one or more unrelated detection. Usually, such events are simply discarded from the acquired data. The image reconstruction in PET is similar to X-ray CT or SPECT, i.e., either by filtered back-projection or by advanced iterative algorithms. Recently, time-of-flight measurement has been made possible by advances in the detection electronic. In these techniques, the time difference between the arrival times of γ-rays at the detector elements could be measured, allowing the localization of the annihilation event along the LOR. The physical limits of the spatial resolution in PET are determined by two factors: the free path length a positron travels until its annihilation, and the small deviation of the emission angle of the γ-rays from 180°. The path length depends on the energy of positron, which differs among the radioisotopes (see below). The statistical deviation of the emission angle results in a small error in the detection of two γ-rays. The resulting geometric deviation depends on the diameter of the detector ring.

4.3.1 Instrumentation

The instrumentation design of PET is similar to SPECT. Principal differences of PET scanners with regard to SPECT systems are the need of detecting significantly higher energies (γ-rays energy being 511 keV) and the replacement of geometrical by electronic collimation requiring the design of a coincidence detection circuitry. Although γ-rays emitted in PET imaging can also be detected by NaI(Tl), the sensitivity of these crystals is about tenfold lower than other crystals that are more sensitive for detection of 511 keV γ-rays. For instance, bismuth germanate (BGO), cerium-doped gadolinium silicate (GSO) or cerium-doped lutetium silicate (LSO) are characterized by higher density and larger effective atomic number than NaI(Tl), and thus result in more interactions between the γ-rays and the crystal; they therefore have a higher detection efficiency. However, there are also other properties that make these materials attractive as scintillation detectors. For instance, a short decay and dead-time of the crystal is required to ensure a short coincidence time window. In addition, the crystal should produce a high light output. Similar to SPECT the emitted light in the scintillation crystal is detected by PMTs. Ideally, coupling each crystal to a separate photomultiplier would give the highest spatial resolution. To reduce the cost of a PET system, usually a number of crystals (e.g., 4×4) are coupled to a separate PMT. In a clinical PET system, the size of such a block is in the order of 3–4 mm, i.e., which determines the intrinsic spatial resolution. Apart from the combination of scintillation crystals with PMTs, direct converters (or solid state detectors) are under development. After the light is converted into an electric signal and amplified, the signal is digitized. The coincidence detection logic is a simple threshold detection of summed signals. If two γ-rays are detected within the coincidence time window, then the added signal of the two detectors exceeds the detection threshold and an event is registered. For a single event the electronic signal will stay below this threshold.

The main advantages of PET with respect to SPECT are higher sensitivity and better spatial resolution. Since PET does not employ geometrical collimation and often uses a detector covering a large fraction of the total space angle, significantly more g-rays are detected. In addition, due to the higher energy of γ-rays in PET (511 keV) absorption by tissue is less relevant and more γ-rays are detected. Sensitivity in PET can be three orders of magnitude higher than in SPECT. Although the theoretical achievable spatial resolution of most positron-emitters is in the order of 1 mm, the spatial resolution of practical PET systems is poorer. It mainly depends on the size of detector elements, and is in the order of 4–8 mm for clinical systems and 2–4 mm for small bore animal systems. Figure 12 shows a PET image of rat obtained with a dedicated animal PET scanner (Philips Moasic). Besides the spatial resolution, the main limitation in clinical PET is the low SNR. This ratio can be increased by using a higher activity of the PET ligand, a longer acquisition time or by improvements in the detection system. With regard to the last point, detectors with improved energy resolution allow the differentiation between scattered γ-rays and those originating from true events, allowing the reduction of background noise. SNR might be improved by making use of advanced detection systems that can measure the differences in arrival times of γ-rays. This information is utilized in time-of-flight PET, where the location of the emission event can currently be determined within 4–10 cm. Including this information can reduce the statistical uncertainty in the reconstructed image and thus yield better images; SNR improvements by one order of magnitude should be feasible. However, time-of-flight PET is still at an experimental stage and not yet ready for widespread clinical use.

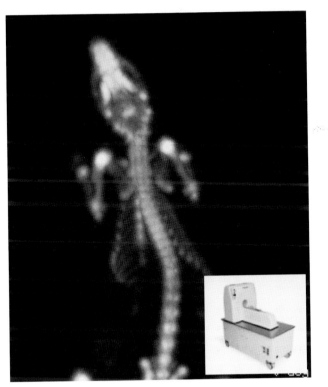

Figure 12.
PET image of a rat obtained with a dedicated small-bore PET system. Use of ^{18}F highlights skeletal structures. (Mosaic, Philips Medical Systems).

4.3.2 PET agents

All radionuclides used in PET imaging are produced by a cyclotron and are synthesized into biological active molecules or highly specific agents. The most commonly used radionuclides are ^{18}F, ^{11}C, ^{15}O and ^{13}N, with the half-life time the energy and positron energy given in Table 2. These radionuclides are produced by proton or deuteron bombardment, protons or deuterons being accelerated in a cyclotron with an energy of 10 MeV or 5 MeV, respectively. Due to the short half-life of all radionuclides, they must be incorporated very rapidly into a radiopharmaceutical. One of the most commonly used PET tracer is 2-fluoro-2-deoxyglucose (FDG), a glucose analog that allows imaging of the glucose metabolism. Since radionuclides used in PET are common building blocks of organic molecules, they can theoretically be inte-

Table 2.
Properties of some important positron emitters

Radionuclide	Half-life time	Max. energy of positrons (keV)
^{18}F	110 min	640
^{11}C	20 min	960
^{13}N	10 min	1190
^{15}O	2 min	1720
^{68}Ga	68 min	1890

grated into a wide range of target structures. This is usually done by isotopic substitution of an atom in the target molecule by its positron-emitting analog, a process that will not affect the biological and chemical behavior of the ligand. A serious disadvantage of PET radionuclides is their short half-life time, which demands on site synthesis and which is to fast for many biological process of interest.

4.3.3 Safety and biological effects

The biological effects encountered in nuclear imaging are same as those discussed for X-ray imaging. Absorption and Compton scattering lead to ionization of atoms in the tissue, which can cause cell damage and/or genetic mutations. The amount of emitted γ-rays depends on the activity of the radionuclide. Typical activities used in nuclear imaging are in the order of 100–1000 MBq. For safety considerations it has to be taken into account that radiopharmaceuticals may accumulate in certain regions or organs; avoidance of too high local activities will limit the overall dose administered.

5 Ultrasound imaging

Ultrasonic imaging is based upon the interaction between acoustic waves and tissue. Typically, sound waves are sent into the body by the imaging system in the form of short-duration pulses that are reflected and scattered from structures/tissue interfaces within the body (Fig. 13). The echoes are then received by the imaging system and reconstructed into an image. The under-

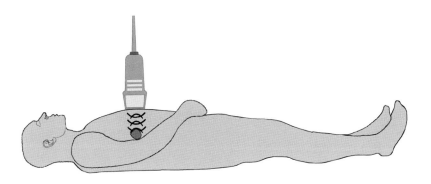

Figure 13.
Principle of ultrasound imaging. A transducer transmits an ultrasound wave into the body and
receives the reflected waves.

lying physical principle that governs the interaction between sound and tissue is that sound is reflected whenever there is a difference in acoustic impedance, which is governed by small-scale differences in density and compress-
ibility of tissue. These differences allow differentiation between tissue types
and in some cases, the distinction between healthy and pathological tissue.
Image reconstruction is accomplished by assuming a constant speed of sound
(about 1540 m/s) in tissue. This assumption along with knowledge of the
time evolved between emission of the pulse and detection of the echo allows
the derivation of geometrical (depth) information and, thus, the reconstruction of an image with physical spatial dimensions. Multiplication the time
delay with the mean velocity and division by two (because the sound has
traveled the distance twice, i.e. back and forth), yields the distance of the
structure from the body surface.

Diagnostic ultrasonic images include a variety of clinical imaging modes
termed A-lines, B-mode, M-mode, and even a less clinically relevant C-scan
mode. The nomenclature is inherited from the world of Radar. In A-line
mode, a one-dimensional profile representing the propagation of sound
along one line of site is recorded. Intensity maxima occur at echogenic structures, typically at tissue interfaces. This principle is currently applied in some
optical applications. B-mode scanning is the most familiar clinical imaging
mode, and is represented by a two-dimensional image. M-mode is the practice of rapidly firing one line of site through a moving organ. This allows the
tracking of motion of a structure such as a cardiac valve or cardiac wall with

high time resolution. Each line can be obtained in less than 100 μs, Therefore, an image consisting of 100 lines can be obtained in less than 10 ms, i.e., real time imaging is possible.

In clinical practice, ultrasound is used for studies of the heart, liver, kidney, ovaries, breast, peripheral vascular, and even portions of the brain through the temporal lobes. In each of these cases, the role of an "acoustic window" allowing the sound waves to reach the tissue of interest is of outmost importance. Ultrasound does not propagate through air and poorly through bone, so that organs that are shielded by these obstructions cannot be imaged.

5.1   Contrast mechanisms

The contrast in ultrasound imaging arises mainly from the propagation properties of the ultrasonic wave through tissue. A key parameter is the acoustic impedance of tissue, which differs for different types of tissue. The degree of reflection is determined by the differences in the acoustic impedances between adjacent structures. When the size of the structure insonified is comparable to the acoustic wavelength, scattering occurs, which will also contribute to image contrast. If the dimension of the structures smaller than the ultrasound wavelength, the dominant process is Rayleigh scattering, which leads to dispersion of the signal in more or less all directions with predicted ultrasonic frequency dependence. The scattering process becomes more complex if the size of the structure is in the same order as the wavelength. Scattering can result in unwanted imaging phenomena called speckle, which describes an interference pattern in an ultrasound image formed by the superposition of many waves scattered by unresolved scatterers. The texture of the observed speckle pattern is not an inherent property of the underlying structure; incoherent speckles rather add to the noise in the image and thus reduce the CNR in ultrasound images. Another technical challenge in clinical ultrasonic imaging is the observation that ultrasonic energy is absorbed by the body, thereby reducing the SNR. The mechanisms for signal attenuation include absorption through the conversion of ultrasonic waves to heat, and also through the scattering of sound into directions away from the transducer/receiver system. The attenuation is characterized by a frequency-dependent exponential decay of the ultrasonic wave intensity that can be approximated by a linear relationship between attenuation (in dB/cm) and the frequency of the ultrasound.

5.1.1 Harmonic tissue imaging

Ultrasound waves propagate through tissue and interact non-linearly with tissue constituents. This phenomenon is due to the small but finite differences in the speed of sound that vary with amplitude of the ultrasonic wave. The result is that the maxima of the pressure wave propagate slightly faster than the minima, resulting in a distortion of the wave. This non-linearity leads to the generation of harmonic frequencies within the wave, which are also reflected and backscattered to the transmitter. In harmonic tissue imaging the fundamental frequency is transmitted, but only its harmonics are received [9]. Usually, the first harmonic is filtered out from all frequencies received. Since harmonic signals originate from within the tissue, the path length traveled is shorter than for the fundamental frequency, which leads to less attenuation. The intensity of the harmonic energy generated is proportional to the square of the energy in the fundamental wave. Most of the harmonic energy results from the strongest part of the beam, with weaker contributions of the beam (e.g. side lobes) generating relatively little harmonic energy, which can result in better focusing. Therefore, harmonic imaging yields a dramatically improved contrast between adjacent tissue structures. In addition, harmonic imaging can be also applied to detect microbubble contrast agents (see below).

5.1.2 Doppler imaging

In addition to imaging of the morphology, ultrasound is also capable of measuring dynamic parameters such as velocity of flowing blood through the Doppler shift in the backscattered frequency. The Doppler effect describes the shift in the frequency, due to a moving source or receiver (Fig. 14). The red blood cells are responsible for scattering the incident ultrasonic waves. Sign and amplitude depend on the predominant flow direction with respect to the ultrasound transducer. If the blood flow is directed towards the Doppler transducer, the echoes from blood reflected back to the transducer will have a

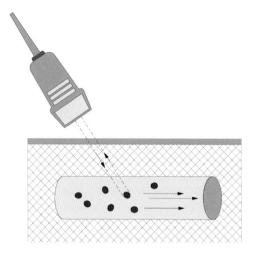

Figure 14.
Principle of Doppler imaging. The movement of the red-blood cells result in a frequency shift of the ultrasound signal that is proportional to the blood velocity.

higher frequency. If the blood flow is directed away from the transducer, the echoes will have a lower frequency than those emitted. The Doppler frequency shift is proportional to the blood flow velocity and thus allows quantification. There are several Doppler modes that are in use in clinical systems. These include pulse wave (PW), continuous wave (CW), and Color Doppler (which also include Power Doppler, Harmonic Power Doppler). PW imaging utilizes a limited number of cycles to determine a Doppler frequency shift at a specific location. This allows, e.g., the measurement of flow patterns across the cardiac valves. CW Doppler does not provide spatial information but is used for detection of flow in situations where there is a dominant flow source. Color Doppler allows qualitative and quantitative measure of two-dimensional spatial distribution of flow. Color Doppler is typically performed using multiple transmitted wave packets and correlating the filtered backscattered signals.

5.2   Instrumentation

An ultrasonic imaging system consists of a transducer, transmitter/detection electronics, a data processing unit and a display. The transducer probe (also

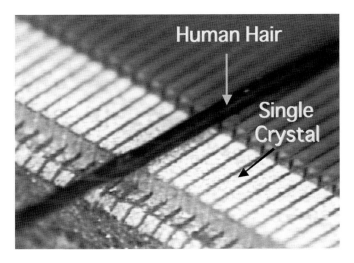

Figure 15.
Electron microcopy image of the piezocrystal array.

called scanhead) is a key component of the ultrasound machine. It sends short pulses of a high frequency sound wave (1–10 MHz) into the body and receives their echoes. The transducer probe generates and receives sound waves using a piezoelectric crystal (Fig. 15). These crystals change their shape rapidly upon application of an oscillating voltage. The most commonly used piezoelectric material is lead zirconate titanate (PZT). The rapid shape changes, or vibrations, of the crystals produce emanating sound waves. The reverse principle is used for detection: an ultrasound wave hitting the crystals causes a distortion and concomitantly a voltage difference across the crystal. Therefore, the same crystals can be used to send and receive sound waves. The probe also contains a sound absorbing substance (called "backing material") to eliminate unwanted reverberations within the probe and to confine the length of ultrasound pulse (Fig. 16). An acoustic lens helps to focus the emitted sound waves and provides improved coupling between the probe and the body surface. Transducer probes come in many shapes and sizes specifically designed for clinical applications. Often, a transducer uses an array of piezoelectric elements to allow for focusing of a sound wave into the body and to differentiate the received echoes from one another. These arrays can consist of a one-dimensional linear arrangement of small piezoelectric crystals (64–512 elements). Since the signals transmitted and the received by the

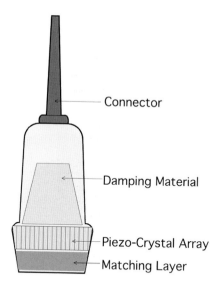

Connector

Damping Material

Piezo-Crystal Array

Matching Layer

Figure 16.
Design of an ultrasound-transducer that consists of a piezocrystal array to steer and to shape ultra-sound beam. A matching layer is used for better coupling of the transducer to the body. The damping material ensures fast decay of the ultrasound wave and thus short ultrasound pulses.

array elements can be individually delayed in time, these probes are also called phased array. The phased array principle allows electronically focusing and steering of the ultrasound beam during the transmit phase. The principle can also be applied for individual echo signal acquisition during the receive phase; so-called "beam-forming". Recently, two-dimensional phased-arrays have been developed that allow true three-dimensional imaging (Fig. 17).

Once the acoustic signal is received by the transducer, converted from pressure waves to electrical signals, and beam-formed, it is then passed on to the rest of the signal conditioning path. One of the key aspects of this path is the compensation for the attenuating affect of propagating sound wave through tissue. This is accomplished through the use of a time-varying (therefore depth-varying) amplification process known as time-gain compensation. The time-gain compensation amplifies those signals proportional to their time delay with respect to the transmitting pulse, i.e. to their depth. Usually, additional depth-depending filtering is applied, because the characteristic spectrum of the noise also changes with the depth. The gain-compensated,

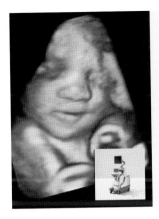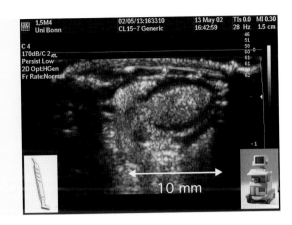

Figure 17.
Three-dimensional ultrasound image of a fetus (left). Two-dimensional ultrasound image of a mouse heart obtained with a clinical ultrasound scanner using a dedicated transducer (right). A microbubble contrast agent provides a high contrast between blood (white) and myocardium (Courtesy of K. Tiemann, University of Bonn, Germany).

filtered, beam-summed signal can then be further processed before finally being scan-converted to provide the operator with a diagnostic image.

When discussing the spatial resolution of an ultrasound system, the three dimensions (axial, lateral, elevation) have to be considered separately. The axial resolution along the propagation direction of the incident acoustic wave is defined as the minimal time difference of two echoes that can be resolved. The minimal distance of two reflecting boundaries that can be resolved depends on the pulse duration and the ultrasound frequency. As the ultrasound frequency increases, the pulse length decreases and the axial resolution improves. However, the use of higher operating frequencies is limited by the fact that the attenuation of the ultrasound in tissue increases at higher frequencies, i.e., the penetration depth decreases. Therefore, lower frequencies (1–3 MHz) are used for studying deep-lying structures, while higher frequencies (5–10 MHz) are superior when imaging regions are close to the body surface. Typical values of the axial resolution are 1–2 mm at 1 MHz and 0.3 mm at 5 MHz. For a single crystal transducer, the lateral width of the ultrasound beam is determined by the size of the aperture. Since the diameter of the transducer is limited (1–5 cm), the intrinsic lateral resolution is not as good as the axial resolution. Therefore, beam-focusing lenses or curved transducer are normally used. Typical values for lateral resolution at the focal plane range between 0.5 to 2 mm for typical clinical scan heads. The elevation dimension is determined by the length of the crystal elements, and is in the order of 2–5 mm for clinical scanners.

The SNR of ultrasound imaging is determined by a number of factors, like the intensity and the frequency of the transmitted wave: the higher the intensity of the transmitted ultrasonic wave, the higher the amplitude of the detected signals. Attenuation increases with the increasing ultrasound frequency, leading to a decrease in SNR. Speckle arising from the phase cancellation of scattering from multiple small scatterers can sometimes obscure small-scale structures. Recently, a composite imaging method (SonoCT®) was developed to reduce these effects [10]. In this technique, several (five to nine) images are acquired using different directions of the transmitted ultrasound wave. The images obtained from the different angles have different speckle patterns. The set of images is then combined to provide a single composite image, which has sharper borders and reduced speckle.

5.3   Ultrasound contrast agents

The detection of blood in small vessels located deep inside the body is difficult. Blood-pool ultrasound contrast agents can be used to increase the delineation of the chambers of the heart or larger vessels and also to detect the perfusion of organs. Two different mechanisms can enhance the CNR for blood in ultrasound. First, differences in the acoustic impedance are increased thereby increasing the backscattering. For instance, a targeted perfluorcarbon emulsion yielded increased backscattering and may be considered as an acoustic mirror [11]. The second mechanism is resonance of so-called microbubbles, which are gas-filled shells, where the shell properties are altered to allow for the desired clinical purpose. Microbubbles possess characteristic resonance frequencies within the frequency range of clinical imaging systems. There are several commercial diagnostic blood pool contrast agents available on the market for ultrasonic diagnostic imaging. Microbubbles are clinically used in perfusion studies [12], and have a great potential for molecular imaging for targeting intravascular targets [13]. Microbubbles show also an increased scattering of the ultrasound wave [14] with non-linear behavior, thereby generating harmonic and sub-harmonic signals. Clinically, this physical phenomenon is exploited to differentiate signals originating from tissue, which has a strong linear and a weak non-linear component from those of the contrast agent, which has a strong non-linear component. Several techniques are utilized by the imaging community to improve the differentiation of contrast agent from tissue. Pulse inversion [15] makes use of the fact that resonant microbubbles do not respond the same way to an incident pulse during the compression phase as they do during the refraction (expanding) phase. The technique sends two pulses that are inverse to each another (opposite phase). The received signals are then added. For linear scatterers such as tissue, the received echoes will cancel, but for signals from non-linear scatterers the sum contains the harmonic component of the signal. There are several other mechanisms exploited for contrast enhancement, such as power modulation, harmonic imaging, ultra-harmonic imaging, and many others that are beyond the scope of this text.

5.4   Safety and biological effects

Diagnostic ultrasound imaging has an established safety record. However, as ultrasonic waves interact with the patient's tissue, they potentially may have some biological effects [16]. In diagnostic imaging, certain safety guidelines have been established that attempt to control the two primary mechanisms for adverse interaction between ultrasound waves and tissue: heat and cavitation. Because the body absorbs ultrasonic energy, there is deposition of energy in the form of heat within tissue. This deposition of heat is rarely a problem in short-time pulse imaging used for two-dimensional imaging as the amount of energy absorbed by the body is small and is quickly conducted by circulation. However, in longer time pulse imaging such as in Doppler modes, there can be finite deposition of heat. The thermal index (TI) was established as a means of quantifying the amount of heat being delivered to tissue. Cavitation refers to the spontaneous formation of gas bubbles in the body due to the ultrasonic pressure wave: if pressure minima are lower than the partial pressure of gases solved in tissue fluid, the gases might actually dissolve. All commercial scanners quantify this risk by keeping the mechanical index (MI) at a sufficiently low value, typically lower than 2.0. The safety metrics, TI and MI, have been chosen such that they provides a considerable safety margin between the values reached in commercial clinical systems and those required to induce adverse biological effects.

6   Magnetic resonance imaging

Magnetic resonance imaging (MRI) is based on the emission of an electro-magnetic wave due to the nuclear resonance effect. MRI is a non-ionizing imaging technique with high soft-tissue contrast, high spatial and good temporal resolution. MRI is capable of exploiting a wide range of endogenous contrast mechanisms that allow the characterization of morphological, physiological, and metabolic information *in vivo*. Therefore, MRI has become the modality of choice for many preclinical and clinical applications.

MRI is based on the NMR effect first described by Bloch and Purcell in 1946. As the three letters in the term NMR indicate, there are three fundamental requirements that have to be fulfilled to measure the NMR effect. The first requirement is that the nucleus of interest possesses a nonzero magnetic moment, a *nuclear spin*. All nuclei with an odd number of protons and/or neutrons have this property and thus behave as small magnets. Typical nuclei used in NMR are, for instance, hydrogen (^{1}H), phosphorus (^{31}P), carbon (^{13}C), sodium (^{23}Na) or fluorine (^{19}F).

The second requirement for NMR is the use of an external static magnetic field, B_0. In the absence of such an external magnetic field, the individual magnetic moments of the atoms in the tissue being examined are randomly oriented and there is no net bulk magnetization. In presence of such a field, the magnetic moments align at a defined angle along or opposed to the external field, as described by the Zeemann interaction. Due to the angel a torque is induced that results in a precessional movement around the B_0 field (Fig. 18). The frequency of precession, also called the *Larmor* frequency, is proportional to B_0, the proportionality constant being the so-called gyromagnetic ratio, which are characteristic for a type of nuclei. Hydrogen plays an important role for preclinical and clinical applications, because of the high abundance of protons in biological tissue (water) and since its gyromagnetic ratio is the largest of all nuclei of relevance. The Larmor frequency of hydrogen spins at an external static magnetic field strength of 1.5 Tesla (T) is approximately 64 MHz. The sign of the rotation depends on orientation of the spins, i.e., some spins have aligned along the B_0 field, whereas others opposed to it. Since an alignment along the B_0 field corresponds to a lower energy state, slightly more nuclei will align along the B_0 field rather than opposed to it. Therefore, the tissue will exhibit a net magnetization parallel to the external magnetic field, which is called longitudinal magnetization.

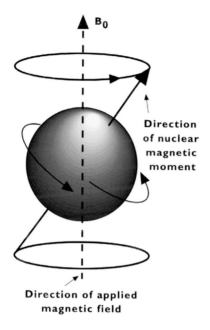

B_0

Direction
of nuclear
magnetic
moment

Direction of applied
magnetic field

Figure 18.
Precession of a nuclear magnetic moment in external applied field B_0.

The percentage of parallel versus opposite orientations of nuclear spins is given by the Boltzmann distribution law and depends on both the temperature and the field strength of the B_0 field. For an applied field of 1.5 T and at room temperature, the excess of magnetic moments that are aligned more along the magnetic field is only 10 in 1 million for hydrogen nuclei. Therefore, the net magnetization, and thus the inherent sensitivity of NMR, is rather small. Application of a higher magnetic field results in a larger net magnetization, thereby increasing the sensitivity of NMR.

The third requirement for measuring the NMR effect is the use of an additional time-varying magnetic field, B_1, applied perpendicular to the static B_0 field and at the resonance condition (i.e., at Larmor frequency,). Radiofrequency (rf) coils are used to produce B_1 field pulses of certain amplitude and duration. Such B_1-pulses flip the longitudinal magnetization to an arbitrary angle with respect to the external static field B_0, the flip angle usually ranging between 10° and 180°. The transverse component of the flipped magnetization precesses around the static B_0 field at the Larmor frequency, and induces a time-varying voltage signal in the rf coil (Fig. 19).

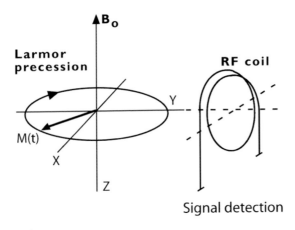

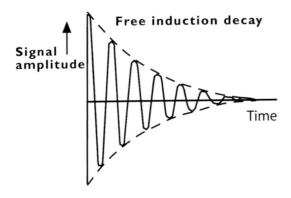

Figure 19.
Signal reception of a free-induction decay (FID).

In order to distinguish magnetization at different locations, magnetic field gradients are applied that cause a linear variation of the magnetic field strength in space. The spatially varying gradient amplitudes $G_{x,y,z}$ determine the difference between the actual field strength at a certain location and the static field B_0, i.e., the precession frequency varies over space. Usually, for three-dimensional encoding, not all gradients are applied simultaneously and the image formation process can be separated into three phases: slice selection, phase encoding and frequency encoding. Slice selection is accomplished using a frequency-selective B_1 pulse applied in the presence of a magnetic field gradient. The position of the slice thickness is determined by frequency of the B_1 pulse, whereas the slice thickness depends on its bandwidth

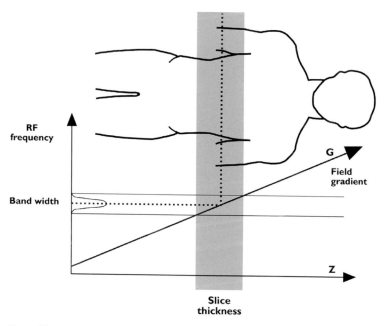

Figure 20.
Principle of slice selection. The use of a gradient field results in a distribution of different resonance frequencies. Only those spins were exited, which frequencies are within the bandwidth of the rf pulse.

and the gradient amplitude (Fig. 20). Having selected a slice, i.e., flipped the longitudinal magnetization within the slice to generate a transverse component, the signal has to be spatially encoded in the remaining two dimensions. One of these directions is encoded by producing a spatially varying phase shift of precessing transverse magnetization. This is achieved by applying a phase-encoding gradient for a short period before signal acquisition. During this gradient pulse, the transverse magnetization components at different locations precess at different frequencies and accumulate location-dependent phase shifts. To achieve full spatial encoding, a number of experiments have to be carried out with step-wise variation of the amplitude of the phase-encoding gradient. Since both amplitude and phase of the NMR signal are detected, the spatial distribution of the magnetization along the phase-encode direction can be determined after performing a Fourier transform. The third spatial dimension is encoded by applying a frequency-encoding gradient during data acquisition. This gradient is changing the precession frequency over space and creates a one-to-one relation between the resonance frequency of the signal and the spatial location of its origin. Performing a Fourier transform of the acquired signal yields the position of the contributing magnetization along the frequency-encode direction.

The spatial resolution in MRI depends on the amplitude of the gradients and the acquisition bandwidth. In addition, smaller voxel sizes result in a lower SNR, as fewer magnetic moments contribute to the acquired signal. Typical values of the spatial resolution of clinical scanners are in the order of 1 mm. Dedicated animal scanner operating at a higher magnetic field strength and applying strong gradients are able to obtain images with voxels smaller than 100 μm. The voxel size achievable also depends on the MR measurement protocol used. A detailed description of the different measurements and the applications of MRI can be found elsewhere [17, 18].

6.1   Contrast mechanisms

6.1.1 Relaxation times

The contrast in MRI is strongly influenced by two relaxation processes. These processes can be described by exponential relationships characterized by the time constants T_1 and T_2, respectively. The relaxation times T_1 and T_2 depend on the specific molecular structure of the analyte, its physical state (liquid or solid) and the temperature; they vary among different tissues and are affected by pathologies.

The longitudinal relaxation time T_1 describes the statistical probability for energy transfer between the excited nuclei and the molecular framework, named the lattice: it is also termed spin-lattice relaxation time. The net magnetization returns to the equilibrium at a rate given by $1/T_1$. Typical T_1 values in biological tissue range from 20 ms to a few seconds. Efficient transfer of energy to the lattice is highly dependent on molecular motion of the lattice, which cause in fluctuations in the local magnetic fields that can induce transitions between the spin states of the nuclei. The motion modes, i.e., rotational, vibrational and translational motion (Fig. 21), depend on the structure and the size of the molecules. The motion of large molecules is characterized by low frequencies, that of medium-sized and small molecules by higher frequencies. Efficient energy transfer (i.e., a short T_1) occurs when the frequency of the fluctuating fields, which is determined by the molecular

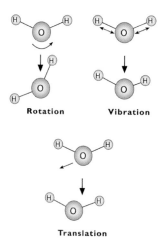

Figure 21.
Different types of molecular motions resulting in fluctuating magnetic fields.

motion, matches the Larmor frequency of the spins. Therefore, the T_1 relaxation time depends on the field strength. Furthermore, T_1 values are generally shorter in solutions than in solids, since vibrational frequencies in solid crystal lattice are typically significantly higher (approximately 10^{12} Hz) than the Larmor frequencies in MRI (approximately 10^{11} Hz). Finally, T_1 relaxation is affected by the presence of macromolecules that possess hydrophilic binding sites, i.e., water protons in tissue relaxing much faster than those in pure water.

Transverse or spin-spin relaxation (T_2) is due to the transfer of energy between magnetic nuclei. Immediately after excitation all spins precess coherently (i.e., in phase). However, interactions between individual magnetic moments result in variations in the precession frequencies of the spins. As a result, a dephasing of the spins occurs, causing an exponential decay of the transverse magnetization. The transverse relaxation time T_2 is influenced by the physical state and the molecular size. Solids and large molecules are characterized by relatively short T_2 times, small molecules by long T_2 values. Therefore, the presence of macromolecules in solution shortens T_2, since the overall molecular motion is reduced, leading to more effective spin-spin interactions. Typical T_2 relaxation times in biological tissue range from a few microseconds in solids to a few seconds in liquids. The T_2 relaxation process is nearly independent of the field strength.

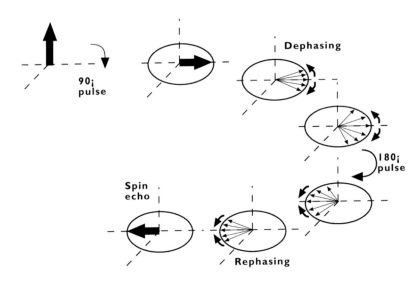

Figure 22.
Principle of the spin echo experiment. After excitation by a 90° pulse the transverse magnetization dephases due to field inhomogeneities. Application of an 180° pulse results in a rephasing of the magnetization and forming of a spin echo.

In addition to the spin-spin interaction, the phase coherence is also influence by local field inhomogeneities in the applied magnetic field. The exponential decay resulting from the combination of T_2 relaxation and field inhomogeneities is referred to as the effective transverse relaxation time T_2^*. The T_2^* relaxation describes the envelope of the time varying signal (Fig. 19), called the free induction decay (FID).

A spin-echo experiment can be used to compensate the influence of B_0 inhomogeneity (Fig. 22) and thus to measure the T_2-decay. In this experiment, two B_1-pulses are applied: the first pulse with a flip angle of 90° tilts all longitudinal magnetization into the transverse plane. The second pulse with a flip angle of 180° refocuses the dephasing caused by B_0 inhomogeneity. Both pulses are separated by a time period of $T_E/2$ and a signal is acquired after T_E (echo delay time). During the first $T_E/2$ period, i.e. between the 90° and 180° pulse, the individual magnetic moments precess at a different Larmor frequencies due to the B_0 inhomogeneity. As a result they obtain different phase shifts, which translate into a dephasing of the bulk magnetization. The 180°-pulse applied at $T_E/2$ inverts the magnetic moments and correspondingly their phases; the phase shift acquired during the following delay

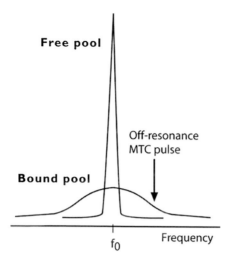

Figure 23.
Principle of MTC. The pool of bound protons is not contributing to the MR signal. An off-resonant rf pulse is used to saturate the protons of the bound pool. The saturated magnetization is exchanged with the magnetization of the free water pool resulting in a reduction of the magnetization of the free pool.

TE/2 exactly compensates the inverted phases shifts acquired during the period prior to the 180° pulse leading to the formation of a so-called spin echo. Its amplitude depends only on the T_2 and the echo time T_E.

6.1.2 Magnetization transfer

The contrast in biological tissue is also affected by exchange of magnetization (cross-correlation) between two main compartments: proton spins in the free water pool and spins that are bound to macromolecules. As discussed, the latter have a very short T_2 and thus cannot be measured. The fast T_2 decay translates into a large range of resonance frequencies, whereas the bulk water is characterized by a long T_2 value and correspondingly a narrow frequency spectrum. The size of the of free and macromolecule-bound water compartments varies for tissues. Free water exchanges its spin state with that of water bound to macromolecules, which leads to apparent relaxation due to loss of coherence. This magnetization transfer can be measured by applying an off-resonant narrow bandwidth rf pulse that saturates the bound water pool prior to the start of the image acquisition. The bulk water pool is not affected by this frequency selective pulse (Fig. 23). Due to the magnetization exchange, this translates into an increased apparent transverse relaxation, the rate being dependent of the exchange rate. This magnetization transfer contrast (MTC) makes tissues that are rich in macromolecules sensitive to this effect (e.g., muscle, cartilage, ligaments), they appear hypointense (darker) in MR images. Tissues like fat, blood and cerebrospinal fluid are hardly affected by MTC.

6.1.3 Chemical shift

As previously described, nuclei of different elements resonate at different Larmor frequencies. It is useful to note that even spins of the same isotope can resonate at different frequencies, if they differ in their molecular environment, i.e., chemical structure. This frequency difference is called chemical shift, and is commonly expressed as a relative measure in parts per million (ppm). MR spectroscopy exploits this effect: recording the NMR signals in optimal homogeneous B_0 field allows resolving the individual resonance frequencies of the molecular constituents in tissue. The comparison of the chemical shifts measured in a sample with values in reference tables allows identification of chemical substances, while the signal intensity is proportional to their concentration. MR spectroscopy of living organisms yields insight into the metabolism of tissue. In particular, MR spectroscopy of the brain is used for grading and staging of tumors, or for the assessment metabolic alterations during ischemia and neurodegenerative diseases. Spectroscopic imaging combines MR spectroscopy with spatial encoding in two or three directions, such that spectroscopic information can be displayed as an image: for each peak in the spectrum the spatial distribution of the integrated peak intensity is displayed. Since the metabolite concentrations in living organisms is four to five orders of magnitude lower than the concentration of water, the voxel size in MR spectroscopy and spectroscopic imaging is usually much larger, and of the order of 1 cm^3.

6.1.4 Flow, perfusion and diffusion

Dynamic processes such as blood flow, tissue perfusion and diffusion constitute an additional contrast mechanism in MRI. All three mechanisms describe the motion of spins on a different time scale. Blood flow is a relatively fast motion restricted to large and medium-sized vessels. Perfusion is slower than blood flow and describes a transport process by which oxygen and nutrients are delivered to tissue through the microvasculature. Diffusion is caused by random thermal motions and due to transport along concentration differences between different compartments. In tissue, barriers lead to a restriction of the diffusion processes and thus to an anisotropy.

In general, the motion of spins causes artifacts in the image due to inconsistencies in the amplitude and phase in the acquisition process. However, the influence of gradient fields on the phase of moving spins during the acquisition process can also be used to obtain information on the velocity and acceleration of moving spins. These methods apply motion-encoding gradients in different directions, resulting in a phase shift of moving spins. The motion-induced phase shift is proportional to the velocity or acceleration of the moving spins and is exploited in phase-contrast angiography (PCA). Another possibility is the exploitation of the effects of motion on the signal amplitude. One option is time-of-flight angiography, which takes advantage of the inflow of fresh, i.e., unsaturated blood into a volume, in which the magnetization due to stationary tissue is saturated. The flow velocity and repetition time T_R determine the amount of unsaturated spins that flow into the imaging volume, greatly increasing the contrast between moving and stationary tissue. A second method involves labeling the spins in blood by changing the state of the longitudinal magnetization using prepulses in the imaging sequence. The labeling is applied to arterial blood in a region upstream of the slice that is imaged, hence the acronym 'arterial spin labeling' (ASL). Usually, two experiments are performed, one with labeling and one without labeling (control scan). From these experiments tissue perfusion rates can be calculated and used to describe the exchange rate between the capillaries and the tissue.

In contrast to flow, diffusion processes are slower and rely on the thermal motion of spins. Random motion in a gradient field causes stochastic phase shifts that cannot be refocused; the signal amplitude is decreased by a factor that depends on the diffusion constant. The apparent diffusion coefficient (ADC) determined from the signal attenuation contains two contributions associated with diffusion of water in the extra- and intracellular compartments. The latter component suffers from restrictions of the diffusion. Therefore, the intracellular diffusion coefficient is smaller than the extracellular one. The rate of water diffusion is often indicative of the status of tissue. For example, brain cells can swell during an ischemic episode (e.g., stroke), which might lead to cell membrane damage. An increase in the intracellular volume leads to a decrease of the ADC value.

To measure the ADC, additional strong gradients are applied to provide high diffusion sensitivity. The ADC value is in general direction dependent, in particular in anisotropic structures such as nerve bundles and fiber tracts. Usually, a number of experiments are performed without and with diffusion gradients in different directions. A detailed description of perfusion and diffusion can be found in [19].

6.1.5 Blood oxygen level-dependent contrast

The signal intensity in MRI is furthermore affected by the oxygenation status of blood. This contrast mechanism is termed blood-oxygen-level-dependent (BOLD) effect [20]. The electron spin of the iron center of blood hemoglobin changes from a diamagnetic to a paramagnetic state during deoxygenation. Therefore, blood deoxygenation results in a reduction of T_2^* relaxation time. This contrast mechanism is exploited in functional brain imaging [21], which allows visualization of activated brain areas. During activation, the blood supply to activated regions exceeds the demand due to the increased oxygen consumption. This leads to an increased concentration of oxygenated hemoglobin in activated brain areas as compared to brain tissue at rest, and thus to a local increase in T_2^*. Using T_2^*-weighted sequences, activated brain areas appear hyperintense, i.e., display increased intensity. By subtracting images acquired during episodes of activation and resting state, activation maps can be computed with activated areas being displayed as bright regions.

6.2 Instrumentation

An MRI system consists of several hardware components: the magnet, the magnetic field gradient system and the rf-transmit/receive system. Currently, magnets field strengths used for clinical MRI systems range between 0.23 and 3 T, and most clinical systems operate at 1.5 T. Recently, a number of research systems for human applications have been installed that work at 7 T or higher. Most animal MRI systems use magnetic field strengths at 4.7 T and 7 T, but systems above 10 T are also available. Although higher field strengths result in a higher signal, the use of such field strengths is hampered by a longer T_1 values and increased rf heating due to rf absorption in tissue. In addition to the magnetic field strength, the magnetic field homogeneity, which must be of the order of 1 ppm within the probe volume, is an important characteristic of the MR magnet. All magnets at higher field strengths are made of superconducting coils that have to be immersed in cryogenic fluids (liquid helium). After installation, the magnet field homogeneity must be optimized, inhomogeneities are accounted for, e.g., by placing pieces of iron in the magnet bore, a procedure is also called passive shimming. In addition, the field homogeneity is optimized for each measurement by applying adequate direct currents to the gradient coils to compensate for field distortions caused by the sample. In a clinical environment, the main magnet field has to be shielded to protect the environment from the effects of the fringe fields; otherwise, devices such as, e.g., neurostimulators and pacemakers might be affected. Magnets can be passively shielded by enclosing the magnet room with tons of iron plating. However, clinical MR magnets are usually actively shielded using two sets of superconducting coil: the inner coil produces the main static field inside the magnet, whereas the outer coil, in which the current flows in the opposite direction, reduces the fringe field.

Spatial encoding requires the use of magnetic field gradients in three orthogonal directions. These weak magnetic field gradients are produced by three coils producing orthogonal fields (Fig. 24) connected to independently controlled gradient amplifiers. The magnetic field gradients generated by these coils should be as linear as possible over the imaging volume. A complicating factor is the occurrence of so-called eddy currents induced in conducting parts of the MR system by temporal switching of the magnetic field gradients. These eddy currents produce unwanted magnetic fields in the imaging volume, resulting in image artifacts. The effects of eddy currents are minimized by designing actively shielded gradient coils. In clinical MR-scanners, the currents applied to the gradient coils are of the order of several hundreds of amperes. Since these currents are flowing inside a static magnetic field, large forces act on the mechanical parts of the gradient coil, leading to oscillations during gradient switching. These oscillations are responsible for the acoustic noise during the MR measurement.

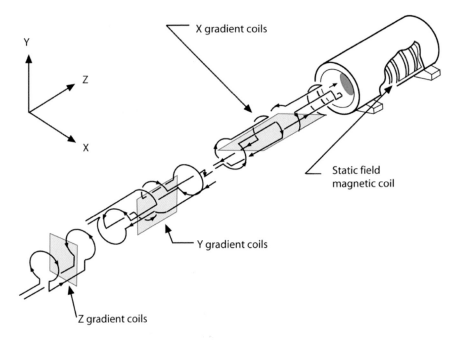

Figure 24.
Geometry of coils form magnetic field gradients in three directions.

Rf coils are used for excitation and signal detection. The coils must be able to produce a uniform or well-defined oscillating field within the imaging volume. The coils are tuned and matched to the resonance frequency of the type of nucleus being observed. Placing of a sample inside the rf coil adds an impedance to the coil circuit, referred to as coil loading, which has to be compensated for (tuning and matching of the coil). At field strengths higher than 0.5 T, the noise introduced by the samples dominates the inherent noise of coil circuit. Often separate coils are used for excitation and detection, i.e., a large volume coil (body coil) is used for excitation, whereas dedicated receive coils are used for detection. Large volume coils yield homogeneous rf excitation, while dedicated receive coils achieve higher sensitivity (Fig. 25) as they are placed close to the region of interest and, in addition, have a better filling factor, i.e., receive less noise. The use of an array of receive coils corresponds to an extension of concept of dedicated receive coils. Each coil element covers a different part of the body and after acquisition the individual images of all coil elements can be combined to large field of view image. In

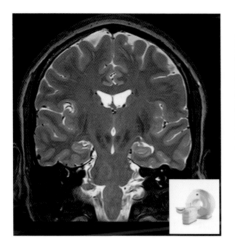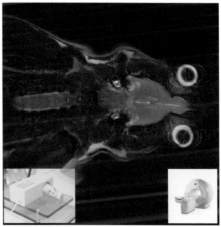

Figure 25.
Left: High-resolution (0.5 mm) brain image obtained on 3-T clinical MR scanner (Philips Medical Systems). Right: High-resolution image (100 µm) of a rat obtained on a 3-T clinical MR scanner image (Courtesy G. Adam UKE Hamburg) using a dedicated solenoid rf coil (Philips Research Hamburg).

addition, the spatial sensitivity of the array coil elements can also be used to speed up the acquisition by means of parallel imaging methods [22].

6.3   MRI contrast agents

In many clinical situations the intrinsic contrast of the tissue might not be sufficient to discriminate pathological from healthy tissue. Therefore, the use of contrast-enhancing agents has become an integral part of MRI investigations. There are two principal classes of MRI contrast agents: paramagnetic and superparamagnetic compounds. Paramagnetic agents primarily shorten the T_1 relaxation time of the tissue, in which they accumulate. Using T_1-weighted imaging sequences such regions can be specifically enhanced. Superparamagnetic agents primarily shorten the T_2 and $T_2{}^*$ values of tissue. A more detail description of MRI contrast agents and the factors determining their behavior can be found elsewhere [23].

Paramagnetic contrast agents are based on metal ions with one or more unpaired electrons. These unpaired electrons result in a very large electron magnetic moment that interacts with the much smaller magnetic moments of the nucleus. Molecular motions result in random fluctuations of this dipolar magnetic interaction, leading to a reduction of both T_1 and T_2 relaxation times. Two mechanisms are responsible for the enhanced relaxation efficacy: 'inner sphere' and 'outer sphere' relaxation. Inner sphere relaxation relies on transient coordination of water molecules to the metal center, resulting in a strong interaction with the magnetic moment of the unpaired electrons. Water molecules that diffuse close to the contrast agent, but do not undergo coordinative binding, experience outer sphere relaxation. Although not as efficient as inner sphere relaxation, it still results in shortening of the relaxation times because a large number of water molecules are affected. For low molecular weight paramagnetic agents, both mechanisms contribute to the same extent. Gadolinium (Gd^{3+}) and manganese (Mn^{2+}) are examples of paramagnetic ions that are used in MR contrast agents. These metal ions are highly toxic, i.e., for biological applications they have to be made inert by coordination to chelating ligands (e.g., diethylene-triamine-pentaacetic acid, DTPA) to form high stability complexes with low probability for dissociation. Most contrast agents used clinically are based on gadolinium, and differ only in the chelating agents, e.g., the most commonly used one is Gd-DTPA (Magnevist®). A typical dose of Gd-DTPA administered to patients is 10 ml at a concentration of 0.5 M, which results in a concentration within the body of approximately 0.1 mmol/kg. The DTPA chelate does not bind to the proteins in the blood, ensuring rapid distribution through the blood stream and fast clearance through the kidneys. For most tissues, except brain, Gd-DTPA accumulates in extracellular space. Paramagnetic agents can be designed specifically to remain in the blood pool for prolonged periods of time. These blood pool agents are either of larger size or bind reversibly to albumin in blood plasma [24]. Recently, a new class of contrast agents was proposed based on the chemical exchange-dependent saturation transfer (CEST) [25]. These agents possess a chemical exchange site, which is selectively saturated (similar to an MTC experiment) and the transfer of saturated magnetization to water is measured. In addition, the biological system is relatively unperturbed by the contrast agent unless the exchange site is specifically saturated. The exchange rate depends on the temperature and pH value, and can therefore be used to measure pH *in vivo*.

Superparamagnetic agents consist of magnetic nanoparticles of iron oxide coated with a polymer matrix such as dextran. The particles are divided into two classes according to the overall particle size: if the diameter is larger than 50 nm they are called superparamagnetic iron oxides (SPIO), for a diameter smaller than this value they are classified as ultrasmall superparamagnetic iron oxides (USPIO). When exposed to an external magnetic field, the magnetic moments of the individual iron oxide particles form a large permanent magnetic moment, significantly larger than that of a paramagnetic ion such as Gd^{3+}. Superparamagnetic contrast agents cause large local field inhomogeneities. The proton magnetic moments of water molecules that diffuse through these inhomogeneous domains undergo rapid dephasing via an outer-sphere mechanism, prompting a decrease in T_2 and/or T_2^* [26]. If the particles are freely dissolved, the extent of the field inhomogeneities is in the order of the diffusion length of the water. As these particles undergo diffusion, i.e., a stochastic motion, the dephasing of the transverse water proton magnetization cannot be refocused; correspondingly T_2 will be affected. If the particles are compartmentalized (e.g., in the vascular bed), the extent of the field inhomogeneities is larger than the diffusion length of the water. Water molecules that diffuse through these field inhomogeneities experience enhanced T_2^* relaxation, which, however, can be refocused. Apart from their strong effect on the T_2- and T_2^*-relaxation times, USPIO particles also have excellent T_1-enhancing properties [27]. In the body, SPIO particles are recognized by the reticuloendothelial system (RES) of the blood and, as a consequence, a large portion of the particles are taken up by the Kupffer cells in the liver and by lymph nodes and spleen. The particles only enter healthy Kupffer cells in the liver and do not accumulate in pathological tissue, hence they are used as contrast agents for the diagnosis of neoplastic liver disease. USPIO particles are not immediately recognized by the RES due to their small size and have, therefore, a longer blood half-life.

6.4   Safety and biological effects

During an MRI examination, the patient is exposed to a strong static magnetic field, switched magnetic field gradients and rf fields. At present, there are no known effects of static magnetic fields on living organisms. During MR procedures, the switched gradient magnetic fields may stimulate nerves or muscles by inducing electric fields in the biological systems. In clinical examinations, current safety standards for gradient magnetic fields provide adequate protection from potential hazards in patients. As discussed, fast switching of gradients may result in a high amplitude acoustic noise. In a clinical environment earplugs or headphones are used to avoid any harmful consequences of the noise exposure to the human ear. The majority of the rf power transmitted for MRI is transformed into heat within the tissues as a result of resistive losses. Rf heating increases with the square of the Larmor frequency used. Therefore, in high field clinical systems, rf heating can exceed regulatory limits, requiring a reduction of the rf power deposited (i.e., a reduction of the flip angle) and/or a reduction of the duty cycle, i.e., a prolongation of the repetition delay (recovery delay in-between subsequent excitations). Apart from these factors, a major risk in all MR exams is the potentially projectile effect of ferromagnetic materials inside the main magnetic field. In addition, conducting wires placed inside the MR system may work as rf antennas and can couple to transmit rf coils. At the resonance condition, high rf power can be received by the rf antennas, resulting in a high electric field and thus high temperature at the tip of the wire.

7 Optical imaging

Optical imaging encompasses a set of imaging technologies that use light from the ultraviolet (UV) over the visible (VIS) to the infrared (IR) region to image the tissue characteristics. Techniques are based on the measurement of the reflectance, the transmission and the emission of light. Optical imaging provides information on structure, physiology, and molecular function. The techniques are established for high-resolution reflectance imaging of surfaces: microscopes are used to characterize pathologies of the skin, whereas endoscopes are introduced into the body to investigate structures inside the body (Fig. 26).

Optical imaging methods can be classified by according to three regions of the electromagnetic spectrum (Fig. 1): the IR, VIS and UV domains. The IR spectral regions (700 nm–1000 nm) can be further classified into a near-IR (NIR: 700–1400 nm) and a far-IR (FIR: 1400 nm–1 mm) domain. The VIS section of the spectrum ranges from about 400–700 nm, whereas the UV radiation covers wavelengths between 200 and 400 nm. In general, optical imaging techniques are applied to surface imaging, since the penetration depth

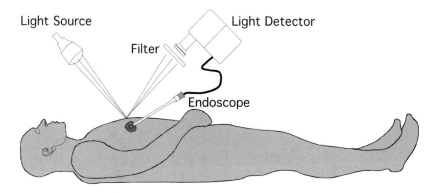

Figure 26.
Principle of optical reflectance imaging.

of the light is very limited. However, light within a small spectral window (600–900 nm) of the NIR region can penetrate about 10 cm into tissue due to the relatively low absorption coefficient at these wavelengths [28]. The lower boundary in this window is given by the high absorption of blood (hemoglobin, methemoglobin), whereas the tissue absorption above 900 nm increases due to the presence of water. For this reason, the NIR part of the spectrum is utilized for non-surface optical imaging. Another factor limiting optical imaging is the strong scattering of light, i.e., photons propagating inside tissue do not follow straight paths, but rather diffuse following random paths. Mathematical modeling of the photon migration in the tissue is required to resolve structures inside the body. Therefore, images with microscopic resolution (sub-micrometer) can be obtained only from surfaces, whereas structures within tissue can be resolved only at low-resolution of the order of several millimeters to a centimeter.

Different techniques can be applied to obtain information from deeper lying tissues. For instance, NIR reflectance imaging can be used to study structures close to the surface, e.g., in small animal imaging. Another class of techniques measures the transmission of light, the light source being located on the other side of the sample [29]; obviously this technique is applicable to small samples (< 10 cm) only. This rather old technique was revisited during the last 20 years due to advances in light sources (e.g., lasers) and detectors (e.g., highly sensitive charged coupled device, CCD, or avalanche photodiodes). There are various types of lasers available for medical use. Lasers are classified by the kind of the lasing medium they use: gas, liquid, solid, semi-

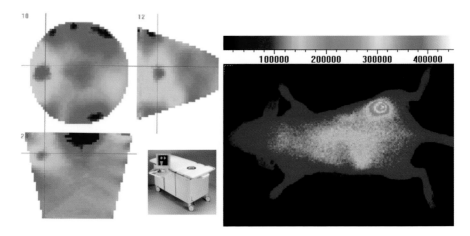

Figure 27.
Left: Multiplanar cross-section images of the right breast of patient obtained with an optical tomography system (Philips Research Eindhoven). The strong attenuation (red) indicates the location of the tumor. Right: Fluorescence images show of a tumor-bearing nude mice 6 h after intravenous injection of a targeted NIR fluorescent probe (Courtesy K. Licha, Schering AG, Berlin).

conductor, or dye lasers. A continuous wave (CW) laser emits a steady beam of light, whereas a pulsed laser emits laser light in an off-and-on manner. The use of short laser pulses allows the selection of ballistic photons, i.e., photons that are not or only weakly scattered, which arrive first on the other side [30]. Another method employs modulated laser light to correct for variations in attenuation [31]. The development of diffuse optical tomography represents a breakthrough in optical imaging. In this technique light is applied from different angles and scattered light is detected from all directions. In contrast to X-ray CT, modeling of the scattering process is essential for image reconstruction in optical imaging. Typically, a numerical solution of the diffusion equation is used to describe the propagation of light photons in diffuse media and to predict the measurements of the experimental set-up (forward problem). Afterwards, model parameters are improved using regression analysis comparing the experimental data with the predictions of the forward approximation, resulting in images [32]. Due to strong influence of scattering and since the reconstruction problem is ill posed, the spatial resolution of optical tomography is rather poor and in the order of 5–10 mm. Diffuse optical tomography has been applied in preclinical (mouse imaging) and clinical applications (breast imaging, Fig. 27). In comparison with transillumination, diffuse optical tomography allows better quantification of absorption, scattering or fluorescence in three dimensions.

7.1   Contrast mechanisms

The contrast in optical imaging relies on endogenous different intrinsic contrast mechanisms like absorption, reflectance, scattering and emission (e.g., luminescence or fluorescence). In particular, light absorption by tissue provides functional information for the tissue, which strongly depends on the wavelength of the light. Measurements at different wavelengths allow the quantification of the water concentration and the oxygenation status of tissue. Oxygenation measurements are used to assess tissue vascularization, an important indicator in cancer diagnosis. Scattering, on the other hand, is associated with the structural properties of tissue. However, as scattering reduces spatial resolution, tissue structures are in general not resolved as such, only indirect structural information is derived from the analysis of scattering parameters.

Absorption and scattering are endogenous properties of tissue. Alternatively, specific information can be derived by administration of exogenous fluorescent compounds. In a fluorescence experiment, energy from an external light source is absorbed by the fluorophore, and almost immediately reemitted at a slightly longer wavelength corresponding to a lower energy. The energy difference between the absorbed and emitted photons is due to intramolecular vibrational relaxation. Tissue contains endogenous fluorescent groups and, therefore, shows autofluorescence, which is usually unspecific and degrades the contrast-to-background ratio. Correlations of intrinsic signals and malignancy have been demonstrated in principle [33], but the specificity achieved so far is low.

7.2   Optical contrast agents

Similar to nuclear imaging, optical imaging is a sensitive modality that can detect very low concentrations of an optical dye; in contrast to PET and SPECT optical imaging does not involve ionizing radiation, the optical probes are in general stable, and the technologies are relatively cheap. Two light generating principles can be differentiated: fluorescence and bioluminescence. In fluorescence imaging a fluorescent probe (optical dye) is activated by an external light source and a signal is emitted at a different wavelength. The fluorescent signal can be resolved with an emission filter and captured, for instance, with a high-sensitivity CCD camera. In the NIR range, indocyanine green (ICG) is a widely used fluorescence agent, which it is safe and approved by the FDA. ICG is an intravascular agent that extravasates through vessels with high permeability [34]. Recently, also ICG derivates with different biodistribution were considered [35]. In addition, the development of semiconductor quantum dots shows high potential for fluorescence imaging, provided that these materials can be made biocompatible [36]. Fluorescent probes have been used in fluorescence reflectance imaging to image superficial structures in microscopy, endoscopy, intravascular or intraoperative imaging studies, as well as in three-dimensional optical tomography to localize and quantify fluorescent probes in deep tissues in small animals [37]. Recently, targeted fluorescent probes have been developed to map specific molecular events, to track cells or to detect gene expression *in vivo*. For example, these probes target specific tumor receptors [38], or tumor angiogenesis [39] or are activated by tumor-associated enzymes (proteases) [40]. The latter probe concept is highly promising, because the probes are only activated in the presence of the targeted enzyme but remain silent otherwise (quenched fluorescence), yielding a 10- to 50-fold fluorescence signal increase in tissues expressing the enzyme. It is expected that clinical application will benefit from the availability of fluorescent probes, especially if targeted probes are developed that can increase the specificity of optical imaging.

In bioluminescence imaging, an enzymatic reaction is used as internal signal source. Luciferases are a class of enzymes (oxgenases) that emit light (bioluminescence) with a broad emission spectra in the presence of oxygen. This reaction is responsible for the glowing effect of fireflies. Also here, the red components of the spectra are the most useful ones for imaging due to minimal absorption by tissue. Bioluminescence signals are commonly detected using highly sensitive CCD cameras. In contrast to fluorescence techniques, there is no inherent background signal in bioluminescence imaging, which results in a high signal-to-background ratio and correspondingly in excellent sensitivity. However, bioluminescence imaging involves genetic engineering of the tissue of interest, which has to express the luciferase reporter gene; hence, the method has only been applied in small animals so far [41].

7.3   Safety and bioeffects

The operation of strong light sources, such as lasers, can lead to potentially hazardous situations. The bioeffect strongly depends on spectrum as well as both average and peak power of the light source. Three mechanisms might lead to tissue damage when using laser light: thermal, acoustic, and photochemical interactions with tissue. Thermal effects are the major cause of laser-induced tissue damage. The amount of thermal damage that can be caused to tissue depends on the thermal sensitivity of the type of tissue. Thermal effects can range from erythema (reddening of the skin) to burning of the tissue. Strong and localized temperature changes cause a localized vaporization of tissue, i.e., of the water contained within the tissue, which in turn can create a mechanical shockwave. This acoustic effect can cause tearing of tissue. Light can also cause induced photochemical reactions in cells, which might lead to harmful effects.

Of most concern in light and laser accidents is the damage to the skin and to the eyes. Skin layers sensitive to light are the epidermis and the dermis. Irradiation with UV-light can cause erythema and blistering. In particular, far-UV (200–300 nm) is a component of sunlight that is thought to have carcinogenic effects on the skin. NIR wavelengths of light are absorbed by the dermis and can cause heating of skin tissue. VIS and NIR wavelengths of light are transmitted through the cornea and lens of the eye, and are absorbed mostly by the retina. The VIS and NIR portions of the spectrum (400–1200 nm) are often referred to as the 'retinal hazard region', because light at these wavelengths can damage the retina. UV and FIR wavelengths of light are predominantly absorbed by the cornea and lens of the eye causing photochemical damage and inflammation.

Lasers are classified into four hazard classes. A class 1 laser is a laser that is incapable of emitting laser radiation higher than 0.4 mW. This applies to very low power devices such as those in semiconductor diode lasers, which are embedded in CD players. Class 2 lasers have low power (1 mW). They normally considered not being hazardous unless an individual were to force himself/herself to stare directly into the beam. Class 3 lasers are medium power lasers (1–500 mW) and are potentially hazardous upon direct exposure of the eye. Class 4 lasers are those devices with power outputs exceeding 500 mW. Most research, medical, and surgical lasers are categorized as class 4.

8   Conclusion

Biomedical imaging modalities differ with respect to the image content, their sensitivity, spatial resolution and time resolution. As described here, the main differences of imaging modalities is the type and amount of energy applied. The interaction of the tissue with energy determines the contrast achievable and thus the image content. X-ray CT is the classical anatomical imaging modality that provides high-resolution structural imaging. One main advantage of CT is its ease of use, because large volume data with high spatial resolution can be acquired rapidly in a push-button mode. However, this technique has a rather poor soft tissue contrast. The use of contrast agents improves the contrast and allows, e.g., the visualization of vessel structures and the measurement of physiological processes such as perfusion. MRI provides superior soft tissue contrast, good spatial resolution and offers a wide range of contrast mechanisms to obtain anatomical, physiological and metabolic information. Due to this flexibility, MRI has become a valuable tool for diagnosis and staging of diseases. The use of MR contrast agents allows the enhancement and quantification of physiological information (e.g., perfusion). The development of targeted MR contrast agents may enable them to be used to study early precursors of diseases in the future. The main disadvantages of MRI are its high cost, its complexity and its inherently low sensitivity. Ultrasound imaging is relatively cheap, easy to use, and the instruments are portable and can be taken to bedside. Ultrasound can provide high-resolution anatomical and functional information in real time. Ultrasound contrast agents are used to enhance the contrast of blood and to measure perfusion. In future, targeted ultrasound contrast agents may allow the detection of early molecular markers in the vascular space. In contrast to the other modalities, which exploit endogenous contrast mechanisms, nuclear imaging techniques such as SPECT and PET are based on the injection of radiopharmaceuticals. Nuclear imaging allows the measurement of the spatial distribution of these tracers over time. There is a wide range of different radiopharmaceuticals available for the characterization of biological processes on a metabolic and molecular level. Although the spatial resolution is poor, the high sensitivity allows the measurement of rare molecular events such as gene-expression processes *in vivo*. Newer optical imaging techniques, like fluorescence imaging, are currently under investigation for their use in clinical use. Due to their high sensitivity, they are already used in biomedical research

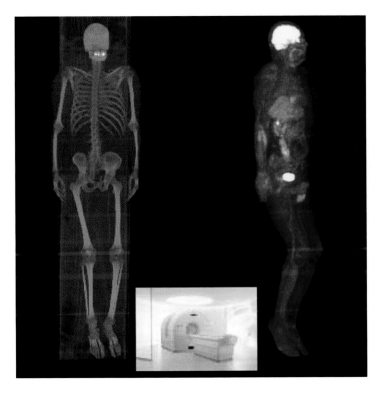

Figure 28.
Combined PET-CT scanner (Gemini, Philips Medical Systems) to obtain anatomical (left) and functional information (right) in one session. The images show whole-body screening of metastasis.

and drug development to detect molecular events in animals. The instrumentation for optical imaging is cheap and the development of optical contrast agents is easier than the synthesis of radiopharmaceuticals.

In general, the different imaging modalities provide different information, and thus can be considered as being complementary rather than competitive. Therefore, the combination of techniques is of high interest. This can be achieved by image processing techniques (i.e., image registration) or using integrated systems. In particular, the combination of structural imaging techniques (like CT) and functional imaging (like nuclear imaging) is of high interest, because it allows the co-registration of anatomy provided by CT with functional and molecular information provided by nuclear imaging. Today, clinical PET-CT (Fig. 28) and SPECT-CT scanner combinations (Fig. 29)

77

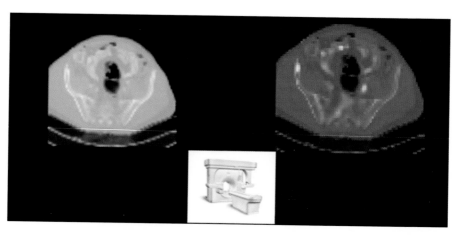

Figure 29.
Combined SPECT-CT scanner (Precedence, Philips Medical Systems) to obtain anatomical (left) and functional information overlaid on anatomy (right) in one session. The images show asymmetric radio-tracer focus for lymph node involvement.

are commercial available, whereas other configurations like PET-MR [42] and optical tomography-MRI [34] are being tested in academic research. Beside the integration of different modalities into one system, the use of a common bed for patients or animal support devices can be used to exchange the patient or animal rapidly between different modalities in a reproducible manner. With this concept the availability of other scanner combinations might be expected in the near future.

Within the last decades extraordinary process was made in the field of bio-medical imaging. In particular, the spatial resolution, sensitivity and acquisition times have been improved tremendously, allowing non-invasive measurement of structural and functional information in animals and humans. Biomedical imaging has become an indispensable tool in clinical practice for diagnosis and staging of diseases, as well as for monitoring of drug response after therapy and in the follow-up process. Recently, advances in the development of targeted contrast agents, which can highlight molecules or molecular pathways, resulted in a new type of imaging [43]. This field of molecular imaging has also a high potential in the field of drug development [44], since it allows the measurement of absorption, distribution and binding of potential drug candidates as well as the assessment of their pharmacodynamic effects. A detailed description of molecular imaging concepts can be found in Chapters 3 and 4. In addition, imaging and especially molecular imaging, has the potential to function as a biomarker, which is an indicator of pathogenic processes or pharmacological responses to a therapy. Monitoring a short-term therapy effect will significantly help in drug development and patient stratification in a clinical setting. With these ongoing developments the range of applications for biomedical imaging will continue to expand.

References

1   Kalender WA (2001) *Computed Tomography: Fundamentals, System Technology, Image Quality, Applications*. MCD Munich
2   Tjuvajev JG, Stockhammer G, Desai R, Uehara H, Watanabe K, Gansbacher B, Blasberg RG (1995) Imaging the expression of transfected genes *in vivo. Cancer Res* 55: 6126–6132
3   Gambhir SS, Barrio JR, Wu L, Iyer M, Namavari M, Satyamurthy N, Bauer E, Parrish C, MacLaren DC, Borghei AR et al (1998) Imaging of adenoviral-directed herpes simplex virus type 1 thymidine kinase reporter gene expression in mice with radiolabeled ganciclovir. *J Nucl Med* 39: 2003–2011
4   Schmidt KC, Turkheimer FE (2002) Kinetic modeling in positron emission tomography. *Q J Nucl Med* 46: 70–85
5   Patlak CS, Blasberg RG (1985) Graphical evaluation of blood-to-brain transfer constants from multiple-time uptake data. Generalizations. *J Cereb Blood Flow Metab* 5: 584–590
6   Cherry SR, Sorenson J, Phelps M (2003) *Physics in Nuclear Medicine*. 3rd edition. W.B. Saunders Company
7   Anger HO (1967) Radioisotope cameras. In: GJ Hine (ed): *Instrumentation in nuclear medicine*, Vol. 1. Academic Press, New York, 485–552
8   Beekman FJ, McElroy DP, Berger F, Gambhir SS, Hoffman EJ, Cherry SR (2002) Towards *in vivo* nuclear microscopy: iodine-125 imaging in mice using micro-pinholes. *Eur J Nucl Med Mol Imaging* 29: 933–938
9   Becher H, Tiemann K, Schlosser T, Pohl C, Nanda NC, Averkiou MA, Powers J, Luderitz B (1998) Improvement in endocardial border delineation using tissue harmonic imaging. *Echocardiography* 15: 511–518
10 Entrekin RR, Porter BA, Sillesen HH, Wong AD, Cooperberg PL, Fix CH (2001) Real-time spatial compound imaging: application to breast, vascular, and musculoskeletal ultrasound. *Semin Ultrasound CT MR*: 22: 50–64
11 Lanza GM, Wallace KD, Scott MJ, Cacheris WP, Abendschein DR, Christy DH, Sharkey AM, Miller JG, Gaffney PJ, Wickline SA (1996) A novel site-targeted ultrasonic contrast agent with broad biomedical application. *Circulation* 94: 3334–3340
12 Lindner JR (2002) Assessment of myocardial viability with myocardial contrast echocardiography. *Echocardiography*19: 417–425
13 Lindner JR (2004) Molecular imaging with contrast ultrasound and targeted microbubbles. *J Nucl Cardiol* 11: 215–221
14 Fritzsch T, Schartl M, Siegert J (1988) Preclinical and clinical results with an ultrasonic contrast agent. *Invest Radiol* 23, Suppl 1: S302–S305

15   Averkiou M, Powers J, Skyba D, Bruce M, Jensen S (2003) Ultrasound contrast imaging research. *Ultrasound Q* 19: 27–37

16   Willams AR (1983) *Ultrasound: Biological Effects and Potential Hazards, Medical Physics Series*. Academic Press, New York

17   Haacke EM, Brown RW, Thomson MR, Venkatesan R (1999) *Magnetic Resonance Imaging, Physical Principles and Sequence Design*. Wiley Liss, New York

18   Vlaardingerbroek MT, den Boer JA (2002) *Magnetic Resonance Imaging, Theory and Practice*,3rd Edition. Springer Verlag, Berlin

19   Le Bihan D (1995) *Diffusion and Perfusion Magnetic Resonance Imaging: Applications to Functional MRI*. Lippincott Williams & Wilkins, New York

20   Ogawa S, Lee TM, Kay AR, Tank DW (1990) Brain magnetic resonance imaging with contrast dependent on blood oxygenation. *Proc Natl Acad Sci USA* 87: 9868–9872

21   Moonen CTW, Bandettini PA (1999) *Functional MRI*. Springer-Verlag, Berlin

22   Pruessmann KP, Weiger M, Scheidegger MB, Boesiger P (1999) SENSE: sensitivity encoding for fast MRI. *Magn Reson Med* 42: 952–962

23   Merbach AE, Toth E (2001) *The Chemistry of Contrast Agents in Medical Magnetic Resonance Imaging*. John Wiley and Sons, New York

24   Lauffer RB, Parmelee DJ, Dunham SU, Ouellet HS, Dolan RP, Witte S, McMurry TJ, Walovitch RC (1998) MS-325: albumin-targeted contrast agent for MR angiography. *Radiology* 207: 529–538

25   Ward KM, Aletras AH, Balaban RS (2000) A new class of contrast agents for MRI based on proton chemical exchange dependent saturation transfer (CEST). *J Magn Reson* 143: 79–87

26   Yablonskiy DA, Haacke EM (1994) Theory of NMR signal behavior in magnetically inhomogeneous tissues: the static dephasing regime. *Magn Reson Med* 32: 749–763

27   Koenig SH, Kellar KE (1995) Theory of 1/T1 and 1/T2 NMRD profiles of solutions of magnetic nanoparticles. *Magn Reson Med* 34: 227–233

28   Cheong WF, Prahl SA, Welch AJ (1990) A review of the optical properties of biological tissues. *IEEE J Quantum Electronics* 26: 2166–2185

29   Cutler M (1929) Transillumination as an aid in the diagnosis of breast lesions. *Surg Gynecol Obstet* 48: 721–729

30   Grosenick D, Wabnitz H, Rinneberg HH, Moesta KT, Schlag PM (1999) Development of a time-domain optical mammograph and first *in vivo* applications. *Applied-Optics* 38: 2927–2943

31   Franceschini MA, Moesta KT, Fantini S, Gaida G, Gratton E, Jess H, Mantulin WW, Seeber M, Schlag PM, Kaschke M (1997) Frequency-domain techniques enhance optical mammography: initial clinical results. *Proc Natl Acad Sci USA* 94: 6468–6473

32   Arridge SR (1999) Optical tomography in medical imaging. *Inverse Problems* 15: R41–R93.

33   Tromberg BJ, Shah N, Lanning R, Cerussi A, Espinoza J, Pham T, Svaasand L, Butler J (2000) Non-invasive *in vivo* characterization of breast tumors using photon migration spectroscopy. *Neoplasia* 2: 26–40

34   Ntziachristos V, Yodh AG, Schnall M, Chance B (2000) Concurrent MRI and diffuse optical tomography of breast after indocyanine green enhancement. *Proc Natl Acad Sci USA* 97: 2767–2772

35   Licha K, Riefke B, Ntziachristos V, Becker A, Chance B, Semmler W (2000) Hydrophilic cyanine dye as contrast agents for nearinfrared tumor imaging: synthesis, photophysical properties and spectroscopic *in vivo* characterization. *Photochem Photobiol* 72: 392–398

36   Gao X, Cui Y, Levenson RM, Chung LW, Nie S (2004) *In vivo* cancer targeting and imaging with semiconductor quantum dots. *Nat Biotechnol* 22: 969–976

37   Ntziachristos V, Tung CH, Bremer C, Weissleder R (2002) Imaging of differential protease expression in breast cancers for detection of aggressive tumor phenotypes. *Nat Med* 8: 757–760

38   Achilefu S, Dorshow RB, Bugaj JE, Rajagopalan R (2000) Novel receptor-targeted fluorescent contrast agents for *in vivo* tumor imaging. *Invest Radiol* 35: 479–485

39   Licha K, Perlitz C, Hauff P, Scholle F-D, Scholz A, Rosewicz, Schirner M (2004) New targeted near-IR fluorescent conjugates for the imaging of tumor angiogenesis. *Proc Society for Molecular Imaging*, 3rd annual meeting: 264

40   Weissleder R, Tung CH, Mahmood U, Bogdanov A (1999) *In vivo* imaging of tumors with protease-activated near-infrared fluorescent probes. *Nature Biotechnol* 17: 375–378

41   Contag PR, Olomu IN, Stevenson DK, Contag CH (1998) Bioluminescent indicators in living mammals. *Nat Med* 4: 245–247

42   Marsden PK, Strul D, Keevil SF, Williams SC, Cash D (2002) Simultaneous PET and NMR. *Br J Radiol* 75, Spec No: S53–S59

43   Weissleder R, Mahmood U (2001) Molecular imaging. *Radiology* 219 : 316–333

44   Rudin M, Weissleder R (2003) Molecular Imaging in Drug Discovery and Development. *Nature Rev Drug Discov* 2: 123–131

Progress in Drug Research, Vol. 62
(Markus Rudin, Ed.)
©2005 Birkhäuser Verlag, Basel (Switzerland)

Magnetic resonance and fluorescence based molecular imaging technologies

By David Sosnovik and
Ralph Weissleder

Center for Molecular Imaging
Research, Massachusetts General
Hospital, Harvard Medical School,
Fruit Street, Boston, MA 02114, USA
<sosnovik@nmr.mgh.harvard.edu>

Glossary of abbreviations

FMT, fluorescence molecular tomography; FRI, fluorescence reflectance imaging
MRS, magnetic relaxation switches, NIRF, near infrared fluorescence, MNP, superparamagnetic
nanoparticles; MRI, magnetic resonance imaging; PET, positron emission tomography; SNR, signal-to-noise ratio; SPECT, single-photon emission computed tomography.

1   Introduction

The traditional role of non-invasive imaging has been to define gross
anatomy and physiology at the level of the whole organ. In the last few years,
however, technological advances have made it possible to characterize molecular expression and physiology at the cellular level with non-invasive
imaging techniques. This emerging field has been broadly termed "molecular imaging" and has the potential to significantly enhance the role of diagnostic imaging in both the basic science and clinical arenas. This review summarizes some of the recent developments in molecular imaging and discusses
their potential impact on several important aspects of drug discovery and
development. We focus our attention in this chapter on optical (fluorescence), and magnetic resonance imaging (MRI) approaches to molecular
imaging. The role of bioluminescence, single-photon emission computed
tomography (SPECT) and positron emission tomography (PET) imaging have
been covered elsewhere in this book.

For a molecular imaging tool to be useful, however, several prerequisites
must be met. It must have a sensitivity high enough to monitor interactions
at the molecular level, a sufficiently high spatial resolution to image mouse
models of human disease and a high degree of specificity for the target of
interest [1]. Each imaging modality has a set of advantages and disadvantages,
and the choice of technique must thus be tailored to the question of interest. For instance, if high-resolution images of myocardial function and con-
traction in a live mouse are desired, MRI is likely to be the modality of choice
[2]. On the other hand, activatable near infrared fluorescence (NIRF) probes
are highly suitable for the detection of enzyme activity within endothelial
membranes and accessible tumors [3, 4].

The use of mouse models of human disease has become increasingly
more important in the era of molecular and genetic medicine [5]. Mouse
models are frequently used in drug development to validate potential tar-

gets, to assess therapeutic efficacy, and to identify and validate biomarkers of drug efficacy and/or safety. The emergence of imaging technology capable of obtaining high quality non-invasive images of mice, *in vivo*, has thus been critical to the development of molecular imaging [6]. Systems that can be housed and operated in basic science laboratories now exist to perform MRI, CT, nuclear imaging, fluorescence and bioluminescence imaging on mice (Tab. 1) [7]. In addition, the cost of these systems is generally less than their clinical counterparts and they are thus likely to become routine tools in the development and assessment of new drugs.

It has become possible recently to combine imaging modalities, and thus exploit the advantages of two techniques. Examples of such combined systems include CT-SPECT imagers, and the combination of MRI with PET and NIRF imaging. Advances in hardware design and image processing have also been accompanied by advances in probe chemistry and design. Many of the recently developed molecular probes are dual modality and thus capable of being detected by these complimentary imaging techniques [7, 8]. A more detailed description of specific imaging modalities and probe designs follows below. The reader is also referred to a number of excellent recent review articles in this area [5, 9–14].

2 General approach to molecular imaging

The characterization of the human genome has led to an intense focus on genetic models of disease. Although theoretically attractive to image, genetic materials such as DNA and RNA generally do not occur in high enough levels to permit robust imaging. The products of these genetic materials, namely the proteins they encode for, however, do exist in large enough quantities to be imaged. Even so, imaging of proteins whether membrane receptors or enzymes, usually requires an amplification strategy to generate an adequate signal. Amplification strategies may be biological, such as the internalization of a nanoparticle after ligand binding to a particular membrane receptor, or chemical such as the used of biotinylated probes. Alternatively reporter probes may be used to indicate the presence of a primary phenomenon with which they are associated. Examples include the use of thymidine kinase to detect gene expression or cell viability by SPECT

Table 1. Overview of high-resolution small-animal imaging systems[a]

Technique	Resolution	Depth	Time	Imaging agents	Sensitivity	Target	Cost[b]	Primary small-animal use	Clinical use
MR imaging	10–100 μm	No limit	Min – hours	Gadolinium, dysprosium, iron oxide particles	~10^{-6} M	A, P, M	$$$	Versatile imaging modality with high soft tissue contrast	Yes
CT imaging	50 μm	No limit	Min	Iodine	~10^{-3} M	A, P	$$	Primarily for lung and bone imaging	Yes
Ultrasound imaging	50 μm	Several cm	Min	Microbubbles	Single microbubble	A, P	$$	Vascular and interventional imaging	Yes
PET imaging	1–2 mm	No limit	Min	^{18}F, ^{11}C, ^{15}O	~10^{-12} M	P, M	$$$	Versatile imaging modality with many different tracers	Yes
SPECT imaging	1–2 mm	No limit	Min	^{99m}Tc, ^{111}In chelates	~10^{-10} M	P, M	$$	Commonly used to image labeled antibodies, peptides, etc.	Yes
Fluorescence reflectance imaging (FRI)	2–3 mm	<1 cm	Sec – min	Photoproteins (GFP) NIR fluorochromes	~$10{-}10$ M	P, M	$	Rapid screening of molecular events in surface-based tumors	Development
Fluorescence mediated tomography (FMT)	1 mm	<10 cm	Sec – min	NIR fluorochromes	~10^{-10} M	P, M	$$	Quantitative imaging of targeted or 'smart' fluorochrome reporters in deep tumors	Development
Bioluminescence imaging	Several mm cm		Min	Luciferins	~10^{-11}– 10^{-12} M	M	$$	Gene expression, cell and bacterial tracking	No No
Intravital microscopy (confocal, multiphoton)	1 μm	<400 μm	Sec – min	Photoproteins (GFP) fluorochromes	~10^{-10} M	P, M	$$$	All of the above at higher resolutions but at limited depths and coverage	Limited development (skin)

[a]Primary area that a given imaging modality interrogates: A, anatomic; P, physiological; M, molecular targets. Reproduced with permission from [6].
[b]Cost of system: $ <100 K; $$ 100–300 K; $$$ >300 K.

imaging, and the use of the transferrin receptor as a reporter gene for MR imaging [15–17].

The performance of an imaging modality may be described by its spatial resolution, signal-to-noise ratio (SNR), contrast-to-noise ratio (CNR), and in the case of dynamic phenomena by its temporal resolution as well. Tissue contrast may be generated by intrinsic differences in the properties of tissues, or may require the administration of an imaging agent or reporter probe. The vast majority of molecular imaging techniques have required the development of probes sensitive to a specific molecular target. The overall performance of the technique is thus determined by a combination of the characteristics of the target, as well as those of the probe and the imaging modality. For instance, the sensitivity of a technique will be influenced by the density and location of the target of interest, the pharmacokinetics of the probe, the vascular and cell membrane permeability of the probe, the affinity of the probe for the desired target, and the physical performance of the imaging modality.

Probes that alter their physical characteristics upon contacting a desired target have recently been developed and are often described as 'activatable'. Examples of such activatable probes include NIRF agents and smart magnetic relaxation switches [18–20]. Activatable NIRF agents exist in a baseline quenched state until cleavage or activation by the desired enzyme produces fluorescence. The relaxation properties of smart magnetic relaxation switches are likewise changed through an interaction with a specific target. In some ways, these probes can therefore be considered pro-drugs whose final product produces an imaging readout.

Randomized clinical studies have become the ultimate standard for evaluating the efficacy of a new drug or therapy. However, to achieve statistically significant results, particularly when hard clinical end-points such as myocardial infarction or death are used, anywhere from hundreds to tens of thousands of patients need to be enrolled in a study. While it is unlikely that the use of molecular imaging will ever make the need for such trials obsolete, molecular imaging has the potential to rationalize the process, reduce the cost of new drug development and ultimately accelerate the introduction of new drugs into clinical practice [6].

3 Magnetic resonance imaging

3.1 General principles

The characteristics of MRI make it a suitable technique for molecular imaging. MRI offers unparalleled soft tissue contrast, can produce images with both a high temporal and spatial resolution, and is non-ionizing. MRI has thus become the imaging modality of choice for studying diseases of the central nervous system such as stroke, neurodegenerative disorders and multiple sclerosis. The role of MRI in the evaluation of cardiovascular disorders is also growing, encompassing the investigation of aortic, carotid and peripheral vascular disease, as well as imaging of the heart itself. MRI is now used routinely to assess ventricular function, detect ischemia and assess myocardial viability [21, 22]. MRI also plays a major role in the evaluation of neoplastic disease, particularly in the pelvis and abdomen, as well as musculoskeletal disease. The broad range of pathologies and organ systems that are imaged with MRI make it an appealing platform for which to develop tools and probes for molecular imaging. In addition, small-bore high-field MRI scanners have been developed to obtain images in small animals such as mice and rats. These small-bore high-field scanners provide the same attributes in the small-animal arena that clinical scanners do in human studies. MRI thus offers the investigator the possibility of composite bench-to-bedside imaging [11].

The role of small-animal MRI scanners in drug development has been recognized by both the pharmaceutical industry and the vendors of small-animal scanners. Actively shielded systems, designed specifically for high-throughput screening in the pharmaceutical setting, have been developed, and do not require the presence of an RF-shielded room, unlike clinical scanners. Cardiovascular imaging in small animals is somewhat more challenging, but high-quality cine images of the heart and great vessels can be readily obtained, as shown in Figure 1.

Several MR-based techniques have been developed to image the cellular and metabolic mileau including, diffusion-weighted MRI and MR spectroscopy. Diffusion-weighted MR is able to detect the acute breakdown of the cell membrane following stroke, and has become the method of choice for the acute detection of cerebro-vascular accidents. Hydrogen MR spectroscopy has been widely used in the diagnosis of demyelinating and neurodegenera-

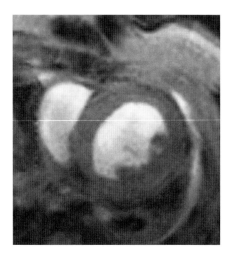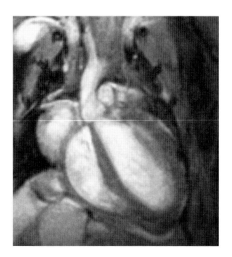

Figure 1.
Cardiac MR images of live mice obtained on a 9.4 T small-bore MR scanner. The images shown were obtained with an in-plane spatial resolution of 150 μm and a temporal resolution of approximately 160 frames per second.

tive diseases of the central nervous system. In addition, MR spectroscopy of high-energy phosphates such as ATP and phospho-creatine has been used to detect abnormal myocardial energetics in heart failure [23]. While these techniques have certainly moved beyond traditional whole-organ imaging, we feel that they cannot truly be classified as molecular imaging techniques since they are not targeted to a specific receptor, protein or pathway. Nevertheless, it is likely that the role of these techniques will continue to grow and perhaps complement the role of targeted MR-based molecular techniques.

The imaging of specific molecular targets by MRI has generally required the development of paramagnetic or superparamagnetic contrast agents directed against a specific molecular target. These agents can be used to enhance the longitudinal relaxation of protons (so-called T1 or relaxivity contrast) or to enhance the transverse relaxation of protons (T2* or susceptibility contrast). Several MR contrast agents, for instance ultra-small superparamagnetic iron oxides, can be used as both relaxivity or susceptibility agents [24–27], while others such as gadolinium are best suited to the imaging of longitudinal relaxation [28].

The critical importance of probe sensitivity in molecular imaging has been alluded to above. The initial parameter of concern in the design of an MR

Table 2.
Examples of polymer-coated magnetic nanoparticles (MNP)

Short-circulating	Comment
Ferumoxides (Feridex)	Approved liver imaging agent
Ferrixan (Resovist)	Approved liver imaging agent

Long-circulating	
Ferumoxtran (Combidex/Sinerem, AMI 227)	Completed Phase 3 trials
Ferumoxytol (AMI 228)	Approved for iron replacement Rx
Feruglose (Clariscan)	Cardiovascular imaging/angiography
Monocrystalline iron oxide (MION)	Experimental MNP [38]
Cross-linked iron oxide (CLIO)	Experimental MNP developed for targeted imaging [105]

contrast agent is thus often the value of its relaxivity. This value refers to the slope of either transverse or longitudinal relaxation rate as a function of probe concentration. Both the R_1 (longitudinal relaxivity) and R_2 (transverse relaxivity) of the paramagnetic contrast agent gadolinium, for instance, are approximately, 4 mMs^{-1} [28]. It should be mentioned, however, that relaxivity may be influenced by field strength and temperature. This is particularly important for T_1 agents since R_1 tends to decrease at progressively higher field strengths [29]. The R_2 of superparamagnetic agents on the other hand tends to plateau at approximately 0.5 T, which is well below the field strengths used in both clinical and small-animal scanners.

Superparamagnetic nanoparticles (MNP) can be classified as either: (a) polymer-coated, (b) targeted, or (c) activatable (Tabs 2 and 3). The latest generation of long-circulating MNP have an R1 and R2 (0.47 T, 40°C) of 40 mMs^{-1} and 150 mMs^{-1}, respectively. The uptake of a given amount of an MNP thus produces a significantly larger change in the MR signal than the uptake of an equivalent amount of gadolinium. Gadolinium-based probes are thus most suited to the imaging of molecular targets with a high degree of biological expression, for instance the presence of fibrin within thombi [30–32]. However, because of its lower intrinsic relaxivity, the imaging of most molecular targets with gadolinium necessitates the construction of larger magnetic nanoparticles and polymers to achieve high magnetic payloads [33]. The safety of such constructs for human use, however, will require extensive further investigation.

Table 3. Examples of targeted and activatable superparamagnetic nanoparticles

Targeted probes	Target	MNP
Anti-myosin [40]	Cardiomyocyte necrosis	MION
AnxCLIO-Cy5.5 [85]	Phosphatidylserine/apoptotic cells	CLIO
E-Selectin [80]	E-Selectin/endothelial inflammation	CLIO
VCAM-1	VCAM-1/endothelial inflammation	CLIO
Activatable probes		
GFP-MRNA	Oligonucleotide	CLIO-MRS
CA-125	Protein	CLIO-MRS
Caspase-3	Protease	CLIO-MRS
HSV-1	Viral particles	CLIO-MRS
L/D tyrosine	Enantiomeric impurities	CLIO-MRS

The use of iron oxide-based MNP for molecular imaging in humans, on the other hand, is based on extensive experience with these agents in humans [27, 34, 35]. These nanoparticles consist of an iron oxide core that is processed by the same pathways that metabolize endogenous and dietary iron [36]. The first MNP to be approved by the FDA for human use was Feridex. This agent consists of an iron oxide core covered by a thin dextran coat, and *in vivo* tends to form large crystal aggregates that are rapidly cleared from the bloodstream by the Kupffer cells [37]. Long-circulating MNP contain more extensive polymer coats that prevent the formation of aggregates *in vivo*, and they are thus not rapidly removed by the reticulo-endothelial system [38]. Several of these agents, including Combidex, Ferumoxytol and Clariscan, have been safely used in humans [24, 27, 39].

3.2   Targeted MR imaging probes

Targeted MR probes generally have a protein, peptide or small-molecule ligand, with affinity for a particular molecular target, attached to the surface of the magnetic nanoparticle. An early example of such a system was the binding of an antibody directed against cardiac myosin to an MNP [40]. This anti-myosin probe was able to image myocardial infarction in rats by *ex vivo* MRI. While antibody-based probes may possess a high degree of specificity, several aspects limit the utility of this construct. Firstly, the large size of whole anti-bodies may limit the bioavailability of the probe beyond the surface of the endothelial membrane. Secondly, whole antibody conjugates are unlikely to be internalized by surface receptors into cells. Finally, whole antibody con-jugates are far more likely to produce adverse reactions in humans than other constructs, and thus will likely face far greater regulatory hurdles prior to approval.

The use of whole antibodies to label magnetic nanoparticles is thus being replaced in many laboratories by the use of antibody fragments, small pro-teins, peptides and peptidomimetics [41]. The smaller size of these labels may allow a probe to be internalized into a cell after ligand binding to the target, which is a biological mechanism for signal amplification. For instance, the conjugation of the HIV-derived Tat peptide to MNP has been shown to pro-mote cell internalization [42, 43]. High-throughput screening libraries are now being used in several laboratories to identify peptides that are not only specific for a particular target but also have physical and chemical properties that promote internalization after binding [44]. A list of targeted MNP, deriva-tized with ligands varying from whole antibodies to peptidomimetics, is pre-sented in Table 3.

The principal disadvantage of ligand-based MR probes, whether large antibodies or small peptides, is the generation of signal from the unbound portion of the probe as well. This background signal produces noise that must be overcome to produce specific images of target uptake. One strategy com-monly used is to wait for washout of the unbound fraction of the probe. This strategy works well for the imaging of subacute and chronic molecular processes, but has obvious limitations for the imaging of acute processes. In these acute situations scavenger systems that selectively alter the properties of unbound probe can be used prior to imaging. Despite the presence of back-ground noise from unbound probe, the use of targeted MR nanoparticles holds much promise, and will remain a vital component of the molecular imaging arsenal for the foreseeable future.

3.3   Activatable probes

Activatable or "smart" MRI probes differ fundamentally from targeted probes in that they undergo chemical or physico-chemical changes upon target

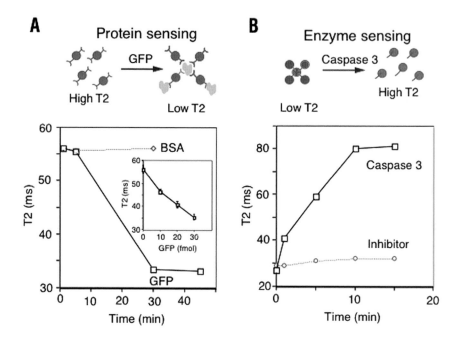

Figure 2.
Assembly/disassembly principle underlying use of superparamagnetic relaxation switches (MRS). (A) Incubation of anti-GFP-P1 nanosensors with GFP or control BSA protein. The transverse relaxation time, T2, decreases as the nanosensor binds to GFP protein. (B) Caspase-3 activity can be detected using an MRS containing the DEVD peptide recognition sequence. The increase in T2 due to caspase-3-mediated disassembly of the MRS is not seen when the caspase-3 inhibitor (N-acetyl-DEVD-CHO) is added. Adapted with permission from [20].

interaction, and thus have a built-in amplification strategy. Increases in signal intensity of up to tenfold above background have been reported with activatable MR imaging compounds [20]. Two broad strategies have been described to "activate" MR contrast probes upon target exposure. The first of these is based on enzymatic conversion of paramagnetic compounds from an inactive into an active form [45]. A gadolinium construct has been developed that is magnetically silent in its baseline form due to the presence of high-affinity chelators blocking the access of water molecules to gadolinium. Cleavage of these chelators by a target enzyme restores the access of the water protons to gadolinium, and results in a detectable increase in R_1. For instance, the presence of lacZ gene expression, which encodes for the enzyme β-galactosidase, was detectable using a construct with chelators sensitive to cleavage by the β-galactosidase enzyme [45].

Enzyme-mediated polymerization has also been used to image nanomolar amounts of peroxidases, which are thought to play a role in predisposing inflamed atherosclerotic plaques to rupture and complication [46, 47]. In the presence of peroxidase, paramagnetic substrates are assembled into oligomers with resultantly higher R_1 values. This assembly/disassembly strategy has also been used recently in the development of superparamagnetic magnetic relaxation switches (MRS). These switches consist of an aggregate of nanoparticles held together by peptide chains containing specific recognition sequences for an enzyme of interest [20]. Exposure to this enzyme results in cleavage of the peptide-linker chains, the disintegration of the nano-assembly into its individual component nanoparticles, and an accompanying reduction in transverse relaxivity.

The use of smart/activatable magnetic contrast agents to image kinases, proteinases and other enzymes involved in disease processes is likely to play an increasingly important role in future drug discovery [48, 49]. A caspase-3-sensitive MRS, containing the DEVD peptide recognition sequence, has been shown to be able to detect caspase-3 activity *in vitro* with a high degree of accuracy (Fig. 2) [20]. Switches capable of detecting oligonucleotides, proteins, viral particles and enatiomeric impurities *in vitro* have also been developed (Tab. 3) [20, 49–52]. A list of proteases, enzymes and other targets suitable for molecular imaging by MR, NIRF, bioluminescence, SPECT and PET is provided in Table 4.

3.4   Future challenges

The principal challenges facing molecular imaging with MR-detectable probes in the near future are likely to be the development of better amplification strategies to differentiate target information from nonspecific background signal, and the development of improved cell-penetrating strategies [53]. The latter will be key if intracellular targets are to be imaged with MRI, and will require extensive studies on the intracellular processing of these potential contrast agents. The flexibility and versatility of MRI remain unparalleled, and it is thus highly likely that MRI will continue to play a central role in all aspects of molecular imaging.

Table 4. Some examples of existing imaging targets/probes used for molecular imaging by MR, NIRF, bioluminescence, SPECT and PET imaging

Proteases	Receptors	Other enzymes
Cathepsin B	Somatostatin	Thymidine kinase (HSV-TK)
Cathepsin D	Bombesin	Farnesyl tranferase
Cathepsin K	Dopamin D2 and D1	Toposiomerase
MMP-1	Serotonin	Cytochrome p450
MMP-2	Benzodiazepine	Hexokinase
MMP-7	Opioid	3-hydroxyacyl-coenzymeA dehydrogenase (HAD)
CMV protease	Acetylcholine	Choline metabolism
HIV protease	Adrenergic	Citrate metabolism
HSV protease	Estrogen	Protein synthesis (amino acids)
HCV protease	Cholecystokinin	Akt kinase
Caspase-1	EGFR	β-Galactosidase
Caspase-3	VEGFR	Glutamate carboxipeptidase
Thrombin	Glycoprotein GP IIb/IIIa	PI3 kinase
	Folate	
	Insulin	
	Neurokinin	
	TGF	
	Asialoglycoprotein	
	Adenosine2	

Angiogenesis	Apoptosis	Cellular tracking
E-selectin	Annexin-V	CD8
$\alpha_5\beta_3$	Caspase-3	CD4
Endostatin	TRAIL, S-TRAIL	CD34
VEGFR	PtdS binding protein	Neural progenitor cells
VCAM-1	Synaptotagmin	Stem cells
CD105		Macrophages
Thrombin		Dendritic cells
		Tumor cell

MMP, matrix metalloprotease; CMV, cytomegalovirus; HIV, human immunodeficiency virus; HSV, herpes simplex virus; HCV, hepatitis C virus; EGFR, epidermal growth factor receptor; VEGFR, vascular endothelial growth factor receptor; TGF, transforming growth factor; HSV-TK, herpes simplex virus thymidine kinase; VCAM1, human vascular cell adhesion molecule; CD105, endoglin; TRAIL, tumor necrosis factor-related apoptosis-inducing ligand. Reproduced with permission from [6].

4   Optical imaging

Optical imaging techniques play a central and well-established role in the *in vitro* study of cell structure and function. Recently however, revolutionary advances in optical imaging technologies have allowed these techniques to be used *in vivo* [54, 55]. The primary facilitating technologies of this remarkable advance have been progress in mathematical modeling of photon prop-agation in tissue, the expanding availability of biologically compatible NIR probes and the development of highly sensitive photon detection technolo-gies [54, 55].

Optical techniques for molecular imaging can be broadly divided into those involving bioluminescence imaging and those that involve fluores-cence imaging. For completeness, it should be noted that there are several other optical techniques being developed, such as NIR spectroscopy [56, 57], *in vivo* Raman spectroscopy [58] or multiphoton imaging [12, 59]. However, the low cost, versatility and high-throughput capability of bioluminescence and fluorescence imaging make them particularly suited to the drug discov-ery and development process. Bioluminescence imaging has been dealt with elsewhere in this text, and we will therefore focus below on fluorescence imaging.

4.1 Technologies for fluorescence imaging

Fluorescence imaging is based on the absorption of energy from an external light source, which is then almost immediately re-emitted at a longer wave-length of lower energy. Many of the fluorochromes used for *in vitro* imaging, for instance green fluorescent protein (GFP), absorb light at wavelengths that fall into the visible spectrum. The use of these fluorochromes for *in vivo* imag-ing, however, is limited by the high absorption coefficient of light within the visible spectrum by body tissues. In addition, tissue autofluorescence tends to be highest at wavelengths within the visible spectrum, thus further com-plicating the use of fluorochromes such as GFP for *in vivo* imaging.

The use of cyanine dyes, with absorption and emission spectra in the NIR range (650–850 nm), has thus been a key advance for fluorescence imaging *in vivo* [60, 61]. Hemoglobin (the principal absorber of visible light), water, and lipids (the principal absorbers of IR light) all have their lowest absorp-tion coefficient in the NIR region of around 650–900 nm. Imaging in the NIR region also has the advantage of minimizing tissue autofluorescence, which is lowest in this range. The use of NIR fluorochromes thus allows deeper struc-tures within the body to be imaged *in vivo*, and provides high target/back-ground ratios. In fact, penetration depths of 7–14 cm are theoretically possi-ble, depending on tissue type.

Fluorescence imaging can be performed at different resolutions and depth penetrations, ranging from micrometers (intravital microscopy [12]) to centimeters (fluorescence molecular tomography, FMT; [62]). Conventional fluorescence reflectance imaging (FRI) is a useful technique to image superficial structures (<5 mm deep), for example in small animals [63], during endoscopy [64–66], dermatological imaging [67], intravascular catheter-based imaging or intraoperative imaging [68]. However, *in vivo* fluorescence imaging of deeper structures has required the development of fluorescence molecular tomographic (FMT) imaging systems. These systems have recently been shown to be able to three-dimensionally localize and quantify fluorescent probes in deep tissues at high sensitivity. FMT of point sources in small animals allowed fluorochrome concentrations to be quantified at femtomolar levels [54], and to be imaged at sub-millimeter spatial resolution [69], as seen in Figure 3.

The imaging principles involved in FMT are similar to X-ray CT, but require the use of a theoretical approach that accounts for the diffuse nature of photons in tissues. At a give time, a single point excitation source illuminates the tissue from a spatially unique position and the photon field distributes in three dimensions along isocontour lines within the tisssue. In each illumination position, the fluorochromes act as secondary sources, emitting energy at a higher wavelength and with an intensity that depends on the position of the light source. The excitation and fluorescence wavelengths are then both collected from multiple points along the surface using appropriate filters [70]. In the near future, FMT techniques are expected to provide even better spatial resolution by utilizing higher-density detector systems and advanced photon technologies, such as modulated intensity light or very short photon pulses.

4.2 Probes for fluorescence imaging

NIRF probes can be divided, much like magnetic nanoparticles, into those agents that are: (a) nonspecific, (b) targeted, and (c) activatable. Indocyanine green, for example, has been used extensively in humans as a nonspecific indicator in dilution estimates of cardiac output. A nonspecific NIRF probe, SF64 (Schering) has also shown promise in phase I trials of optical mammography in women. Targeted NIRF probes are constructed by attaching a fluorochrome to an affinity ligand, much in the same way as a targeted mag-

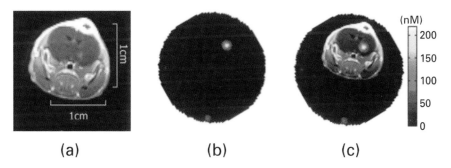

Figure 3.
In vivo FMT of cathepsin B expression in stereotactically implanted 9L gliosarcomas. The images shown are: (a) gadolinium-enhanced axial image of the tumor. The area of gadolinium enhancement is shown in green. (b) FMT image of the tumor after intravenous injection of a cathepsin B activatable NIRF probe. (c) Fusion of MR and FMT images after appropriate scaling of the MR image. Adapted with permission from [62].

netic nanoparticle is constructed [65, 71, 72]. However, targeted NIR fluorochromes tend to be quite similar in size to the actual ligand, while targeted magnetic nanoparticles tend to be significantly larger than the ligand alone. The difference in these two constructs may thus have important implications for probe delivery and pharmacokinetics.

Activatable NIRF probes have recently been developed, and have become central to the field of molecular imaging. These probes, in their baseline state, contain fluorochromes in close physical proximity to each other, resulting in the quenching of any fluorescence. The critical components of these probes can thus be designed to be held in close physical approximation to each other by peptide linkers, such as polylysine chains, that are susceptible to cleavage by a specific enzyme or kinase [18]. Exposure of a quenched activatable fluorochrome to the target enzyme results in cleavage at the recognition site, and hence the production of fluorescence. These activatable agents produce no background signal until they come into contact with the enzyme of interest, and thus constitute an extremely robust amplification strategy. Increases in signal intensity of up to 100-fold above background have been reported with the use of activatable caged NIR fluorochromes.

Activatable NIR imaging agents can be used to identify potential enzymes and kinases for therapeutic inhibition, and subsequently as tools for the objective assessment of therapeutic efficiency [73, 74]. In one such study, the efficacy of a matrix metalloproteinase-2 (MMP-2) inhibitor at varying dosing and timing was assessed with an MMP-2-targeted imaging probe [73]. Small-molecule–induced target inhibition could be externally imaged as shortly as 8 h after therapeutic drug administration. It is clear that many similar imaging agents will be developed to image the growing array of different drug targets, and play an important role in drug discovery and development.

Recently, the potential of a new class of nanoparticles, quantum dots, for fluorescence imaging has also been realized [75]. These nanoparticles consist of a semiconductor core surrounded by an outer shell, and have several unique properties. Subtle changes in the size of a quantum dot can significantly change both the absorption and emission wavelengths of the particle, and they are thus "tunable". These agents are also generally far more stable than conventional fluorochromes, and emit significantly more energy. Unfortunately, most of the current quantum dot constructs contain highly toxic core substances such as cadmium, selenide and arsenic. Future research will focus on the development of quantum dots containing safer materials in their semiconductor core, and the development of more biocompatible outer shells that are optimized for bioconjugation [76].

5 MR and NIRF imaging in specific disease states

The use of unlabeled NIR fluorochromes and ultra-small iron oxide nanoparticles may in its own right be extremely useful in certain applications. For instance, iron oxide nanoparticles have shown significant promise for use in MR angiography, cardiac MR imaging and for the detection of lymph node metastases in certain cancers [25–27]. The applications described below, however, focus purely on the use of targeted and activatable NIRF and MR probes. The reader is also referred to Table 2 and several excellent reviews for additional lists of potential targets for molecular imaging.

5.1 Cardiovascular disease

5.1.1 Thrombosis

Thrombosis plays a central role in both venous thromboembolism and the acute coronary syndromes. Numerous targets for molecular imaging exist on both platelets and the clotting factors involved in the coagulation cascade. Gadolinium-based probes have been developed for the detection of fibrin using various affinity ligands [30–32, 77]. A targeted NIRF probe to factor XIIIa and an activatable NIRF probe for thrombin activity have also been developed [78, 79]. Receptors on the surface of platelets, such as the II_bIII_a receptor are also suitable targets for affinity-based probes. The use of these probes should facilitate the development of new anti-thrombotic therapies, and allow their efficacy *in vivo* to be assessed.

5.1.2 Endothelial inflammation

The role of endothelial inflammation in the initiation of atherosclerotic plaques is being increasingly recognized. Early in the process, adhesion molecules such as VCAM-1, ICAM-1 and E-selectin are expressed on the endothelial membrane [80]. Antibodies and peptides that bind to these inflammatory molecules have been developed for conjugation to magnetic nanoparticles and NIR fluorochromes. In addition, an activatable NIRF probe to cathepsin D has been shown to be able to detect proteolytic activity in atherosclerotic plaques [81]. Myoperixidase activity in atherosclerotic plaques may also be detectable using an activatable paramagnetic MR contrast agent [47].

5.1.3 Angiogenesis

Angiogenesis may play an important role in plaque stability and the development of collateral vessels in ischemic myocardium. Targeted magnetic nanoparticle probes have been developed to detect integrins ($\alpha_5\beta_3$) involved in the angiogenesis process [82–84]. Targeted probes to VCAM-1 and E-Selectin will also be of relevance in this situation [80]. These probes have the potential to facilitate the development of novel angiogenic therapies.

5.1.4 Cardiomyocyte apoptosis

Cardiomyocyte apoptosis is thought to play an important role in several diseases involving the heart, including ischemia, reperfusion injury and heart failure. Fluorescent, magnetic and combined magneto-optical probes have been developed for apoptosis imaging. Annexin V and synaptotagmin have beeen conjugated to magnetic nanoparticles and NIR fluorochromes for the detection phoshatidylserine on the surface of apoptotic cardiomyocytes [85]. MRSs and activatable fluorochromes have been used to detect caspase-3 activity, which is the terminal kinase in the apoptotic cascade [20]. The use of these probes should provide a clearer insight into the role of apoptosis in cardiovascular disease, and facilitate the development of new cardioprotective therapies.

5.1.5 Myocardial matrix remodeling

The remodeling process in heart failure involves, amongst other processes, the degredation of the connective tissue matrix in the myocardium by matrix metallo-proteinases (MMPs), principally MMP 2 and MMP9. The activity of these MMPs can be detected with activatable NIR probes and followed serially [63, 86]. This has the potential to facilitate the development of novel anti-remodeling therapeutic strategies.

5.1.6 Myocardial inflammation

The use of currently available non-invasive imaging modalities to diagnose myocarditis and cardiac transplant rejection has generally been unrewarding. The use of long-circulating MNP has allowed myocardial inflammation to be imaged in animal models of myocarditis and transplant rejection [87]. The accumulation of the nanoparticles in the myocardium results, presumably, both from the increased vascular permeability associated with the inflammation and from the inflammatory cells themselves. There is currently intense interest in the use of the agents to detect myocarditis and transplant rejection in humans. The availability of a robust non-invasive technique with which to image the degree of myocardial inflammation could be of considerable use in the design and testing of new therapeutic agents for patients with myocarditis and transplant rejection.

5.2 Neoplastic disease

5.2.1 Early detection of cancer

The early detection of adenomatous colonic polyps is central to the prevention of colon cancer. NIRF endoscopic systems that allow mucosal surfaces in the bowel, bladder and lung to be imaged with FRI have recently been developed [66]. The use of protease-activatable NIRF probes has been shown to allow adenomatous polyps to be detected at an earlier stage than is possible by conventional light imaging techniques [88]. The use of high-through-put screening libraries also allows peptides with surface specificity for neoplastic mucosal cells to be identified. A targeted fluorescent probe, for instance, with specificity for colonic cancer has been successfully developed [72]. Malignant cells may also overexpress the transferrin receptor on their surface allowing for early detection with iron oxide nanoparticles.

5.2.2 Molecular characterization of cancer

While the size and location of tumors can be assessed with traditional imaging modalities, serial molecular characterization of tumors *in vivo* would likely have important therapeutic implications. For instance breast cancers with high protease activity, imaged with a cathepsin-activated protease probe, were shown to be more invasive than those with low protease activity [74]. Elevated telomerase levels are also found in many cancers and may have important diagnostic and therapeutic implications. An activatable MRS, capable of imaging telomerase activity and its phosphorylation state, has been developed [89]. This may prove a useful tool in the design of new chemotherapeutic agents. The potential of a tumor to spread locally and distally may be related to the level of MMP activity within the tumor. An activatable NIRF probe has been shown to be able to image MMP activity in tumors implanted into mice and, moreover, image the pharmacological inhibition of MMPs in these tumors [63, 86].

5.2.3 Accurate staging/detection of metastases

MNP have been used to detect lymph node metastases in abdominal, pelvic and prostate cancers [27, 90]. The use of this technique has been shown to accurately detect even small lymphatic metastases and may thus prove an extremely useful tool in the assessment of the efficacy of new chemotherapeutic agents. An NIR fluorochrome attached to a protected graft polymer was also able to detect lymph node metastases after either intravenous or subcutaneous injection in mice [91]. Certain tumors, such as nasopharyngeal tumors, overexpress folate receptors, that can be detected by both targeted MR and NIR probes, on their surface. Pancreatic neuroendocrine tumors may be difficult to diagnose by traditional techniques but are thought to overexpress somatostatin and bombesin in high levels. Targeted probes have been developed against these receptors and may allow for earlier detection and improved monitoring of therapy.

5.2.4 Monitoring of response to therapy

The efficacy of chemotherapy in solid tumors is currently judged by assessing a reduction in tumor volume after several cycles of drug therapy. Many tumors, however, undergo apoptosis soon after the initiation of a chemotherapeutic agent, if they are sensitive to it. Both NIRF and magnetic Annnexin-based probes have been used to image tumor apoptosis following the initiation of chemotherapy in small-animal models [92, 93]. Importantly, the quantification of tumor apoptosis with an NIRF probe has been shown to be significantly more accurate with FMT than with FRI [93]. The ability to assess the early response of a tumor to new therapies should greatly aid the development of new chemotherapeutic agents.

5.3 Targets in inflammatory/autoimmune disease

5.3.1 Imaging of protease activity in rheumatoid arthritis

Disease activity in rheumatoid arthritis can be imaged *in vivo* with protease-activated NIR probes [94]. The use of these probes allows inflammatory activity in the joint to be followed and the response to disease-modifying drugs to be monitored.

5.3.2 Pancreatic beta cells in diabetes

Type 1 diabetes is caused by inflammation of the pancreatic islets and a reduction in beta cell mass. Pancreatic inflammation can be detected *in vivo* by imaging the accumulation of long-circulating MNP in the pancreas. The accumulation of these nanoparticles reflects the increased vascular permeability and monocyte infiltration associated with pancreatic islet inflamtion [95]. In addition, ligands with affinity for specific receptors on the surface of beta cells have been developed and allow beta cell mass to be quantified non-invasively [96]. The ability to do this may allow novel therapies for type 1 diabetes to be developed.

5.3.3 Imaging of viral proteases

A fluorescent probe specific for the HIV-1 protease has recently been reported [97]. This probe could successfully image the inhibition of the protease by the HIV-1 protease inhibitor indinavir. The ability to image HIV-protease activity *in vivo* would allow the efficacy of drug therapy to be assessed directly *in vivo*.

5.4   Cell survival, tracking and gene expression

There is intense interest in the use of stem cells to regenerate lost myocardium, nervous tissue and pancreatic beta cells. Iron oxide nanoparticles are being used by many investigators to label and track these stem cells with serial MRI studies over time [98, 99]. A highly derivatized form of cross-linked iron oxide has also been used to track cytotoxic lymphocyte homing to tumors, and may provide valuable insights for the development of immune-based therapies in certain cancers [100]. There is also significant interest in the promise of gene therapy. Both magnetic nanoparticles and NIRF agents can be used to detect reporter genes whose expression is driven by the primary gene of interest. For MR imaging, overexpression of an engineered transferrin receptor can lead to significantly greater uptake of iron oxide by cells expressing the transgene than by those cells that do not, thus providing a useful reporter mechanism [101, 102]. Genes encoding for specific proteases can also serve as useful reporters of primary transgene expression through the use of activatable NIRF probes.

6 Issues in molecular imaging trial design

6.1 Level of target expression

In general, the most suitable targets for molecular imaging are those with the highest degree of selective expression. For instance, the effect of a drug on an upstream factor in the coagulation cascade may be more accurately assessed by imaging the downstream activity of fibrin, which is highly expressed in thrombi, than by imaging the activity of the upstream factor itself. The initial step in the design of a molecular imaging trial must, therefore, be the identification of the target with the highest level of expression, which nevertheless provides relevant information on the target against which the drug is directed.

Targets with fairly low levels of expression may be more suitable for detection with radiolabeled and fluorescently labeled probes than with MR-detectable probes. However, the higher sensitivity of these radiolabeled and NIRF probes must be balanced against the low spatial resolution obtainable with these techniques. If high resolution imaging is required, for instance to resolve the transmural extent of a molecular process within the myocardium, then MRI is likely to be the procedure of choice. Paramagnetic contrast agents, however, will likely only be able to detect targets which are highly expressed. Superparamagnetic contrast agents have significantly higher relaxivities than paramagnetic ones, but are still less sensitive than radiolabeled and NIRF probes. The need for high spatial resolution must, therefore, be balanced against the SNR and CNR obtainable with a particular technique and be tailored to the specific question of interest.

6.2   Target location

Many targets relevant to drug design are located within the cell. The imaging of these targets, however, is somewhat more challenging than the imaging of extracellular targets. Due to their smaller size, radiolabeled and NIRF probes are best able to penetrate the cell membrane, and are thus most suited to the imaging of intracellular targets. At the present time the use of cell-penetrating superparamagnetic contrast agents is still investigational, and their use in clinical trials of drug efficacy is thus still premature.

Advances in the design of endoscopes will likely allow NIRF imaging to be performed routinely in endoscopic studies of the gastrointestinal, urogenital and respiratory systems. The use of both targeted and activatable NIRF agents to interrogate these systems thus offers the possibility of both tomographic or endoscopic detection, and is likely to be of considerable use. Intravascular devices capable of NIRF imaging have been developed and are likely to be used in combination with either intravascular ultrasound or optical coherence tomography. This approach may allow the effects of investigational drugs on plaque morphology and composition to be imaged with a high degree of accuracy.

6.3   Stability of probe delivery

Alterations in the level of probe delivery over time can significantly complicate the interpretation of molecular imaging studies of novel therapies. The signal intensity from a particular target in a tumor, for instance, can be altered both by the direct effect of the drug on the tumor itself, or by a secondary effect on tumor vascularity. Studies designed to serially image the expression of a molecular target in a tumor over time, therefore, generally require a strategy to compensate for this potential effect. Dual wavelength imaging with either NIRF agents or radio-isotopes is one such strategy that can be used to normalize the molecular image of the tumor to its perfusion image [103, 104]. An unlabeled isotope or fluorochrome with a wavelength distinct from the labeled probe is injected simultaneously into the animal and used to create the perfusion map. Perfusion maps can also be created by MRI using endogenous contrast mechanisms such as arterial spin labeling or exogenous contrast agents such as gadolinium.

6.4   Imaging of enzyme levels/activity

Many drugs currently in development are directed against specific proteases and kinases involved in important metabolic pathways. The use of activatable NIRF probes, particularly with tomographic systems, is likely to be the most promising technique with which to image enzyme activity. Activatable MR contrast agents have been developed and, as in the case of targeted agents, provide higher spatial resolution at the cost of lower sensitivity. At the present time, however, the use of activatable MR agents, *in vivo*, remains investigational and their use *in vivo* has not yet been adequately validated. Radiolabeled inhibitors of enzyme activity have also been used to image enzyme distribution. This technique depends on the labeled inhibitor having both a high degree of specificity and affinity for the enzyme of interest. These radiolabeled probes also do not have the built-in amplification strategy that is produced by continuous activation of NIRF probes. Nevertheless, until NIRF systems for large animal and human imaging become more available, the use of radiolabeled enzyme inhibitors has the potential to play an important role.

6.5   Imaging of acute processes

The imaging of molecular phenomena that are acute or transient is significantly more challenging than the imaging of chronically expressed targets with stable or increasing levels of expression over time. The use of targeted contrast agents in this situation is often limited by high levels of signal from the unbound fraction of the probe shortly after injection. Thus, for targeted agents to be of use in this situation they require both a very high affinity for the target of interest and fairly rapid elimination of the unbound portion of the probe. An alternative strategy is the use of activatable probes which produce low levels of background signal in the absence of specific activation. It is likely, however, that initial molecular imaging trials of drug efficacy will involve the imaging of chronic stable targets.

6.6   Human trials

Although certain gadolinium chelates and polymer-coated iron oxides are already approved for use in humans, once a targeted ligand is added to these particles their use in humans becomes experimental and subject to the full range of regulatory procedures for any new agent. Extensive data regarding the biodistribution, elimination and toxicity of the labeled agent would need to be acquired in animals prior to the use of the probes in humans. Initial constructs of activatable NIRF probes are likely to receive FDA approval in the near future as well, but any change in the construct will once again require full investigation. The list of both MR-detectable and NIRF probes that are approved for human use is likely to grow over the next several years but this issue will still need to be taken into account in the design of trials where human involvement is considered essential.

7   Conclusion

Molecular imaging has the potential to revolutionize both the drug discovery process and the practice of medicine. MRI and NIRF imaging are well suited to the molecular imaging mission. They are non-ionizing and provide a mechanism for both targeted and activatable imaging strategies. Moreover, both modalities can be applied in small animals and humans, fulfilling the need for bench-to-bedside translation. Rapid improvements in both probe design and detector hardware are being made, which will allow imaging readouts to be performed with both greater sophistication and accuracy. The full realization of the potential of these modalities, however, will require an active collaborative effort between the hardware manufacturers, biosynthetic chemists, biologists and physician scientists.

References

1   Weissleder R, Mahmood U (2001) Molecular imaging. *Radiology* 219: 316–333
2   Ruff J, Wiesmann F, Hiller KH, Voll S, von Kienlin M, Bauer WR, Rommel E, Neubauer S, Haase A (1998) Magnetic resonance microimaging for noninvasive quantification of myocardial function and mass in the mouse. *Magn Reson Med* 40: 43–48
3   Funovics MA, Weissleder R, Mahmood U (2004) Catheter-based *in vivo* imaging of enzyme activity and gene expression: feasibility study in mice. *Radiology* 231: 659–666

4   Mahmood U, Tung CH, Bogdanov A Jr., Weissleder R (1999) Near-infrared optical imaging of protease activity for tumor detection. *Radiology* 213: 866–870

5   Weissleder R (2002) Scaling down imaging: molecular mapping of cancer in mice. *Nat Rev Cancer* 2: 11–18

6   Rudin M, Weissleder R (2003) Molecular imaging in drug discovery and development. *Nat Rev Drug Discov* 2: 123–131

7   Josephson L, Kircher MF, Mahmood U, Tang Y, Weissleder R (2002) Near-infrared fluorescent nanoparticles as combined MR/optical imaging probes. *Bioconjug Chem* 13: 554–560

8   Kircher MF, Mahmood U, King RS, Weissleder R, Josephson L (2003) A multimodal nanoparticle for preoperative magnetic resonance imaging and intraoperative optical brain tumor delineation. *Cancer Res* 63: 8122–8125

9   Weissleder R, Ntziachristos V (2003) Shedding light onto live molecular targets. *Nat Med* 9: 123–128

10   Rudin M, Beckmann N, Porszasz R, Reese T, Bochelen D, Sauter A (1999) *In vivo* magnetic resonance methods in pharmaceutical research: current status and perspectives. *NMR Biomed* 12: 69–97

11   Beckmann N, Mueggler T, Allegrini PR, Laurent D, Rudin M (2001) From anatomy to the target: contributions of magnetic resonance imaging to preclinical pharmaceutical research. *Anat Rec* 265: 85–100

12   Jain RK, Munn LL, Fukumura D (2002) Dissecting tumour pathophysiology using intravital microscopy. *Nat Rev Cancer* 2: 266–276

13   Phelps ME (2000) Inaugural article: positron emission tomography provides molecular imaging of biological processes. *Proc Natl Acad Sci USA* 97: 9226–9233

14   Fischman AJ, Alpert NM, Rubin RH (2002) Pharmacokinetic imaging: a noninvasive method for determining drug distribution and action. *Clin Pharmacokinet* 41: 581–602

15   Tjuvajev JG, Stockhammer G, Desai R, Uehara H, Watanabe K, Gansbacher B, Blasberg RG (1995) Imaging the expression of transfected genes *in vivo*. *Cancer Res* 55: 6126–6132

16   Gambhir SS, Barrio JR, Phelps ME, Iyer M, Namavari M, Satyamurthy N, Wu L, Green LA, Bauer E, MacLaren DC et al. (1999) Imaging adenoviral-directed reporter gene expression in living animals with positron emission tomography. *Proc Natl Acad Sci USA* 96: 2333–2338

17   Moore A, Josephson L, Bhorade RM, Basilion JP, Weissleder R (2001) Human transferrin receptor gene as a marker gene for MR imaging. *Radiology* 221: 244–250

18   Tung CH, Bredow S, Mahmood U, Weissleder R (1999) Preparation of a cathepsin D sensitive near-infrared fluorescence probe for imaging. *Bioconjug Chem* 10: 892–896

19   Weissleder R, Tung CH, Mahmood U, Bogdanov A Jr (1999) *In vivo* imaging of tumors with protease-activated near-infrared fluorescent probes. *Nat Biotechnol* 17: 375–378

20   Perez JM, Josephson L, O'Loughlin T, Hogemann D, Weissleder R (2002) Magnetic relaxation switches capable of sensing molecular interactions. *Nat Biotechnol* 20: 816–820

21   Kim RJ, Wu E, Rafael A, Chen EL, Parker MA, Simonetti O, Klocke FJ, Bonow RO, Judd RM (2000) The use of contrast-enhanced magnetic resonance imaging to identify reversible myocardial dysfunction. *N Engl J Med* 343: 1445–1453

22   Earls JP, Ho VB, Foo TK, Castillo E, Flamm SD (2002) Cardiac MRI: recent progress and continued challenges. *J Magn Reson Imaging* 16: 111–127

23   Neubauer S, Beer M, Landschutz W, Sandstede J, Seyfarth T, Lipke C, Kostler H, Pabst TKenn W, Meininger M, von Kienlin M et al (2000) Absolute quantification of high

energy phosphate metabolites in normal, hypertrophied and failing human myocardium. *Magma* 11: 73–74

24   Bjerner T, Johansson L, Ericsson A, Wikstrom G, Hemmingsson A, Ahlstrom H (2001) First-pass myocardial perfusion MR imaging with outer-volume suppression and the intravascular contrast agent NC100150 injection: preliminary results in eight patients. *Radiology* 221: 822–826

25   Stillman AE, Wilke N, Jerosch-Herold M (1997) Use of an intravascular T1 contrast agent to improve MR cine myocardial-blood pool definition in man. *J Magn Reson Imaging* 7: 765–767

26   Paetsch I, Thiele H, Schnackenburg B, Bornstedt A, Muller-York A, Schwab J, Fleck E, Nagel E (2003) Improved functional cardiac MR imaging using the intravascular contrast agent CLARISCAN. *Int J Cardiovasc Imaging* 19: 337–343

27   Harisinghani MG, Barentsz J, Hahn PF, Deserno WM, Tabatabaei S, van de Kaa CH, de la Rosette J, Weissleder R (2003) Noninvasive detection of clinically occult lymph-node metastases in prostate cancer. *N Engl J Med* 348: 2491–2419

28   Lauffer RB (1990) Magnetic resonance contrast media: principles and progress. *Magn Reson Q* 6: 65–84

29   Chapon C, Franconi F, Lemaire L, Marescaux L, Legras P, Saint-Andre JP, Denizot B, Le Jeune JJ (2003) High field magnetic resonance imaging evaluation of superparamagnetic iron oxide nanoparticles in a permanent rat myocardial infarction. *Investigative Radiology* 38: 141–146

30   Lanza GM, Lorenz CH, Fischer SE, Scott MJ, Cacheris WP, Kaufmann RJ, Gaffney PJ, Wickline SA (1998) Enhanced detection of thrombi with a novel fibrin-targeted magnetic resonance imaging agent. *Acad Radiol* 5, Suppl 1: S173–S176; discussion S183–S184

31   Winter PM, Caruthers SD, Yu X, Song SK, Chen J, Miller B, Bulte JW, Robertson JD, Gaffney PJ, Wickline SA, Lanza GM (2003) Improved molecular imaging contrast agent for detection of human thrombus. *Magn Reson Med* 50: 411–416

32   Botnar RM, Perez AS, Witte S, Wiethoff AJ, Laredo J, Hamilton J, Quist W, Parsons EC Jr, Vaidya A, Kolodziej A et al. (2004) *In vivo* molecular imaging of acute and subacute thrombosis using a fibrin-binding magnetic resonance imaging contrast agent. *Circulation* 109: 2023–2029

33   Morawski AM, Winter PM, Crowder KC, Caruthers SD, Fuhrhop RW, Scott MJ, Robertson JD, Abendschein DR, Lanza GM, Wickline SA (2004) Targeted nanoparticles for quantitative imaging of sparse molecular epitopes with MRI. *Magn Reson Med* 51: 480–486

34   Weissleder R, Liver MR (1994) imaging with iron oxides: toward consensus and clinical practice. *Radiology* 193: 593–595

35   Johansson LO, Bjerner T, Bjornerud A, Ahlstrom H, Tarlo KS, Lorenz CH (2002) Utility of NC100150 injection in cardiac MRI. *Acad Radiol* 9, Suppl 1: S79–S81

36   Weissleder R, Stark DD, Engelstad BL, Bacon BR, Compton CC, White DL, Jacobs P, Lewis J (1989) Superparamagnetic iron oxide: pharmacokinetics and toxicity. *AJR Am J Roentgenol* 152: 167–173

37   Josephson L, Groman E, Weissleder R (1991) Contrast agents for magnetic resonance imaging of the liver. *Targeted Diagn Ther* 4: 163–187

38   Shen T, Weissleder R, Papisov M, Bogdanov A Jr., Brady TJ (1993) Monocrystalline iron oxide nanocompounds (MION): physicochemical properties. *Magn Reson Med* 29: 599–604

39   Bunce, N.H. et al. (2001) Improved cine cardiovascular magnetic resonance using Clar-iscan (NC100150 injection). *J Cardiovasc Magn Reson* 3: 303–310

40   Weissleder R, Lee AS, Khaw BA, Shen T, Brady TJ (1992) Antimyosin-labeled monocrys-talline iron oxide allows detection of myocardial infarct: MR antibody imaging. *Radiol-ogy* 182: 381–385

41   Schellenberger EA, Reynolds F, Weissleder R, Josephson L (2004) Surface-functionalized nanoparticle library yields probes for apoptotic cells. *Chembiochem* 5: 275–279

42   Lewin M, Carlesso N, Tung CH, Tang XW, Cory D, Scadden DT, Weissleder R (2000) Tat peptide-derivatized magnetic nanoparticles allow *in vivo* tracking and recovery of prog-enitor cells. *Nat Biotechnol* 18: 410–414

43   Wunderbaldinger P, Josephson L, Weissleder R (2002) Tat peptide directs enhanced clearance and hepatic permeability of magnetic nanoparticles. *Bioconjug Chem* 13: 264–268

44   Hogemann D, Ntziachristos V, Josephson L, Weissleder R (2002) High throughput mag-netic resonance imaging for evaluating targeted nanoparticle probes. *Bioconjug Chem* 13: 116–121

45   Louie AY, Huber MM, Ahrens ET, Rothbacher U, Moats R, Jacobs RE, Fraser SE, Meade TJ (2000) *In vivo* visualization of gene expression using magnetic resonance imaging. *Nat Biotechnol* 18: 321–325

46   Bogdanov A Jr., Matuszewski L, Bremer C, Petrovsky A, Weissleder R (2002) Oligomer-ization of paramagnetic substrates result in signal amplification and can be used for MR imaging of molecular targets. *Mol Imaging* 1: 16–23

47   Chen JW, Pham W, Weissleder R, Bogdanov A Jr (2004) Human myeloperoxidase: a potential target for molecular MR imaging in atherosclerosis. *Magn Reson Med* 52: 1021–1028

48   Capdeville R, Buchdunger E, Zimmermann J, Matter A (2002) Glivec (STI571, imatinib), a rationally developed, targeted anticancer drug. *Nat Rev Drug Discov* 1: 493–502

49   Perez JM, Josephson L, Weissleder R (2004) Use of magnetic nanoparticles as nanosen-sors to probe for molecular interactions. *Chembiochem* 5: 261–264

50   Perez JM, O'Loughin T, Simeone FJ, Weissleder R, Josephson L (2002) DNA-based mag-netic nanoparticle assembly acts as a magnetic relaxation nanoswitch allowing screen-ing of DNA-cleaving agents. *J Am Chem Soc* 124: 2856–2857

51   Perez JM, Simeone FJ, Saeki Y, Josephson L, Weissleder R (2003) Viral-induced self-assem-bly of magnetic nanoparticles allows the detection of viral particles in biological media. *J Am Chem Soc* 125: 10192–10193

52   Tsourkas A, Hofstetter O, Hofstetter H, Weissleder R, Josephson L (2004) Magnetic relax-ation switch immunosensors detect enantiomeric impurities. *Angew Chem Int Ed Engl* 43: 2395–2399

53   Tung CH, Weissleder R (2003) Arginine containing peptides as delivery vectors. *Adv Drug Deliv Rev* 55: 281–294

54   Ntziachristos V, Weissleder R (2002) Charge-coupled-device based scanner for tomogra-phy of fluorescent near-infrared probes in turbid media. *Med Phys* 29: 803–809

55   Ntziachristos V, Bremer C, Weissleder R (2003) Fluorescence imaging with near-infrared light: new technological advances that enable *in vivo* molecular imaging. *Eur Radiol* 13: 195–208

56   Tromberg BJ, Shah N, Lanning R, Cerussi A, Espinoza J, Pham T, Svaasand L, Butler J

(2000) Non-invasive *in vivo* characterization of breast tumors using photon migration spectroscopy. *Neoplasia* 2: 26–40

57   Chance B (2001) Near-infrared (NIR) optical spectroscopy characterizes breast tissue hormonal and age status. *Acad Radiol* 8: 209–210

58   Hanlon EB, Manoharan R, Koo TW, Shafer KE, Motz JT, Fitzmaurice M, Kramer JR, Itzkan I, Dasari RR, Feld MS (2000) Prospects for *in vivo* Raman spectroscopy. *Phys Med Biol* 45: R1–59

59   Brown EB (2001*) In vivo* measurement of gene expression, angiogenesis and physiological function in tumors using multiphoton laser scanning microscopy. *Nat Med* 7: 864–868

60   Lin Y, Weissleder R, Tung CH (2002) Novel near-infrared cyanine fluorochromes: synthesis, properties, and bioconjugation. *Bioconjug Chem* 13: 605–610

61   Lin Y, Weissleder R, Tung CH (2003) Synthesis and properties of sulfhydryl-reactive near-infrared cyanine fluorochromes for fluorescence imaging. *Mol Imaging* 2: 87–92

62   Ntziachristos V, Tung CH, Bremer C, Weissleder R (2002) Fluorescence molecular tomography resolves protease activity *in vivo*. *Nat Med* 8: 757–760

63   Bremer C, Tung CH, Weissleder R (2001*) In vivo* molecular target assessment of matrix metalloproteinase inhibition. *Nat Med* 7: 743–748

64   Marten K, Bremer C, Khazaie K, Sameni M, Sloane B, Tung CH, Weissleder R (2002) Detection of dysplastic intestinal adenomas using enzyme-sensing molecular beacons in mice. *Gastroenterology* 122: 406–414

65   Ito S, Muguruma N, Kusaka Y, Tadatsu M, Inayama K, Musashi Y, Yano M, Bando T, Honda H, Shimizu I et al. (2001) Detection of human gastric cancer in resected specimens using a novel infrared fluorescent anti-human carcinoembryonic antigen antibody with an infrared fluorescence endoscope *in vitro*. *Endoscopy* 33: 849–853

66   Funovics MA, Alencar H, Su HS, Khazaie K, Weissleder R, Mahmood U (2003) Miniaturized multichannel near infrared endoscope for mouse imaging. *Mol Imaging* 2: 350–357

67   Zonios G, Bykowski J, Kollias N (2001) Skin melanin, hemoglobin, and light scattering properties can be quantitatively assessed *in vivo* using diffuse reflectance spectroscopy. *J Invest Dermatol* 117: 1452–1457

68   Kuroiwa T, Kajimoto Y, Ohta T (2001) Development and clinical application of near-infrared surgical microscope: preliminary report. *Minim Invasive Neurosurg* 44: 240–242

69   Graves EE, Ripoll J, Weissleder R, Ntziachristos V (2003) A submillimeter resolution fluorescence molecular imaging system for small animal imaging. *Med Phys* 30: 901–911

70   Graves EE, Culver JP, Ripoll J, Weissleder R, Ntziachristos V (2004) Singular-value analysis and optimization of experimental parameters in fluorescence molecular tomography. *J Opt Soc Am A Opt Image Sci Vis* 21: 231–241

71   Becker A, Hessenius C, Licha K, Ebert B, Sukowski U, Semmler W, Wiedenmann B, Grotzinger C (2001) Receptor-targeted optical imaging of tumors with near-infrared fluorescent ligands. *Nat Biotechnol* 19: 327–331

72   Kelly K, Alencar H, Funovics M, Mahmood U, Weissleder R (2004) Detection of invasive colon cancer using a novel, targeted, library-derived fluorescent peptide. *Cancer Res* 64: 6247–6251

73   Bremer C, Bredow S, Mahmood U, Weissleder R, Tung CH (2001) Optical imaging of matrix metalloproteinase-2 activity in tumors: feasibility study in a mouse model. *Radiology* 221: 523–529

74   Bremer C, Tung CH, Bogdanov A Jr., Weissleder R (2002) Imaging of differential protease

expression in breast cancers for detection of aggressive tumor phenotypes. *Radiology* 222: 814–818

75 Dubertret B, Skourides P, Norris DJ, Noireaux V, Brivanlou AH, Libchaber A (2002) *In vivo* imaging of quantum dots encapsulated in phospholipid micelles. *Science* 298: 1759–1762

76 Jaiswal JK, Simon SM (2004) Potentials and pitfalls of fluorescent quantum dots for biological imaging. *Trends Cell Biol* 14: 497–504

77 Flacke S, Fischer S, Scott MJ, Fuhrhop RJ, Allen JS, McLean M, Winter P, Sicard GA, Gaffney PJ, Wickline SA, Lanza GM (2001) Novel MRI contrast agent for molecular imaging of fibrin: implications for detecting vulnerable plaques. *Circulation* 104: 1280–1285

78 Jaffer FA, Tung CH, Wykrzykowska JJ, Ho NH, Houng AK, Reed GL, Weissleder R (2004) Molecular imaging of factor XIIIa activity in thrombosis using a novel, near-infrared fluorescent contrast agent that covalently links to thrombi. *Circulation* 110: 170–176

79 Jaffer FA, Tung CH, Gerszten RE, Weissleder R (2002) *In vivo* imaging of thrombin activity in experimental thrombi with thrombin-sensitive near-infrared molecular probe. *Arterioscler Thromb Vasc Biol* 22: 1929–1935

80 Kang HW, Josephson L, Petrovsky A, Weissleder R, Bogdanov A Jr (2002) Magnetic resonance imaging of inducible E-selectin expression in human endothelial cell culture. *Bioconjugate Chemistry* 13: 122–127

81 Chen J, Tung CH, Mahmood U, Ntziachristos V, Gyurko R, Fishman MC, Huang PL, Weissleder R (2002) *In vivo* imaging of proteolytic activity in atherosclerosis. *Circulation* 105: 2766–2771

82 Winter PM, Morawski AM, Caruthers SD, Fuhrhop RW, Zhang H, Williams TA, Allen JS, Lacy EK, Robertson JD, Lanza GM, Wickline SA (2003) Molecular imaging of angiogenesis in early-stage atherosclerosis with alpha(v)beta3-integrin-targeted nanoparticles. *Circulation* 108: 2270–2274

83 Sipkins DA, Cheresh DA, Kazemi MR, Nevin LM, Bednarski MD, Li KC (1998) Detection of tumor angiogenesis *in vivo* by alphaVbeta3-targeted magnetic resonance imaging. *Nat Med* 4: 623–626

84 Anderson SA, Rader RK, Westlin WF, Null C, Jackson D, Lanza GM, Wickline SA, Kotyk JJ (2000) Magnetic resonance contrast enhancement of neovasculature with alpha(v)beta(3)-targeted nanoparticles. *Magn Reson Med* 44: 433–439

85 Schellenberger EA, Sosnovik D, Weissleder R, Josephson L (2004) Magneto/optical annexin V, a multimodal protein. Bioconjug Chem 15: 1062–1067

86 Bremer C, Tung CH, Weissleder R (2002) Molecular imaging of MMP expression and therapeutic MMP inhibition. *Acad Radiol* 9, Suppl 2: S314–S315

87 Kanno S, Wu YJ, Lee PC, Dodd SJ, Williams M, Griffith BP, Ho C (2001) Macrophage accumulation associated with rat cardiac allograft rejection detected by magnetic resonance imaging with ultrasmall superparamagnetic iron oxide particles. *Circulation* 104: 934–938

88 Mahmood U (2004) Near infrared optical applications in molecular imaging. Earlier, more accurate assessment of disease presence, disease course, and efficacy of disease treatment. *IEEE Eng Med Biol Mag* 23: 58–66

89 Grimm J, Perez JM, Josephson L, Weissleder R (2004) Novel nanosensors for rapid analysis of telomerase activity. *Cancer Res* 64: 639–643

90 Harisinghani MG, Saini S, Weissleder R, Hahn PF, Yantiss RK, Tempany C, Wood BJ, Mueller PR (1999) MR lymphangiography using ultrasmall superparamagnetic iron

oxide in patients with primary abdominal and pelvic malignancies: radiographic-pathologic correlation. *AJR Am J Roentgenol* 172: 1347–1351

91   Josephson L, Mahmood U, Wunderbaldinger P, Tang Y, Weissleder R (2003) Pan and sentinel lymph node visualization using a near-infrared fluorescent probe. *Mol Imaging* 2: 18–23

92   Petrovsky A, Schellenberger E, Josephson L, Weissleder R, Bogdanov A Jr. (2003) Near-infrared fluorescent imaging of tumor apoptosis. *Cancer Res* 63: 1936–1942

93   Ntziachristos V, Schellenberger EA, Ripoll J, Yessayan D, Graves E, Bogdanov A Jr, Josephson L, Weissleder R (2004) Visualization of antitumor treatment by means of fluorescence molecular tomography with an annexin V-Cy5.5 conjugate. *Proc Natl Acad Sci USA* 101: 12294–12299

94   Wunder A, Tung CH, Muller-Ladner U, Weissleder R, Mahmood U (2004*) In vivo* imaging of protease activity in arthritis: a novel approach for monitoring treatment response. *Arthritis Rheum* 50: 2459–2465

95   Denis MC, Mahmood U, Benoist C, Mathis D, Weissleder R (2004) Imaging inflammation of the pancreatic islets in type 1 diabetes. *Proc Natl Acad Sci USA* 101: 12634–12639

96   Moore A, Bonner-Weir S, Weissleder R (2001) Noninvasive *in vivo* measurement of beta-cell mass in mouse model of diabetes. *Diabetes* 50: 2231–2236

97   Shah K, Tung CH, Chang CH, Slootweg E, O'Loughlin T, Breakefield XO, Weissleder R (2004*) In vivo* imaging of HIV protease activity in amplicon vector-transduced gliomas. *Cancer Res* 64: 273–278

98   Weissleder R, Cheng HC, Bogdanova A, Bogdanov A Jr (1997) Magnetically labeled cells can be detected by MR imaging. *J Magn Reson Imaging* 7: 258–263

99   Hill JM, Dick AJ, Raman VK, Thompson RB, Yu ZX, Hinds KA, Pessanha BS, Guttman MA, Varney TR, Martin BJ et al (2003) Serial cardiac magnetic resonance imaging of injected mesenchymal stem cells. *Circulation* 108: 1009–1014

100   Kircher MF, Allport JR, Graves EE, Love V, Josephson L, Lichtman AH, Weissleder R (2003*) In vivo* high resolution three-dimensional imaging of antigen-specific cytotoxic T-lymphocyte trafficking to tumors. *Cancer Res* 63: 6838–6846

101   Hogemann D, Josephson L, Weissleder R, Basilion JP (2000) Improvement of MRI probes to allow efficient detection of gene expression. *Bioconjug Chem* 11: 941–946

102   Ichikawa T, Hogemann D, Saeki Y, Tyminski E, Terada K, Weissleder R, Chiocca EA, Basilion JP (2002) MRI of transgene expression: correlation to therapeutic gene expression. *Neoplasia* 4: 523–530

103   Kircher MF, Josephson L, Weissleder R (2002) Ratio imaging of enzyme activity using dual wavelength optical reporters. *Mol Imaging* 1: 89–95

104   Kircher MF, Weissleder R, Josephson L (2004) A dual fluorochrome probe for imaging proteases. *Bioconjug Chem* 15: 242–248

105   Wunderbaldinger P, Josephson L, Weissleder R (2002) Crosslinked iron oxides (CLIO): a new platform for the development of targeted MR contrast agents. *Acad Radiol* 9, Suppl 2: S304–S306

Progress in Drug Research, Vol. 62
(Markus Rudin, Ed.)
©2005 Birkhäuser Verlag, Basel (Switzerland)

Studying molecular and cellular processes in the intact organism

By Olivier Gheysens and
Sanjiv S. Gambhir

Molecular Imaging Program at
Stanford (MIPS)
Departments of Radiology and
Bioengineering
Bio-X Program
Stanford University
318 Campus Dr.
Clark Center, E-150
Stanford, CA 94305, USA
<sgambhir@stanford.edu>

Glossary of abbreviations

BLI, bioluminescence imaging; CCD, charge-coupled device; FBP, filtered back projection; FDG, 2'-fluoro-2'-deoxyglucose; FHBG, 9-(4-fluoro-3-hydroxymethylbutyl) guanine; FLT, fluorothymidine; FMAU, fluoromethyluracil; HSV1-TK, herpes simplex virus type 1 thymidine kinase; MRI, magnetic resonance imaging; NIR, near infrared; NIS, sodium iodide symporter; PET, positron emission tomography; PRG, PET reporter genes; PRP, PET reporter probes; SPECT, single-photon emission computed tomography.

1   Introduction

Recent years have witnessed a revolution in the field of biological imaging, from a discipline that was focused on anatomy and physiology to one that is able to image the molecular basis of disease. The genome of higher organisms (human and mouse) has been sequenced and a large number of biological assays are now available for molecular biology researchers. Most of these assays have exquisite sensitivity and spatial resolution at the cellular level; however, they cannot be used to obtain the same information from cells deep within the intact whole animal. Longitudinal non-invasive imaging of animal models with molecular imaging probes can be used to characterize biological processes and interactions at the cellular level under physiological conditions, before, during and after intervention. This field has generally been termed "molecular imaging" and focuses on the visualization of molecular and cellular interactions in whole organisms [1]. This review focuses on the recent developments in molecular imaging and discusses the applications for drug development and testing. We highlight in this chapter the optical (bioluminescence), positron emission tomography (PET) and single-photon emission computed tomography (SPECT) approaches to molecular imaging. Other imaging modalities, such as fluorescence and magnetic resonance imaging (MRI) are discussed in Chapter 3 of this book.

The visualization of molecular targets in whole organisms is achieved using imaging modalities based on radionuclides, magnetic resonance, ultrasound, or the visible-near infrared (NIR) region of the electromagnetic spectrum [1]. Molecularly, signal for these different imaging modalities is generated either by introduction of exogenous probes targeted to endogenous molecules or through transgene expression. Examples of exogenous delivered probes consist of those that are trapped after transport (e.g., glucose analogs) or those binding to cell surface receptors (somatostatin, melanotropin, dopamine) [2–5]. Transgenes that have been used in molecular imaging include genes encoding non-mammalian enzymes that either trap (herpes simplex virus type 1 thymidine kinase, HSV1-tk) or internalize the probe (sodium iodide symporter, NIS) and optical reporter proteins (e.g., luciferases, fluorescent proteins) [6–10]. Because none of the imaging modalities combines high sensitivity, specificity, temporal and spatial resolution, the preferred imaging technique depends on the biological question one wants to answer.

Recently, multimodality molecular imaging has become of major interest because it allows combining the advantages of several imaging modalities. The combination of anatomical imaging using MRI/CT with functional imaging using PET/SPECT should facilitate the development of various imaging assays. One can achieve this goal by co-registration of both anatomical and functional images. Recently, combined small-animal SPECT/CT systems have become commercially available and the development of joint PET/MRI systems in the near future may allow more accurate interpretation and validation of new imaging assays [11–13].

Imaging techniques (PET, SPECT, MRI, CT, optical fluorescence/bioluminescence, ultrasound) and multimodality molecular probes are under intense investigation, and are constantly being optimized to assess molecular targets in living animals with higher precision and information density. Because many of these molecular imaging modalities have counterparts that are already being used in the clinics, one can use these systems for drug testing and validation, first in animal models of specific diseases and then eventually in patients. The use of mouse models simulating human diseases is of growing interest in the field of molecular imaging, and one promise of this effort is the eventual translation from animal work to the clinic [14, 15].

2 Positron emission tomography

2.1 General principles

The recent developments in molecular biology have led to a rapidly increasing knowledge of potential cellular/molecular targets. Taking advantage of the identification of these targets, molecular imaging probes can be developed to non-invasively image cellular/molecular events in small animals and humans with PET [15, 16]. These molecular probes are also referred to as reporter probes or tracers, and can be used to evaluate cell surface receptor density (e.g., dopamine type 2 (D2) receptor), measurement of cytoplasmic enzyme expressions (e.g., hexokinase, thymidine kinase), and monitoring of mRNA levels.

PET is routinely used in clinical settings, and is the modality of choice for studying neoplastic diseases in terms of staging, differentiating benign from malignant lesions, and evaluation of therapeutic response [15]. The role of PET in neurological and cardiovascular diseases is increasingly being recognized for the evaluation of brain tumors, Alzheimer's disease, and myocardial viability. PET is also being utilized for the evaluation of inflammatory diseases such as vasculitis and fever of unknown origin [17, 18].

During the last decade, smaller PET cameras have been developed and optimized to allow for monitoring of molecular events in small animals (e.g., mice). These small-animal PET scanners open the possibility for developing and testing new drugs in preclinical animal models before conducting clinical trials. Before the era of small-animal PET scanners, the opportunity to perform PET studies in preclinical small-animal models was limited. Now studies of drug biodistribution, efficacy as measured by a PET tracer, and many other applications are possible. The development of small-animal PET scanners therefore serves as a catalyst to further accelerate the role of PET in drug development.

Small-animal PET scanners have a resolution of ~2 mm^3, with the newest generation scanner attaining ~1 mm^3, compared to the most recent clinical PET scanners having a spatial resolution of 5–6 mm^3 [19, 20]. The sensitivity of both small-animal and clinical PET scanners is relatively high, on the order of 10^{-11} to 10^{-12} M, compared to other imaging modalities. The sensitivity of radionuclide imaging techniques is less affected by tissue depth in contrast to optical imaging techniques, where there is a loss of sensitivity as a function of depth and location (discussed below). Thus, PET imaging provides quantitative information on the detailed location and time-kinetics of molecular probe accumulation in small animals.

For molecular probes to be detectable with PET imaging, they need to be labeled with a positron-emitting radioisotope. A variety of natural biological molecules such as glucose, thymidine and peptides have been labeled with radioisotopes to study various biological processes. These radiolabeled probes can take on many names such as molecular beacons, reporter probes, or tracers [1]. The radioisotopes used with PET are positron emitters, in contrast to SPECT imaging in which the isotopes used are γ-emitters. The most commonly used positron emitter is ^{18}F, followed by ^{11}C, ^{13}N, ^{15}O, ^{64}Cu and ^{124}I, in no particular order. The generation of most isotopes takes place in a cyclotron, which accelerates charged particles for collision with a target to create isotopes having a relatively short half-life (e.g., ^{18}F has a half-life of 110 min) [21]. Because of the relatively short half-life of positron emitters, production of isotope-labeled molecules requires great efficiency and has to be in relative close vicinity of the animal research or clinical facility. In this regard, only centers having a cyclotron have the capabilities to perform imaging using isotopes with a short half-life such as ^{11}C and ^{13}N (half-life of 20 and 10 min, respectively).

Following synthesis of the radionuclide and labeling the molecule of interest with an isotope, systemic delivery of the radioactive probe then allows one to study the distribution of the probe. Following systemic delivery, the molecular probe distributes in most cases from the intravascular compartment to the extravascular compartment, and then in some cases to the intracellular compartment. The positron-emitting moiety of this molecular probe decays by emitting a positron from its nucleus. This positron annihilates with an electron of a neighboring atom and produces two 511-keV photons, which travel in almost exactly opposite directions (see Chapter 2, Fig. 12). These two γ-rays are then detected by a coincidence counting detection system [22]. The detection of one γ-ray results in the opening of an electronic time window during which detection of a γ-ray in another detector results in the counting of a coincident event. To be detectable, this coincidence event must have occurred along a straight line connecting the two detectors. Following acquisition, mathematical reconstruction algorithms of the coincident lines such as filtered back projection (FBP), ordered subset of expectation maximization (OSEM) or maximum a posteriori (MAP) give the location(s) of the isotope. Tomographic images can be obtained in the sagittal, coronal and transverse planes and quantitative information deduced from the images is related to the underlying biological process. However, several corrections for Compton scatter and tissue attenuation have to be made to achieve absolute quantitation. For a more detailed description of PET technology the reader is referred to Chapter 2 of this volume.

PET imaging is quantitative and, due to the short half-life of isotopes, repetitive imaging in the same living subject is feasible, which allows performing longitudinal studies [5, 23–25]. One should keep in mind that radiolabeled probes also have some limitations. Radiolabeled probes (for PET and SPECT imaging) produce signal constantly through the decay of the radioisotope and can not be turned "on and off". Therefore, a time-delay between injection of the radiolabeled probe and imaging allows the untrapped probe to clear. Most of the untrapped radiolabeled probes are cleared through the urinary and/or hepatobiliary tracts. This physiological excretion route of the probes makes them less suitable for imaging molecular processes in these organ systems. To image in or near routes of clearance the use of longer-lived isotopes (e.g., ^{124}I; $t_{1/2} = \sim 4$ days) can be useful because one can image long after clearance of the tracer has occurred.

2.2   PET imaging probes

Currently, several commonly used clinical PET tracers are also used for small-animal imaging, e.g., 2'-fluoro-2'-deoxyglucose (FDG), 3'-deoxy-3'-[^{18}F]fluoro-thymidine (FLT), and [^{13}N]ammonia. Recently, there are also different PET reporter probes (PRP) specifically developed to image PET reporter genes (PRG) [e.g., 9-(4-fluoro-3-hydroxymethylbutyl) guanine (FHBG)] for imaging the *HSV1-tk* gene product (HSV1-TK). These reporter genes can encode for an enzyme or a receptor and are designed to accumulate the molecular probe intracellularly or on the surface of cells expressing the reporter gene. The amount of injected probe for PET is very low, in the nanogram to microgram range, and does not have any measurable pharmacological effect [26].

   PET offers two great advantages for drug testing compared to other molecular imaging techniques. First, the low mass levels required for PET imaging makes the translation into humans easier, and second, the availability of positron-emitting atoms such as C, F, N, O allows labeling of drug candidates, resulting in a molecule that is close to or identical to the actual parent drug.

   PET opens the possibility of non-invasively monitoring the pharmacokinetics of potential drugs in living subjects. PET technology can address several important steps in drug development and testing, including biodistribution of the drug by radiolabeling the actual drug [27]. However, the power of PET as a tool for drug discovery goes beyond studying drug biodistribution, it provides a means to investigate the mechanism of drug action *in vivo*, and contributes to a better understanding of diseases. Discussed below are different PET tracers and PRG/PRP systems that have potential applications in drug development and evaluation.

2.2.1 PET probes for imaging endogenous proteins

Several radiotracers have been developed to provide information on cell metabolism. One prominent example of such a tracer is FDG, which has been the most widely used tracer in the field of PET. FDG is a deoxyglucose analogue which can be metabolically trapped following phosphorylation by the hexokinase enzyme [28]. Thus, the amount of FDG trapped in tissues reflects both the expression of glucose transporter and hexokinase enzyme. FDG normally accumulates in the brain, heart, skeletal muscle, and brown fat. FDG is cleared through the urinary tract because, unlike glucose, it is not reabsorbed in the distal renal tubules. This leads to a low background signal relative to target tissues, allowing for good imaging characteristics.

The most prevalent use of FDG consists of imaging glucose utilization in tumors, which is dependent on cell function and proliferation. As a result, drugs which alter tumor metabolism should also affect the amount of FDG trapped in the cells. Several studies have assessed the feasibility of non-invasive metabolic monitoring of chemotherapy using FDG [29–31]. It was also reported that quantitative FDG-PET scans of primary breast cancer showed a fast and significant decline in glucose metabolism after efficient treatment, even before a reduction in tumor size was detected. These findings were absent in non-responders and, therefore, FDG-PET has its value as an early metabolic marker for therapeutic efficacy [30]. Another recent application of FDG-PET to evaluate early response on chemotherapy is the use of Gleevec® for gastrointestinal stromal tumors (GIST) [32, 33]. Major changes in GIST tumor volume, evaluated by CT, tend to occur rather late after the start of therapy, which could impair therapeutic management in the case of non-responders. In contrast, FDG-PET is a sensitive method to evaluate early response and is helpful for prognostication and follow-up.

Besides metabolism, cell proliferation is another important marker providing information on the growth rate of cells. There are several PET-based cell proliferation markers available such as [11C]fluoromethyluracil (FMAU) and FLT [34–36]. FLT is a deoxy analogue of thymidine that is phosphorylated by

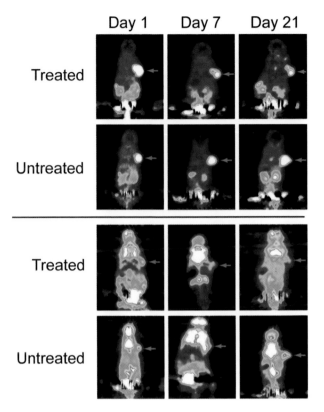

Figure 1.
Representative microPET images of mouse treated with daily administration of vehicle or protein kinase inhibitor-166 (PKI-166) for 3 weeks. Arrows indicate the location of the subcutaneous A431 (human epidermoid carcinoma) tumor. Treatment with PKI-166 lowered tumor [^{18}F]FLT uptake by 79% within 1 week. [^{18}F]FLT uptake (upper panel) significantly correlated with the tumor proliferation index. Tumor [^{18}F]FDG uptake (lower panel) generally paralleled the changes seen for [^{18}F]FLT. These results suggest that [^{18}F]FLT may be used to non-invasively monitor the anti-proliferative effects of PKI. Reproduced by permission of the Society of Nuclear Medicine from: Waldherr C, Mellinghoff I.K., Tran C, et al. Monitoring Antiproliferative Responses to Kinase Inhibitor Therapy in Mice with 3'-deoxy-3'-18F-Fluorothymidine PET. *J Nucl Med* 2005;46-114-120, Figure 1 B.) [39].

mammalian thymidine kinase. Because the fluorine is placed in the 3'-position on the sugar, [^{18}F]FLT can work as a terminator of the growing DNA chain. Only a small fraction of [^{18}F]FLT is actually accumulated in DNA; most of it is retained intracellularly after phosphorylation [35, 37, 38]. Thus, FLT is a marker for the evaluation of tumor growth, and can be used as a non-invasive tracer to evaluate the effect of an anti-proliferative drug [39, 40] (Fig. 1).

PET imaging has also enlarged our understanding of the function of the basal ganglia, and Parkinson's disease is the neurodegenerative disorder that has been best studied. ^{11}C-labeled raclopride is a widely used PET tracer for measurement of striatal D2 dopamine receptor binding characteristics and for quantification of thalamic D2 receptor binding. The accumulation of tracer in the thalamus and nigrostriatal system reflects the density of dopamine receptors [41]. ^{11}C-labeled raclopride has the ability to detect changes in synaptic dopamine levels based on the competition of dopamine with ^{11}C-labeled raclopride for D2/D3 receptor binding [42]. These changes can be induced by pharmacologic interventions, and the difference between baseline and post-therapy ^{11}C-labeled raclopride binding can then be used as a measure of dopamine release [43, 44].

PET ligands targeting endogenous receptors can be used in multiple ways during the drug discovery process. Pharmacokinetic evaluation includes parameters such as biodistribution, absorption, and metabolism as well as drug delivery issues. Receptor occupancy studies are a powerful tool for evaluating the mechanism of action and dose regimen. Furthermore, PET can be used to compare a new drug versus the gold standard therapy, and to evaluate different analogs before further development. With regards to clinical applications, the pharmacokinetic evaluation obtained with PET can be used to adjust dosage and further optimize trials.

Information of pharmacokinetic properties of a drug candidate in target tissues is important since inhomogenous distribution in the target tissue might limit therapeutic efficiency. Analysis of the distribution of a radiolabeled compound following various routes of administration is relatively straightforward, and provides highly useful information [45]. For example, it was shown that pulmonary deposition of FDG-labeled inhaled powder particles was predominantly present in the central lung regions in patients with chronic obstructive lung disease, compared to homogenous deposition in normal persons [46].

Another important pharmacokinetic parameter that can be monitored with PET is the plasma binding of a drug. Some drugs (e.g., L-703717) have a very poor penetration through the blood-brain barrier because of binding to plasma proteins. It was reported that inhibition of protein binding resulted in increased blood-brain barrier permeability, which was detected with PET [47]. Finally, radionuclide-labeled drugs could be used to demonstrate that a particular drug-delivery device is working as designed [48].

Site-specific occupancy studies are one way to determine dose regimens for a particular drug [49, 50]. The level of receptor occupancy is estimated by comparing the PET scans of the tracer alone and experiments done with the unlabeled drug compound. The study with tracer alone gives information about target regions (receptor expression) versus regions lacking receptors, resulting in a target/non-target ratio. The second scan is performed with the same tracer following administration of the unlabeled drug that has affinity for the receptor. In this condition, there is a competition between the unlabeled drug and the tracer for the binding sites, resulting in a lower target/non-target ratio. The decrease in this ratio reflects the fraction of binding sites occupied with the drug. The receptor occupancy data obtained in normal human volunteers can be used to determine the dosage for early clinical trials, thereby avoiding doses with a risk of major side-effects. Several drugs have been extensively investigated with PET in terms of receptor occupancy [51–53]. Thus, the quantitative relation between these receptor occupancy data *in vivo* and pharmacodynamic effects in patients can be used to optimize the dose regimen [54].

2.2.2 PET reporter genes/PET reporter probe systems

Reporter genes can be used as a powerful tool to validate molecular interactions (i.e., protein-protein interactions) and to provide insights into the underlying pathophysiology of diseases. Validation of molecular targets in living subjects is an important step in the drug development process. More recently, alternative therapeutic approaches, such as cell and gene therapy, for various disorders have been developed. These therapies can be significantly aided by the ability to determine the location and magnitude of transgene expression as well as monitoring cell survival. Current clinical methods (serum markers, histology, anatomical-based imaging, and physical exam) have difficulties answering fundamental questions such as: did the vector reach its target, was the gene expressed, or are the cells still viable? These questions should be addressed quite early after the start of therapy to change the management in case of non-responders. Molecular imaging has the ability to answer these questions using reporter gene technology in living subjects. Reporter genes can be coupled to a therapeutic gene to monitor the efficacy of gene delivery [55, 56] and track gene expression. Alternatively, cells can be transfected with these reporter genes to track the location of cells and cell survival [57]. Discussed below are several examples of transgenes that have been utilized for reporter gene imaging.

2.2.2.1 Herpes simplex virus type 1 thymidine kinase

The *HSV1-tk* gene is an example of a transgene that can be used both as a reporter gene and a therapeutic gene. When *HSV1-tk* is used as the therapeutic gene, it is referred to as a suicide gene [58]. Alternatively, *HSV1-tk* can also serve as a stand-alone reporter gene. The gene product (HSV1-TK protein) can be imaged with PET. There are two different subtypes of mammalian thymidine kinase: a cytosolic and a mitochondrial form that phosphorylate thymidine for its incorporation into DNA during cell replication [59]. The viral thymidine kinase (HSV1-TK) has a broad substrate specificity and is able to phosphorylate acycloguanosine, guanosine and thymidine derivatives that are trapped intracellularly after phosphorylation [60]. When delivered with a pro-drug such as acyclovir, ganciclovir or penciclovir, the *HSV1-tk* gene acts as a suicide gene since the incorporation of phosphorylated nucleoside analogs into DNA cause chain termination and also inhibition of both the viral and the cellular DNA polymerases.

Mutated forms of the *HSV1-tk* gene, such as the *HSV1-sr39tk* have been developed and have greater sensitivity as compared to the wild-type for acycloguanosine substrates [61]. The HSV1-sr39TK protein is more adept at phosphorylating ganciclovir, and has lower affinity for the endogenous competitor thymidine compared to HSV1-TK. There are two categories of reporter probes to image *HSV1-tk/HSV1-sr39tk* reporter gene expression. The first category consist of thymidine derivatives, such as 5-iodo-2'-fluoro-2'-deoxy-1-β-D-arabinofuranosyl-5-iodouracil (FIAU), and the second group is the acycloguanosine group, e.g., 9-(4-fluoro-3-hydroxymethylbutyl)guanine (FHBG), which is a derivative of penciclovir.

Recently, several other PET tracers, 2'-fluoro-2'-deoxyarabino-furanosyl-5-ethyluracil (FEAU) and 1-(2'-fluoro-2'-deoxy-D-arabinofuranosyl)-5-methyluracil (FMAU), have been developed for monitoring *HSV1-tk* expression. [^{3}H]FEAU was found to be the most selective *in vitro* in both *HSV1-tk*- and *HSV1-sr39tk*-expressing cells compared to FIAU and FMAU. It was also shown that accumulation was the highest and most selective for FEAU, which makes radiolabeled FEAU a promising candidate for monitoring the *HSV1-tk* expression in small animals [62]. The reader is also referred to a number of excellent articles that review the details of the synthesis and kinetics of these radiolabeled analogs [6, 63–67].

HSV1-sr39TK phosphorylates all of the above probes with [^{18}F]FHBG as the most efficient substrate for the mutant HSV1-sr39TK compared to the wild-type HSV1-TK (threefold improvement of trapping the reporter probe). Mammalian thymidine kinase, HSV1-TK and HSV1-sr39TK each show a different pattern of substrate specificity, which can be used for therapeutic and imaging strategies. Since the endogenous mammalian thymidine kinase has very low affinity for phosphorylating the probe, only cells expressing the reporter gene, *HSV1-tk* can phosphorylate a sufficient amount of the probe and can be detected.

HSV1-tk has been used as a PET reporter gene in many applications, and also recently as a suicide gene in a human adenoviral gene therapy trial [68]. *HSV1-tk* transgene expression was monitored with [^{18}F]FHBG-PET-CT in patients with hepatocellular carcinoma (HCC) after intratumoral injection using varying titers of a replication incompetent adenovirus in which *HSV1-tk* is driven by the CMV promoter. At 48 h after adenovirus administration, transgene expression was detected in the treated tumors, as evidenced by FHBG uptake. Serial studies during treatment with the pro-drug ganciclovir showed the ability for FHBG to monitor the location(s), and time variation of *HSV1-tk* gene expression. Further imaging studies should help to significantly help gene therapy optimization. Another clinical gene-therapy trial was performed using a liposomal vector to deliver *HSV1-tk* transgene intratumorally [69]. *HSV1-tk* transgene expression was monitored with [^{124}I]FIAU-PET. Ganciclovir treatment was done 4 days after vector delivery, and treatment response was evaluated with [^{124}I]FIAU, [^{18}F]FDG, [^{11}C]methionine and MRI for anatomical co-registration. Transgene expression was only observed in one out of five patients, the other four patients were found to have a low mitotic index in their tumors. Only the patient with detectable transgene expression on PET showed a therapeutic response, as evidenced by signs of necrosis on FDG and [^{11}C]methionine-PET in the region of FIAU uptake before treatment. Thus, non-invasive monitoring of transgene expression over time is very important and will further help to optimize gene therapy protocols and safe vector applications.

2.2.2.2 Dopamine type-2 receptor

The dopamine type 2 receptor reporter (*D2R*) gene is an example of a receptor-based reporter gene [5]. D2R is an endogenous, cell-surface receptor predominantly expressed in the striatum and the pituitary glands. Activation of D2R causes G-protein-coupled reduction of cAMP because of inhibition of adenylate cyclase. Dopamine binding to the D2R can thus modulate cyclic AMP levels, potentially compromising the usefulness of the *D2R* as a reporter gene *in vivo*. To overcome potential deleterious effects due to ectopic D2R activation by circulating endogenous ligands, a mutant *D2R* reporter gene (*D2R80A*) has been generated [24]. The D2R80A has the same affinity for its substrate compared to the wild type and it eliminates potential reduced efficacy due to modulation of cAMP. The D2R/[^{18}F]FESP {3-(2'-[^{18}F]-fluoroethyl)spiperone} imaging assay has been developed and extensively investigated. [^{18}F]FESP, a radiolabeled D2R antagonist (spiperone) serves as the receptor ligand and accumulates intracellularly and on the cell surface of D2R-expressing tissues [5].

This D2R/[^{18}F]FESP reporter gene system has several advantages compared to *HSV1-tk* reporter gene. D2R is an endogenous protein and, therefore, it is not immunogenic. The fact that [^{18}F]FESP has the ability to cross the blood-brain barrier and cell membranes makes it more appropriate for imaging the central nervous system (for sites other than the striatum) compared to [^{18}F]FHBG, which is not as efficient in crossing the blood-brain barrier. In contrast to [^{18}F]FHBG, which has to cross the cell membrane to interact with the target enzyme and is subjected to transport kinetics, [^{18}F]FESP can easier reach its target, which is the cell surface and intracellular receptor. It is worth mentioning that the sensitivity of both D2R/[^{18}F]FESP and HSV1-sr39TK/[^{18}F]FHBG are nearly equivalent. It is possible that newer substrates for HSV1-sr39TK (e.g., FEAU) may lead to greater sensitivity for the *HSV1-sr39tk* reporter gene as compared to the *D2R* reporter gene.

2.2.2.3 Sodium-iodide symporter

The human sodium-iodide symporter (NIS) is a membrane protein, predominantly expressed in the thyroid, stomach and salivary glands, which translocates and concentrates iodide within the thyroid [70, 71]. Radioisotope uptake through the NIS has been routinely used in the diagnosis and therapy of thyroid diseases [58, 71–76]. Recent cloning of the symporter gene has permitted the investigation of its role as both a reporter gene for PET and SPECT imaging and a therapeutic gene [77–79].

The use of NIS as a reporter and therapeutic gene offers several advantages. The reporter probe is relatively simple to produce and commercially available, and there is no need for specialized radiochemistry compared to *HSV1-tk* system. Since NIS is a human gene, there is no immune response to the protein and the toxicity and biodistribution for several isotopes has been well validated in clinical use. The NIS transgene can either be imaged with PET (^{124}I) or SPECT (^{123}I) for diagnostic purpose or ^{131}I for therapeutic purposes [9, 10, 80]. The main limitation of the NIS reporter gene system is that radioiodine is not only localized in the target cells, but also in normal tissues that express physiological levels of endogenous NIS such as the thyroid, salivary glands, breast, and stomach.

3   Single photon emission computed tomography

3.1   General principles

SPECT imaging with a γ-camera is very similar to PET imaging, but the radioisotope emits a single γ-ray instead of a positron. SPECT has become the imaging modality of choice for studying skeletal diseases, such as degenerative osteo-articular disorders, and detection of bone metastasis. The role of SPECT in evaluating cardiovascular and neurological disorders has been well established and is used to investigate myocardial and brain perfusion as well as measuring cardiac ejection fraction. SPECT also plays a major role in several neoplastic diseases, such as thyroid cancer and neuro-endocrine tumors. SPECT can be used to evaluate a broad range of diseases, making the development of different probes for molecular imaging a very interesting project.

Recently, small-animal SPECT scanners have been developed that provide the same information as clinical scanners, and which allow the translation from bench to bedside. The development of SPECT-CT imaging systems exploits the advantages of both systems, and gives both anatomical and functional information. Small-animal SPECT systems have a resolution about 1 mm^3 compared to 2 mm^3 for small-animal PET. Besides better resolution, SPECT can be used to image two radioisotopes with different energies simultaneously, allowing two probes to be distinguished within the same study.

This is not possible with PET systems because all positron emitters lead to 511-keV γ-rays. Although γ-camera imaging ("planar imaging") is much more accessible and affordable than PET imaging, the diminished sensitivity due to the loss of many decay events is one major disadvantage. Another limitation of planar imaging is the overlap of different foci/organs, resulting in poor spatial resolution. The latter can be overcome using SPECT, which acquires volumetric data by rotating the γ-camera around the subject and using a multi-detector system [81]. The loss of sensitivity can be partially compensated by injecting more radiolabeled probe to increase signal-to-noise.

Similar to PET, a variety of molecules can be labeled with a radioisotope that emits a photon with characteristic energies, such as ^{99m}Tc (140 keV), ^{111}In (171 and 245 keV) and ^{125}I (27–35 keV). The half-life of these isotopes is much longer compared to most PET radioisotopes (from several hours to days for SPECT tracers compared to minutes for PET), which makes it more accessible than PET and does not require a cyclotron facility. After systemic delivery, imaging is performed with a γ-camera, a scintillation detector (sodium iodide crystal) and several photomultiplier tubes (see Chapter 2, Figs 7 and 8). During decay, the probes emit a γ-ray at their specific energy, some of which scatter, lose energy or never reach the camera. Scattered γ-rays are absorbed by the collimator, while photons that come in parallel with the collimator are detected and converted into photons of light by the crystal. These photons are then converted into an electrical signal that is proportional to the energy of the γ-ray; γ-rays of lower energy are likely to result from scattering and therefore have lost their geometrical information. The result is a two-dimensional image from a three-dimensional subject ("planar imaging"), which has some disadvantages as mentioned above. Thus, SPECT imaging has the advantage of quantitative and repetitive imaging in the same living subject. SPECT has a better resolution than PET, but the sensitivity is an order of magnitude lower. Similar to PET, the excretion of the probe through the hepatobiliary or urinary tract makes SPECT imaging less suitable for evaluating cellular/molecular events in these organ systems [5, 23–25].

3.2 SPECT imaging probes

The most commonly used SPECT isotopes are metals such as ^{99m}Tc or ^{111}In. Labeling analogues of drug candidates with these isotopes requires the presence of a chelating moiety. These chelates in small molecules often alter the physical properties of the drug candidate, and it also limits the use for determining the specific binding of the drug at its target. Despite these restraints, ^{99m}Tc-TRODAT is a radiolabeled molecule suited for imaging the dopamine transporter status [82]. Labeling molecules with iodine (^{123}I) also alters the specific characteristics of a drug analogue, but several radiotracers based on iodine are available and clinically used (e.g., ^{123}I-beta-CIT to image the dopamine transporter status) [83]. In analogy with PET, these SPECT tracers can also be used to evaluate pharmacokinetic measurements such as biodistribution of a drug candidate.

Currently, there is evidence that most chemotherapeutic agents cause tumor cell death by induction of apoptosis, and that resistance to anticancer treatment involves suppression of several mechanisms controlling apoptosis [84]. This theory has increased the importance of being able to predict whether cancer cells could undergo apoptosis in response to chemotherapeutic treatment. The development of a non-invasive technique to detect treatment-induced apoptosis could provide important information on early therapeutic response. Annexin V is a protein that has a high binding affinity for phosphatidylserine (PS), which externalizes during early apoptosis. To detect apoptosis *in vivo*, a radiolabeled annexin V with ^{99m}Tc has been developed for SPECT imaging [85, 86]. ^{99m}Tc-annexin V has been used to assess the effectiveness of chemotherapy in rodents with hepatoma [87]. This would allow one to screen different anticancer drugs before clinical trials.

A first phase I clinical trial conducted with ^{99m}Tc recombinant human annexin V showed the safety and the feasibility of annexin V to study treatment-induced apoptosis [88, 89]. It was reported that a significant post-treatment increase in annexin V uptake above pretreatment levels predict at least a partial response to chemotherapy. However, the timing of annexin V imaging after initial therapy is of major importance. A recent small-animal study shows there is a biphasic response after treatment with a first peak of ^{99m}Tc-annexin V uptake within 1–5 h after treatment, followed by a second peak at 9–24 h post treatment, corresponding with the actual cell loss [90]. Thus, non-invasive monitoring of cell death *in vivo* has the potential to evaluate the success of treatment on an individual basis, supporting clinical decision making, and could further facilitate screening of different drugs before clinical testing.

Neuroreceptor imaging is also a promising area of brain imaging used to investigate various neurodegenerative and neuropsychiatric disorders. In the research setting, radiopharmaceuticals targeted to specific areas of the brain are used along with SPECT to assess and analyze functional mechanisms within brain structures. The information obtained from these studies may aid in the development of drug therapies to relieve symptoms [91].

4   Optical imaging

There are essentially two different types of optical-based molecular imaging techniques: fluorescence imaging that uses fluorophores such as green fluorescent protein (GFP), wavelength-shifted GFP mutants (eGFP), red fluorescent protein (DSRED), red-shifted mutants (monomeric RFP, mRFP), fluorescent dyes (e.g., Cy5.5), "smart" NIR fluorescent (NIRF) probes and secondly bioluminescence imaging (BLI), which utilizes systems such as firefly luciferase (FL)/D-luciferin or *Renilla* luciferase (RL)/coelenterazine [92, 93]. Imaging modalities based on optics are rapid, sensitive and easily accessible techniques for *in vivo* molecular imaging with relatively low instrumentation costs. Therefore, these modalities may be a useful tool for drug development and testing. This chapter focuses on BLI, since fluorescence imaging has been extensively dealt with in Chapter 3.

4.1   Bioluminescence imaging technologies

BLI is based on the interaction between the luciferase enzyme and its substrate generating visible light via a chemiluminescent reaction. The generated light can then be detected externally as an indicator of a biological/molecular process. Thus, light is generated after an injectable substrate is delivered to the subject and specific conditions are met depending on the system that has been used (discussed below). The emitted light can be detected with a cooled charge-coupled device (CCD) camera, since its wavelength lies within the range of the visible spectrum (400–750 nm). Recent advances in the development of these cameras have significantly increased their sensitivity since optical methods for *in vivo* imaging have to deal with the limited transmission of light through deep tissues. These cameras are very sensitive to low

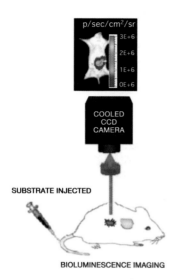

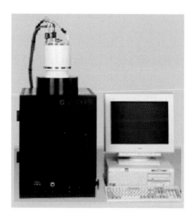

Figure 2.
Basic principles of optical CCD imaging: bioluminescence. BLI utilizes systems such as firefly luciferase/D-luciferin or Renilla luciferase/coelenterazine. Bioluminescent systems generate light *de novo* when the appropriate substrates/co-factors are made available. In that case, light emitted from either system can be detected with a thermoelectrically cooled CCD camera since they emit light in the visible light range (400–700 nm) to NIR range (~800 nm). Cooled to –120° to –150°C, these cameras can detect weakly luminescent sources within a light-tight chamber. Being exquisitely sensitive to light, these desktop camera systems allow for quantitative analysis of the data (shown on the right). The method of imaging bioluminescent sources in living subjects with a CCD camera is relatively straightforward: the animal is anesthetized, subsequently injected with the substrate and immediately placed in the light-tight chamber. A light photographic image of the animal is obtained which is followed by a bioluminescence image captured by the cooled CCD camera positioned above the subject within the confines of the dark chamber. The two images are subsequently superimposed on one another by a computer, and relative location of luciferase activity is inferred from the composite image.

light levels and allow for quantitative analysis. BLI in living subjects with these desktop cameras is easy and fast: following the injection of substrate intraperitoneally (D-luciferin) or intravenously (coelenterazine), the anesthetized animal is then placed in a light-tight chamber for several seconds to minutes (Fig. 2). Subsequently, a standard photographic image is acquired followed by a bioluminescence image that is detected by the CCD camera. The software superimposes both acquired images so that the location of the bioluminescent signal with regard to the overall anatomy can be deduced from the superimposed image. This signal can be quantified as absolute photons per second per cm^2 per steradian (a measure of solid angle). Thus, the whole procedure to perform BLI is very straightforward and allows for high through-put.

Recently, significant progress has been made in spectral imaging of different wavelengths. Multi-spectral imaging has predominantly been applied to fluorescence imaging since it can be used to remove autofluorescence. In addition to autofluorescence removal, spectral imaging opens the possibility of imaging multiple fluorescence-labeled molecules or cells at the same time (multiplexing) [94, 95]. This technique can likely be extended to BLI, allowing for simultaneously imaging bioluminescent reporter proteins with different emission spectra (e.g., FL and RL) instead of sequentially imaging (discussed below).

There are important differences between optical-based imaging technologies and other small-animal imaging modalities such as PET, SPECT and MRI. BLI systems are at least one order of magnitude more sensitive compared to PET and SPECT at limited depths [8]. Another advantage of BLI modalities consist of being very rapid and straightforward, and being very accessible for *in vivo* analysis with relatively low instrumentation costs. In contrast to radionuclide-based and MRI-based imaging modalities, there is significantly less spatial resolution obtained with BLI. The spatial resolution is approximately equal to the depth of the signal. Since the emission of light is limited by the tissue depth from which the signal has been generated, the sensitivity decreases with increasing depth.

Light transmission in living subjects is limited due to both tissue scatter and absorbance [96]. Scattering occurs at the cell membrane, whereas absorbance mainly depends on the presence of tissue hemoglobin or melanin [96]. The absorption due to hemoglobin occurs predominantly in the green-blue spectrum (400–600 nm), but less in the red region, and that is one of the reasons to develop more red-shifted fluorophores [97]. Both tissue absorption and scatter are less in nude or white mice because of the lower amount of melanin. Light absorption by water molecules is also a limiting factor but only at longer wavelength (> 900 nm). However, sufficient amounts of emitted light can be detected by the camera even though only a small fraction of the light escapes tissue absorption and scattering. The development of red-shifted mutants together with recent advances in optics and sensor technologies provides good quality optical images [96, 98, 99]. Another limitation of BLI is the oxygen requirement of the luciferases because these are oxygenases. This oxygen requirement can limit the use of luciferases in anaerobic environments but in most cases the oxygen requirement to produce significant amounts of light is far below the oxygen levels found in cells of living subjects.

4.2 Reporter probes for BLI

The most commonly used bioluminescence reporter genes are firefly (*Fluc*) and Renilla (*Rluc*) luciferases. *Fluc* encodes for the monomeric protein FL derived from *Photinus pyralis*, the North-American firefly [99]. Light emission is achieved by catalyzing D-luciferin into oxyluciferin in the presence of oxygen, ATP and Mg^{2+} as cofactor, resulting in a peak emission wavelength at 562 nm. To make *Fluc* more suitable for imaging mammalian tissues, several modifications to the gene have been made. The first one consists of the removal of a peroxisomal targeting site, resulting in increased expression and cytosolic localization, and the second modification consists of changing the amino acid sequence so the peak emission is shifted toward the red region of the visible spectrum above 600 nm, making it more suitable for *in vivo* imaging [8].

The *Rluc* gene is another bioluminescent system encoding for a monomeric protein RL, which has been tested in small animals [93]. In contrast to FL, RL does not require ATP and Mg^{2+} to oxidize the substrate (coelenterazine) and the peak emission occurs at 480 nm.

Both substrates, D-luciferin and coelenterazine, are very specific for FL and RL, respectively, and there is no cross-reaction between the substrates and the luciferase enzymes. Because there is no cross-reaction and since the enzyme kinetics of RL are much faster as compared to FL, both reporter genes can be used simultaneously. Imaging both reporter genes can be performed sequentially, the first images are acquired after injection of coelenterazine followed by injection of D-luciferin and a second image acquisition [92]. It is important to note that some of the substrates such as coelenterazine may also be pumped out of cells by P-glycoprotein and this needs to be taken into account in specific applications (e.g., tumor studies).

To make these reporter genes more suitable for *in vivo* imaging, modifications to these genes are under intense investigation. Because FL is relatively thermolabile at *in vivo* temperatures, with half-lives around 1 h *in vivo*, mutants have been created with higher thermostability and longer half-lives (two- to fivefold compared to wild type) [100]. It was shown that thermosta-bilization achieved by the specific mutations led to a higher accumulation of enzyme *in vivo*. In consequence, fewer cells can be detected accurately (up to 100 cells compared to 1000 cells with the wild type), resulting in increased sensitivity [100–102].

More recently, a synthetic Renilla luciferase reporter gene (*hRluc*), that has been codon optimized, has been utilized; this has a higher sensitivity than the native *Rluc* [103]. It was shown that hRL can yield a higher signal when compared to native RL, both in cell culture studies and in living mice. Muta-tions of *Rluc* are also under active investigation to make this reporter pro-tein more suitable for small-animal imaging since by having the excitation and emission wavelength more red-shifted, it would allow for better pene-tration and less tissue scatter. Recently, several *Rluc* mutants have been screened and the best were combined in a single protein (RL8) [104, 105]. Compared to the native RL, RL8 has a much longer serum stability half-life (105 h versus 0.7 h), a small red-shift of 5 nm, and a fivefold higher light output. The higher serum stability together with the increased light output of RL8 is a major improvement to image bioluminescence-labeled ligands in living subjects; e.g., if a probe is used in which a targeting sequence is fused to a mutant RL protein [106]. These developments should further facilitate the use of these reporter genes for small-animal imaging and enlarge the applications of BLI.

Monitoring total number of viable cells is the most common application for bioluminescence reporter genes. Viable cell number correlates linearly with optical signal intensity, assuming all other parameters including the location of the bioluminescent source to be identical, and therefore changes in viable cell number could be inferred from optical signal intensity. This method can be used to evaluate the efficacy of different drugs (e.g., anti-tumor therapy). The evaluation and testing of anti-tumor therapies, espe-cially against minimal disease or micrometastasis, requires highly sensitive imaging systems to assess efficacy. The advantage of using molecular imag-ing techniques to evaluate the therapeutic effect of a drug is that this method provides a measure of only viable cells. Conventional methods rely on tumor size, which does not reflect viable cells only since there could be necrotic and inflammatory regions. Edinger et al. [107] labeled cervical cancer cells with a luciferase reporter gene and monitored their proliferation in irradiated ani-mals, indicating that chemotherapy or immunotherapy for labeled cells could be followed sensitively in small animals using BLI. The *Fluc* reporter gene was also used to screen different potential anti-tumor agents in living subjects [108–110]. This allows a very sensitive and quantitative screening of different drugs in a high-throughput manner, and could facilitate a rapid and efficient optimization of treatment regimens.

Another important application of optical BLI is to non-invasively monitor cell trafficking. Imaging can be used to follow different aspects of trafficking, including cell transplantation, metastasis and host response to infection. Optical imaging has been used to detect metastasis in a prostate cancer model [111]. Following systemic administration of a prostate-specific adenovirus vector carrying *Fluc*, metastasis could be detected in the lung and spine. Homing of T cells using BLI was shown in a lymphoma model [112]. Using this approach, an immune-based strategy based on the tumoricidal activity of T cells could be monitored. Such applications enable a better understanding of the disease process and the response of neoplastic and immune cells to therapeutics.

DNA-based therapies for genetic diseases and cancer are under intense investigation, and the effective development of these novel therapeutic strategies is very dependent on high-throughput testing in animal models. Therefore, BLI is well suited for the analysis and evaluation of these novel therapeutics because it is a rapid and accessible imaging modality. Several examples of how BLI can contribute to and accelerate the evaluation of DNA-based therapies have been reported, and have proven the value of BLI [113–115]. Another example using BLI for DNA-based therapy is the use of a bispecific antibody to target adenoviral infection specifically to angiotensin-converting enzyme (ACE), which is preferentially expressed on pulmonary capillary endothelium and which may thus enable gene therapy for pulmonary vascular disease [116]. Optical reporter genes can be used to non-invasively monitor both gene delivery and efficacy. TRAIL (tumor necrosis factor-related apoptosis induced ligand)-induced apoptosis could be monitored in a glioma tumor model [56]. The efficacy of the delivered gene was inferred from the drop in optical signal since the optical signal intensity correlates with the number of viable cells.

There is currently a great interest in developing pharmaceuticals that can specifically alter dysfunctional protein-protein interactions in cancer cells [117]. The study of small-molecule-mediated interactions is important for understanding the pathophysiology of cancer, and could play a major role

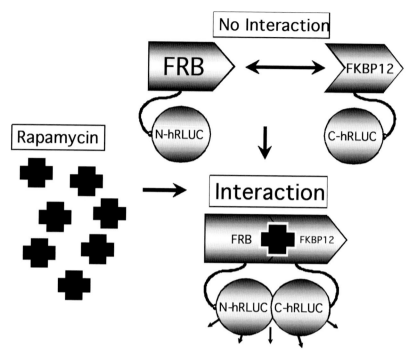

Figure 3.
Schematic of a drug-mediated synthetic Renilla luciferase (hRLUC) protein fragment-assisted complementation strategy. In this strategy, N-terminal and C-terminal portions of hRLUC fragments are attached to proteins X and Y, respectively, through a short peptide linker GGGGSGGGGS. The N and C portions of hRLUC fragments are closely approximated by the dimerization of proteins FRB and FKBP12 only in the presence of the small molecule rapamycin, and this, in turn, leads to recovered activity of the hRLUC protein. The recovered activity of the hRLUC protein can then be detected with a cooled CCD camera after injection of coelenterazine i.v. This system can then be used to screen and test different drugs that inhibit the interaction of both proteins X and Y, resulting in a loss of signal since there is no recovery of the functional hRluc. This mechanism has been illustrated by simultaneous administration of rapamycin (agonist) and ascomycin (antagonist) of the interaction of both proteins FRB and FKB12. Reproduced with permission from [118].

in drug development and validation. Molecular imaging of drug-modulated protein-protein interactions can be the first step towards drug testing. The heterodimerization of the human proteins FRB and FKB12 mediated by rapamycin based on protein fragment-assisted complementation of split RL has been studied (Figs 3 and 4). It was reported that this system could be easily titrated by changing the concentration of the different interacting molecules in living subjects, which is essential for drug screening and testing [118].

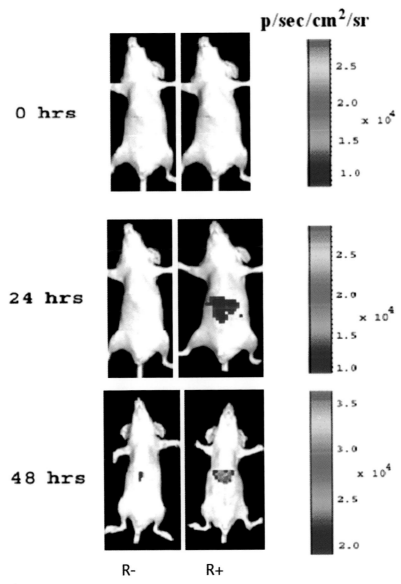

$$p/sec/cm^2/sr$$

Figure 4.
Optical charged coupled device imaging of living mice carrying i.v. injected 293T cells transiently cotransfected with Nhrluc-FRB and FKBP12-Chrluc. The animals not receiving rapamycin showed only a mean background signal of 4×10^3 p/s/cm^2/sr at all of the time points studied. The animals receiving repeated injections of rapamycin emitted signals, originating from the region of the liver, that were threefold (mean, 1.6×10^4 p/s/cm^2/sr) and fivefold (mean, 3.0×10^4 p/s/cm^2/sr) higher than background (P < 0.05) at 24 h and 48 h after the injection of rapamycin, respectively. (R-, animals not receiving rapamycin; R+, animals receiving rapamycin). Reproduced with permission from [118].

The development of this technique allows the ability to screen a variety of molecules (agonists as well as antagonists) that play a role in protein-protein interaction in a living animal model of cancer. This split imaging reporter complementation system can further be extrapolated to every other protein-protein interaction, and therefore the screening of dimerizer drugs for protein interactions is possible. This system will give more insights into the signaling pathways involved in cancer and allow testing of new drugs designed to modulate those pathways.

Another approach is based on studying homodimeric protein-protein interactions that are of critical importance to most cellular functions in living subjects. It was reported that an *in vivo* protein fragment-assisted complementation assay based on split RL reporter gene can be used to study homodimerization of HSV1-TK in living subjects. The high sensitivity of this assay for detection and quantifying homodimerization of proteins should make it a valuable tool for developing novel drugs based on the inhibition of active protein interactions [119].

5 Outlook

The field of molecular imaging has made significant progress in developing assays for imaging molecular events in living subjects, which can be applied both in preclinical models and clinical trials. Both optical and PET/SPECT imaging can be useful for preclinical models, and PET in particular can be very useful in clinical trials with new therapeutics. The development of multimodality reporters and generalizable reporters/probes will enable researchers to significantly speed up and simplify the process from *in vitro* to *in vivo* evaluation, and allow the study of more complex biological processes. Several challenges remain to make the routine use of imaging into the drug optimization and evaluation process. These include:

(1) Incorporating molecular imaging earlier into the drug development process. As lead candidates are identified, imaging should start to be utilized in the preclinical setting so that appropriate imaging probes (including labeled drug itself) can be utilized in a clinical trial.

(2) Assessment of what is important to imaging drug efficacy should be evaluated early in the process. Is a more upstream measure, such as drug interacting directly with the target, important or is a more downstream mea-

sure, such as apoptosis, more important to understanding therapeutic efficacy?

(3) The testing of pharmacokinetics of the radiolabeled drug in man earlier in the development process needs to be routinely done so that certain candidates can be excluded early in the testing process if needed.

(4) Education is critical, and teams in both the preclinical and clinical divisions of a pharmaceutical group need a better understanding of all the different roles imaging can play.

(5) Because the strategies described in this chapter require injection of substrates into living subjects, even though often at very low doses, regulatory concerns (e.g., filing of an investigational new drug for the molecular imaging agent) need to be tackled early on so that administration to patients does not become a limiting factor. Although still a long way from being routinely utilized, it is likely that molecular imaging including optical and radionuclide technologies will play increasing roles in drug development in the years to come.

References

1   Massoud TF, Gambhir SS (2003) Molecular imaging in living subjects: seeing fundamental biological processes in a new light. *Genes Dev* 17: 545–580

2   Chen J, Cheng Z, Miao Y, Jurisson SS, Quinn TP (2002) Alpha-melanocyte-stimulating hormone peptide analogs labeled with technetium-99m and indium-111 for malignant melanoma targeting. *Cancer* 94: 1196–1201

3   Chaudhuri TR, Rogers BE, Buchsbaum DJ, Mountz JM, Zinn KR (2001) A noninvasive reporter system to image adenoviral-mediated gene transfer to ovarian cancer xenografts. *Gynecol Oncol* 83: 432–438

4   Barrio JR, Huang SC, Phelps ME (1997) Biological imaging and the molecular basis of dopaminergic diseases. *Biochem Pharmacol* 54: 341–348

5   MacLaren DC, Gambhir SS, Satyamurthy N, Barrio JR, Sharfstein S, Toyokuni T, Wu L, Berk AJ, Cherry SR, Phelps ME et al (1999) Repetitive, non-invasive imaging of the dopamine D2 receptor as a reporter gene in living animals. *Gene Ther* 6: 785–791

6   Iyer M, Barrio JR, Namavari M, Bauer E, Satyamurthy N, Nguyen K, Toyokuni T, Phelps ME, Herschman HR, Gambhir SS (2001) 8-[18F]Fluoropenciclovir: an improved reporter probe for imaging HSV1-tk reporter gene expression *in vivo* using PET. *J Nucl Med* 42: 96–105

7   Tjuvajev JG, Doubrovin M, Akhurst T, Cai S, Balatoni J, Alauddin MM, Finn R, Bornmann W, Thaler H, Conti PS et al (2002) Comparison of radiolabeled nucleoside probes (FIAU, FHBG, and FHPG) for PET imaging of HSV1-tk gene expression. *J Nucl Med* 43: 1072–1083

8   Contag CH, Bachmann MH (2002) Advances in *in vivo* bioluminescence imaging of gene expression. *Annu Rev Biomed Eng* 4: 235–260

9   Groot-Wassink T, Aboagye EO, Glaser M, Lemoine NR, Vassaux G (2002) Adenovirus biodistribution and noninvasive imaging of gene expression *in vivo* by positron emission tomography using human sodium/iodide symporter as reporter gene. *Hum Gene Ther* 13: 1723–1735

10   Groot-Wassink T, Aboagye EO, Wang Y, Lemoine NR, Reader AJ, Vassaux G (2004) Quantitative imaging of Na/I symporter transgene expression using positron emission tomography in the living animal. *Mol Ther* 9: 436–442

11   Shao Y, Cherry SR, Farahani K, Meadors K, Siegel S, Silverman RW, Marsden PK (1997) Simultaneous PET and MR imaging. *Phys Med Biol* 42: 1965–1970

12   Kastis GK, Barber HB, Barrett HH, Gifford HC, Pang IW, Patton DD, Sain JD, Stevenson G, Wilson DW (1998) High resolution SPECT imager for three-dimensional imaging of small animals. *Journal of Nuclear Medicine* 39: 9P

13   Sharma V, Luker GD, Piwnica-Worms D (2002) Molecular imaging of gene expression and protein function *in vivo* with PET and SPECT. *J Magn Reson Imaging* 16: 336–351

14   Weissleder R, Mahmood U (2001) Molecular imaging. *Radiology* 219:316-33.

15   Gambhir SS (2002) Molecular imaging of cancer with positron emission tomography. *Nat Rev Cancer* 2: 683–693

16   Cherry SR, Gambhir SS (2001) Use of positron emission tomography in animal research. *Ilar J* 42: 219–232

17   Blockmans D (2003) The use of (18F)fluoro-deoxyglucose positron emission tomography in the assessment of large vessel vasculitis. *Clin Exp Rheumatol* 21: S15–S22

18   Meller J, Becker W (2001) [Nuclear medicine diagnosis of patients with fever of unknown origin (FUO)]. *Nuklearmedizin* 40: 59–70

19   Chatziioannou A, Tai YC, Doshi N, Cherry SR (2001) Detector development for microPET II: a 1 microl resolution PET scanner for small animal imaging. *Phys Med Biol* 46: 2899–2910

20   Chatziioannou AF (2002) Molecular imaging of small animals with dedicated PET tomographs. *Eur J Nucl Med Mol Imaging* 29: 98–114

21   Strijckmans K (2001) The isochronous cyclotron: principles and recent developments. *Comput Med Imaging Graph* 25: 69–78

22   Phelps ME, Hoffman EJ, Mullani NA, Ter-Pogossian MM (1975) Application of annihilation coincidence detection to transaxial reconstruction tomography. *Journal of Nuclear Medicine* 16: 210–224

23   Yu Y, Annala AJ, Barrio JR, Toyokuni T, Satyamurthy N, Namavari M, Cherry SR, Phelps ME, Herschman HR, Gambhir SS (2000) Quantification of target gene expression by imaging reporter gene expression in living animals. *Nat Med* 6: 933–937

24   Liang Q, Satyamurthy N, Barrio JR, Toyokuni T, Phelps MP, Gambhir SS, Herschman HR (2001) Noninvasive, quantitative imaging in living animals of a mutant dopamine D2 receptor reporter gene in which ligand binding is uncoupled from signal transduction. *Gene Ther* 8: 1490–1498

25   Herschman HR, MacLaren DC, Iyer M, Namavari M, Bobinski K, Green LA, Wu L, Berk AJ, Toyokuni T, Barrio JR et al (2000) Seeing is believing: non-invasive, quantitative and repetitive imaging of reporter gene expression in living animals, using positron emission tomography. *J Neurosci Res* 59: 699–705

26   Gambhir SS, Herschman HR, Cherry SR, Barrio JR, Satyamurthy N, Toyokuni T, Phelps ME, Larson SM, Balatoni J, Finn R et al (2000) Imaging transgene expression with radionuclide imaging technologies. *Neoplasia* 2: 118–138

27   Foster KA, Roberts MS (2000) Experimental methods for studying drug uptake in the head and brain. *Curr Drug Metab* 1: 333–356

28   Pauwels EK, Ribeiro MJ, Stoot JH, McCready VR, Bourguignon M, Maziere B (1998) FDG accumulation and tumor biology. *Nucl Med Biol* 25: 317–322

29   Romer W, Hanauske AR, Ziegler S, Thodtmann R, Weber W, Fuchs C, Enne W, Herz M, Nerl C, Garbrecht M et al (1998) Positron emission tomography in non-Hodgkin's lymphoma: assessment of chemotherapy with fluorodeoxyglucose. *Blood* 91: 4464–4471

30   Wahl RL, Zasadny K, Helvie M, Hutchins GD, Weber B, Cody R (1993) Metabolic monitoring of breast cancer chemohormonotherapy using positron emission tomography: initial evaluation. *J Clin Oncol* 11: 2101–2111

31   Findlay M, Young H, Cunningham D, Iveson A, Cronin B, Hickish T, Pratt B, Husband J, Flower M, Ott R (1996) Noninvasive monitoring of tumor metabolism using fluorodeoxyglucose and positron emission tomography in colorectal cancer liver metastases: correlation with tumor response to fluorouracil. *J Clin Oncol* 14: 700–708

32   Stroobants S, Goeminne J, Seegers M, Dimitrijevic S, Dupont P, Nuyts J, Martens M, van den Borne B, Cole P, Sciot R et al (2003) 18FDG-Positron emission tomography for the early prediction of response in advanced soft tissue sarcoma treated with imatinib mesylate (Glivec). *Eur J Cancer* 39: 2012–2020

33   Jager PL, Gietema JA, van der Graaf WT (2004) Imatinib mesylate for the treatment of gastrointestinal stromal tumours: best monitored with FDG PET. *Nucl Med Commun* 25: 433–438

34   Conti PS, Alauddin MM, Fissekis JR, Schmall B, Watanabe KA (1995) Synthesis of 2'-fluoro-5-[11C]-methyl-1-beta-D-arabinofuranosyluracil ([11C]-FMAU): a potential nucleoside analog for *in vivo* study of cellular proliferation with PET. *Nucl Med Biol* 22: 783–789

35   Shields AF (2003) PET imaging with 18F-FLT and thymidine analogs: promise and pitfalls. J Nucl Med 44: 1432–1434

36   Mankoff DA, Shields AF, Krohn KA (2005) PET imaging of cellular proliferation. Radiol Clin North Am 43: 153–167

37   Shields AF, Grierson JR, Dohmen BM, Machulla HJ, Stayanoff JC, Lawhorn-Crews JM, Obradovich JE, Muzik O, Mangner TJ (1998) Imaging proliferation *in vivo* with [F-18]FLT and positron emission tomography. *Nat Med* 4: 1334–1336

38   Grierson JR, Schwartz JL, Muzi M, Jordan R, Krohn KA (2004) Metabolism of 3'-deoxy-3'-[F-18]fluorothymidine in proliferating A549 cells: validations for positron emission tomography. *Nucl Med Biol* 31: 829–837

39   Waldherr C, Mellinghoff IK, Tran C, Halpern BS, Rozengurt N, Safaei A, Weber WA, Stout D, Satyamurthy N, Barrio J et al (2005) Monitoring antiproliferative responses to kinase inhibitor therapy in mice with 3'-deoxy-3'-18F-fluorothymidine PET. *J Nucl Med* 46: 114–120

40   Barthel H, Cleij MC, Collingridge DR, Hutchinson OC, Osman S, He Q, Luthra SK, Brady F, Price PM, Aboagye EO (2003) 3'-deoxy-3'-[18F]fluorothymidine as a new marker for monitoring tumor response to antiproliferative therapy *in vivo* with positron emission tomography. *Cancer Res* 63: 3791-3798

41   Volkow ND, Fowler JS, Wang GJ, Dewey SL, Schlyer D, MacGregor R, Logan J, Alexoff D, Shea C, Hitzemann R et al (1993) Reproducibility of repeated measures of carbon-11-raclopride binding in the human brain. *J Nucl Med* 34: 609–613

42   Volkow ND, Wang GJ, Fowler JS, Logan J, Schlyer D, Hitzemann R, Lieberman J, Angrist

B, Pappas N, MacGregor R et al (1994) Imaging endogenous dopamine competition with [11C]raclopride in the human brain. *Synapse* 16: 255–262

43   Piccini P, Brooks DJ, Bjorklund A, Gunn RN, Grasby PM, Rimoldi O, Brundin P, Hagell P, Rehncrona S, Widner H et al (1999) Dopamine release from nigral transplants visualized *in vivo* in a Parkinson's patient. *Nat Neurosci* 2: 1137–1140

44   Piccini P, Pavese N, Brooks DJ (2003) Endogenous dopamine release after pharmacological challenges in Parkinson's disease. *Ann Neurol* 53: 647–653

45   Salazar DE, Fischman AJ (1999) Central nervous system pharmacokinetics of psychiatric drugs. *J Clin Pharmacol* Suppl: 10S–12S

46   Yanai M, Hatazawa J, Ojima F, Sasaki H, Itoh M, Ido T (1998) Deposition and clearance of inhaled 18FDG powder in patients with chronic obstructive pulmonary disease. *Eur Respir J* 11: 1342–1348

47   Haradahira T, Zhang M, Maeda J, Okauchi T, Kawabe K, Kida T, Suzuki K, Suhara T (2000) A strategy for increasing the brain uptake of a radioligand in animals: use of a drug that inhibits plasma protein binding. *Nucl Med Biol* 27: 357–360

48   Berridge MS, Heald DL (1999) *In vivo* characterization of inhaled pharmaceuticals using quantitative positron emission tomography. *J Clin Pharmacol* Suppl: 25S–29S

49   Farde L, Wiesel FA, Halldin C, Sedvall G (1988) Central D2-dopamine receptor occupancy in schizophrenic patients treated with antipsychotic drugs. *Arch Gen Psychiatry* 45: 71–76

50   Waarde A (2000) Measuring receptor occupancy with PET. Curr Pharm Des 6: 1593–1610

51   Bench CJ, Lammertsma AA, Grasby PM, Dolan RJ, Warrington SJ, Boyce M, Gunn KP, Brannick LY, Frackowiak RS (1996) The time course of binding to striatal dopamine D2 receptors by the neuroleptic ziprasidone (CP-88,059-01) determined by positron emission tomography. *Psychopharmacology (Berl)* 124: 141–147

52   Nyberg S, Farde L, Eriksson L, Halldin C, Eriksson B (1993) 5-HT2 and D2 dopamine receptor occupancy in the living human brain. A PET study with risperidone. *Psychopharmacology (Berl)* 110: 265–272

53   Hode Y, Reimold M, Demazieres A, Reischl G, Bayle F, Nuss P, Hameg A, Dib M, Macher JP (2005) A positron emission tomography (PET) study of cerebral dopamine D(2) and serotonine 5-HT(2A) receptor occupancy in patients treated with cyamemazine (Tercian). *Psychopharmacology (Berl)* Mar 15; [Epub ahead of print]

54   Farde L (1996) The advantage of using positron emission tomography in drug research. *Trends Neurosci* 19: 211–214

55   Wu JC, Chen IY, Wang Y, Tseng JR, Chhabra A, Salek M, Min JJ, Fishbein MC, Crystal R, Gambhir SS (2004) Molecular imaging of the kinetics of vascular endothelial growth factor gene expression in ischemic myocardium. *Circulation* 110: 685–691

56   Shah K, Tang Y, Breakefield X, Weissleder R (2003) Real-time imaging of TRAIL-induced apoptosis of glioma tumors *in vivo*. *Oncogene* 22: 6865–6872

57   Wu JC, Chen IY, Sundaresan G, Min JJ, De A, Qiao JH, Fishbein MC, Gambhir SS (2003) Molecular imaging of cardiac cell transplantation in living animals using optical bioluminescence and positron emission tomography. *Circulation* 108: 1302–1305

58   Yaghoubi SS, Barrio JR, Namavari M, Satyamurthy N, Phelps ME, Herschman HR, Gambhir SS (2005) Imaging progress of herpes simplex virus type 1 thymidine kinase suicide gene therapy in living subjects with positron emission tomography. *Cancer Gene Ther* 12: 329–339

59   Arner ES, Eriksson S (1995) Mammalian deoxyribonucleoside kinases. *Pharmacology and Therapeutics* 67: 155–186

60   De Clercq E (1993) Antivirals for the treatment of herpesvirus infections. *J Antimicrob Chemother* 32: 121–132

61   Gambhir SS, Bauer E, Black ME, Liang Q, Kokoris MS, Barrio JR, Iyer M, Namavari M, Phelps ME, Herschman HR (2000) A mutant herpes simplex virus type 1 thymidine kinase reporter gene shows improved sensitivity for imaging reporter gene expression with positron emission tomography. *Proc Natl Acad Sci USA* 97: 2785–2790

62   Kang K, Min J, Chen X, Gambhir SS (2005) Comparison of [14C]FMAU, [3H]FEAU, [14C]FIAU, and [3H]PCV accumulation in cells expressing wild type or mutant Herpes Simplex Virus type 1 thymidine kinase reporter genes (A). *Mol Imaging Biol* 7: 138

63   Tjuvajev JG, Finn R, Watanabe K, Joshi R, Oku T, Kennedy J, Beattie B, Koutcher J, Larson S, Blasberg RG (1996) Noninvasive imaging of herpes virus thymidine kinase gene transfer and expression: a potential method for monitoring clinical gene therapy. *Cancer Res* 56: 4087–4095

64   Yaghoubi S, Barrio JR, Dahlbom M, Iyer M, Namavari M, Satyamurthy N, Goldman R, Herschman HR, Phelps ME, Gambhir SS (2001) Human pharmacokinetic and dosimetry studies of [(18)F]FHBG: a reporter probe for imaging herpes simplex virus type-1 thymidine kinase reporter gene expression. *J Nucl Med* 42: 1225–1234

65   Alauddin MM, Conti PS (1998) Synthesis and preliminary evaluation of 9-(4-[18F]-fluoro-3-hydroxymethylbutyl)guanine ([18F]FHBG): a new potential imaging agent for viral infection and gene therapy using PET. *Nucl Med Biol* 25: 175–180

66   Alauddin MM, Conti PS, Mazza SM, Hamzeh FM, Lever JR (1996) 9-[(3-[18F]-fluoro-1-hydroxy-2-propoxy)methyl]guanine ([18F]-FHPG): a potential imaging agent of viral infection and gene therapy using PET. *Nucl Med Biol* 23: 787–792

67   Namavari M, Barrio JR, Toyokuni T, Gambhir SS, Cherry SR, Herschman HR, Phelps ME, Satyamurthy N (2000) Synthesis of 8-[(18)F]fluoroguanine derivatives: *in vivo* probes for imaging gene expression with positron emission tomography. *Nucl Med Biol* 27: 157–162

68   Penuelas I, Mazzolini G, Boan JF, Sangro B, Marti-Climent J, Ruiz M, Satyamurthy N, Qian C, Barrio J, Phelps ME et al (2005) Positron emission tomography imaging of adenoviral-mediated transgene expression in liver cancer patients. *Gastroenterology* 128: 1787–1795

69   Jacobs A, Voges J, Reszka R, Lercher M, Gossmann A, Kracht L, Kaestle C, Wagner R, Wienhard K, Heiss WD (2001) Positron-emission tomography of vector-mediated gene expression in gene therapy for gliomas. *Lancet* 358: 727–729

70   Riedel C, Dohan O, De la Vieja A, Ginter CS, Carrasco N (2001) Journey of the iodide transporter NIS: from its molecular identification to its clinical role in cancer. *Trends Biochem Sci* 26: 490–496

71   Dohan O, De la Vieja A, Paroder V, Riedel C, Artani M, Reed M, Ginter CS, Carrasco N (2003) The sodium/iodide Symporter (NIS): characterization, regulation, and medical significance. *Endocr Rev* 24: 48–77

72   Eichler O, Hess H, Linder F, Schmeiser K (1951) [Radioiodine therapy of thyroid carcinoma.]. *Langenbecks Arch Klin Chir Ver Dtsch Z Chir* 269: 19–36

73   Horst W (1951) [Diagnostic use of radioiodine 131.]. *Strahlentherapie* 85: 183–186

74   Klain M, Ricard M, Leboulleux S, Baudin E, Schlumberger M (2002) Radioiodine therapy for papillary and follicular thyroid carcinoma. *Eur J Nucl Med Mol Imaging* 29, Suppl 2: S479–S485

75   Manders JM, Corstens FH (2002) Radioiodine therapy of euthyroid multinodular goitres. *Eur J Nucl Med Mol Imaging* 29, Suppl 2: S466–S470

76   Reiners C, Schneider P (2002) Radioiodine therapy of thyroid autonomy. *Eur J Nucl Med Mol Imaging* 29, Suppl 2: S471–S478

77   Mandell RB, Mandell LZ, Link CJ Jr (1999) Radioisotope concentrator *Gene Thera*py using the sodium/iodide symporter gene. *Cancer Res* 59: 661–668

78   Spitzweg C, Dietz AB, O'Connor MK, Bergert ER, Tindall DJ, Young CY, Morris JC (2001) *In vivo* sodium iodide symporter *Gene Thera*py of prostate cancer. *Gene Ther* 8: 1524–1531

79   Spitzweg C, O'Connor MK, Bergert ER, Tindall DJ, Young CY, Morris JC (2000) Treatment of prostate cancer by radioiodine therapy after tissue-specific expression of the sodium iodide symporter. *Cancer Res* 60: 6526–6530

80   Haberkorn U, Henze M, Altmann A, Jiang S, Morr I, Mahmut M, Peschke P, Kubler W, Debus J, Eisenhut M (2001) Transfer of the human NaI symporter gene enhances iodide uptake in hepatoma cells. *J Nucl Med* 42: 317–325

81   Rosenthal MS, Cullom J, Hawkins W, Moore SC, Tsui BM, Yester M (1995) Quantitative SPECT imaging: a review and recommendations by the Focus Committee of the Society of Nuclear Medicine Computer and Instrumentation Council. *J Nucl Med* 36: 1489–1513

82   Mozley PD, Stubbs JB, Plossl K, Dresel SH, Barraclough ED, Alavi A, Araujo LI, Kung HF (1998) Biodistribution and dosimetry of TRODAT-1: a technetium-99m tropane for imaging dopamine transporters. *J Nucl Med* 39: 2069–2076

83   Kuikka JT, Akerman K, Bergstrom KA, Karhu J, Hiltunen J, Haukka J, Heikkinen J, Tiihonen J, Wang S, Neumeyer JL (1995) Iodine-123 labelled N-(2-fluoroethyl)-2 beta-carbomethoxy-3 beta-(4-iodophenyl)nortropane for dopamine transporter imaging in the living human brain. *Eur J Nucl Med* 22: 682–686

84   Evan GI, Vousden KH (2001) Proliferation, cell cycle and apoptosis in cancer. *Nature* 411: 342–348

85   Blankenberg FG, Katsikis PD, Tait JF, Davis RE, Naumovski L, Ohtsuki K, Kopiwoda S, Abrams MJ, Darkes M, Robbins RC et al (1998) *In vivo* detection and imaging of phosphatidylserine expression during programmed cell death. *Proc Natl Acad Sci USA* 95: 6349–6354

86   Blankenberg FG, Katsikis PD, Tait JF, Davis RE, Naumovski L, Ohtsuki K, Kopiwoda S, Abrams MJ, Strauss HW (1999) Imaging of apoptosis (programmed cell death) with 99mTc annexin V. *J Nucl Med* 40: 184–191

87   Mochizuki T, Kuge Y, Zhao S, Tsukamoto E, Hosokawa M, Strauss HW, Blankenberg FG, Tait JF, Tamaki N (2003) Detection of apoptotic tumor response *in vivo* after a single dose of chemotherapy with 99mTc-annexin V. *J Nucl Med* 44: 92–97

88   Belhocine T, Steinmetz N, Green A, Rigo P (2003) *In vivo* imaging of chemotherapy-induced apoptosis in human cancers. *Ann NY Acad Sci* 1010: 525–529

89   Belhocine T, Steinmetz N, Hustinx R, Bartsch P, Jerusalem G, Seidel L, Rigo P, Green A (2002) Increased uptake of the apoptosis-imaging agent (99m)Tc recombinant human Annexin V in human tumors after one course of chemotherapy as a predictor of tumor response and patient prognosis. *Clin Cancer Res* 8: 2766–2774

90   Mandl SJ, Mari C, Edinger M, Negrin RS, Tait JF, Contag CH, Blankenberg FG (2004) Multi-modality imaging identifies key times for annexin V imaging as an early predictor of therapeutic outcome. *Mol Imaging* 3: 1–8

91   Ross SA, Seibyl JP (2004) Research applications of selected 123I-labeled neuroreceptor SPECT imaging ligands. *J Nucl Med Technol* 32: 209–214

92   Bhaumik S, Gambhir S (2002) Optical Imaging of Renilla luciferase reporter gene expression in living mice. *Proc Natl Acad Sci USA* 99: 377–382

93   Contag CH, Ross BD (2002) It's not just about anatomy: *in vivo* bioluminescence imaging as an eyepiece into biology. *J Magn Reson Imaging* 16: 378–387

94   Levenson R, Mansfield JR, Gossage KW (2005) Hardware and software for optimized multispectral imaging *in vivo* (A). *Mol Imaging Biol* 7: 106

95   Gao X, Cui Y, Levenson RM, Chung LW, Nie S (2004) *In vivo* cancer targeting and imaging with semiconductor quantum dots. *Nat Biotechnol* 22: 969–976

96   Rice BW, Cable MD, Nelson MB (2001) *In vivo* imaging of light-emitting probes. *J Biomed Opt* 6: 432–440

97   Tromberg BJ, Shah N, Lanning R, Cerussi A, Espinoza J, Pham T, Svaasand L, Butler J (2000) Non-invasive *in vivo* characterization of breast tumors using photon migration spectroscopy. *Neoplasia* 2: 26–40

98   Contag CH, Spilman SD, Contag PR, Oshiro M, Eames B, Dennery P, Stevenson DK, Benaron DA (1997) Visualizing gene expression in living mammals using a bioluminescent reporter. *Photochem Photobiol* 66: 523–531

99   Contag PR, Olomu IN, Stevenson DK, Contag CH (1998) Bioluminescent indicators in living mammals. *Nat Med* 4: 245–247

100   Baggett B, Roy R, Momen S, Morgan S, Tisi L, Morse D, Gillies RJ (2004) Thermostability of firefly luciferases affects efficiency of detection by *in vivo* bioluminescence. *Mol Imaging* 3: 324–332

101   Leclerc GM, Boockfor FR, Faught WJ, Frawley LS (2000) Development of a destabilized firefly luciferase enzyme for measurement of gene expression. *Biotechniques* 29: 590–591, 594-6, 598 passim

102   Contag CH, Jenkins D, Contag PR, Negrin RS (2000) Use of reporter genes for optical measurements of neoplastic disease *in vivo*. *Neoplasia* 2: 41–52

103   Bhaumik S, Lewis XZ, Gambhir SS (2004) Optical imaging of Renilla luciferase, synthetic Renilla luciferase, and firefly luciferase reporter gene expression in living mice. *J Biomed Opt* 9: 578–586

104   Loening AM, Wu AM, Gambhir SS (2005) Improved mutants of Renilla luciferase for imaging application in living subjects (A). *Mol Imaging Biol* 7: 143

105   Loening AM, Paulmurugan R, Wu AM, Gambhir SS (2003) A novel renilla luciferase/epidermal growth factor fusion protein as an optical molecular probe for cancer imaging (A). *Mol Imaging* 2 (3): 132

106   Park JM, Gambhir SS (2005) Multimodality radionuclide, fluorescence, and bioluminescence small-animal imaging. *Proceedings of the IEEE* 93: 771–783

107   Edinger M, Sweeney TJ, Tucker AA, Olomu AB, Negrin RS, Contag CH (1999) Noninvasive assessment of tumor cell proliferation in animal models. *Neoplasia* 1: 303–310

108   Shin JH, Chung JK, Kang JH, Lee YJ, Kim KI, So Y, Jeong JM, Lee DS, Lee MC (2004) Non-invasive imaging for monitoring of viable cancer cells using a dual-imaging reporter gene. *J Nucl Med* 45: 2109–2115

109   Sweeney TJ, Mailander V, Tucker AA, Olomu AB, Zhang W, Cao Y, Negrin RS, Contag CH (1999) Visualizing the kinetics of tumor-cell clearance in living animals. *Proc Natl Acad Sci USA* 96: 12044–12049

110   Rehemtulla A, Stegman LD, Cardozo SJ, Gupta S, Hall DE, Contag CH, Ross BD (2000) Rapid and quantitative assessment of cancer treatment response using *in vivo* bioluminescence imaging. *Neoplasia* 2: 491–495

111   Adams JY, Johnson M, Sato M, Berger F, Gambhir SS, Carey M, Iruela-Arispe ML, Wu L

(2002) Visualization of advanced human prostate cancer lesions in living mice by a targeted gene transfer vector and optical imaging. *Nat Med* 8: 891–897

112   Edinger M, Cao YA, Verneris MR, Bachmann MH, Contag CH, Negrin RS (2003) Revealing lymphoma growth and the efficacy of immune cell therapies using *in vivo* bioluminescence imaging. *Blood* 101: 640–648

113   Costa GL, Sandora MR, Nakajima A, Nguyen EV, Taylor-Edwards C, Slavin AJ, Contag CH, Fathman CG, Benson JM (2001) Adoptive immunotherapy of experimental autoimmune encephalomyelitis via T cell delivery of the IL-12 p40 subunit. *J Immunol* 167: 2379–2387

114   Lipshutz GS, Gruber CA, Cao Y, Hardy J, Contag CH, Gaensler KM (2001) In utero delivery of adeno-associated viral vectors: intraperitoneal gene transfer produces long-term expression. *Mol Ther* 3: 284–292

115   Nakajima A, Seroogy CM, Sandora MR, Tarner IH, Costa GL, Taylor-Edwards C, Bachmann MH, Contag CH, Fathman CG (2001) Antigen-specific T cell-mediated *Gene Therapy* in collagen-induced arthritis. *J Clin Invest* 107: 1293–1301

116   Reynolds PN, Zinn KR, Gavrilyuk VD, Balyasnikova IV, Rogers BE, Buchsbaum DJ, Wang MH, Miletich DJ, Grizzle WE, Douglas JT et al (2000) A targetable, injectable adenoviral vector for selective gene delivery to pulmonary endothelium *in vivo*. *Mol Ther* 2: 562–578

117   Veselovsky AV, Ivanov YD, Ivanov AS, Archakov AI, Lewi P, Janssen P (2002) Protein-protein interactions: mechanisms and modification by drugs. *J Mol Recognit* 15: 405–422

118   Paulmurugan R, Massoud TF, Huang J, Gambhir SS (2004) Molecular imaging of drug-modulated protein-protein interactions in living subjects. *Cancer Res* 64: 2113–2119

119   Massoud TF, Paulmurugan R, Gambhir SS (2004) Molecular imaging of homodimeric protein-protein interactions in living subjects. *Faseb J* 18: 1105–1107

Progress in Drug Research, Vol. 62
(Markus Rudin, Ed.)
©2005 Birkhäuser Verlag, Basel (Switzerland)

Disease phenotyping: structural and functional readouts

By R. Mark Henkelman,
X. Josette Chen
and John G. Sled

Mouse Imaging Centre (MICe)
Hospital for Sick Children
University of Toronto
555 University Avenue
Toronto, Ontario,
Canada M5G 1X8
<mhenkel@phenogenomics.ca>

Glossary of abbreviations

Bpm, beats per minute; CAD, computer-aided diagnosis; CSI, chemical shift imaging; CT, computed tomography; fMRI, functional MR imaging; FSE, fast spin echo; MICe, Mouse Imaging Centre; MMMRI, multiple mouse MR imaging; MR, magnetic resonance; OPT, optical projection tomography; PET, positron emission tomography; SNR, signal-to-noise ratio; SPECT, single photon emission computed tomography; UBM, ultrasound biomicroscopy; US, ultrasound.

1   Introduction

Animal models have always been important in drug discovery and testing. However, with completion of the human genome sequence in the 1990s [1], and now the availability of the mouse genome sequence [2], animal models will have an even more important role. The ability to modify the mouse genome provides for a rich and growing array of mouse models of human diseases. Also, the mouse mammalian model is well suited to the study of disease associated with aging populations because of the short life span and rapid reproductive cycle; helping control the high costs of animal research. Furthermore, the growing awareness that the individual's genome affects not only the beneficial response to drugs, but also any side effects or adverse reactions, has lead to the new field of pharmacogenetics (see for example the new journal published by Nature Publishing Group entitled: The Pharmacogenetics Journal). Animal research into pharmacogenetics is greatly facilitated by the availability of inbred mouse strains and the wide selection of techniques available for specifically modifying the mouse genome. Thus, much of the animal research in drug discovery and evaluation is now concentrated on the mouse.

Over the same period that genetic models have become important in pharmaceutical research, clinical medicine has seen a surge in the importance of imaging in medical diagnosis, evaluation of disease progression, and response to treatments. This importance is illustrated by the awarding of Nobel prizes in medicine for computed tomography (CT) in 1979 and magnetic resonance (MR) in 2003. Just as imaging is essential in clinical medicine, it is being recognized that it has a major role to play in animal research. In particular, mouse imaging is becoming a requisite technology for drug discovery and evaluation.

There are many advantages that arise from the use of imaging technology in animal-based pharmacological research [3]. The use of non-invasive imag-

153

ing on live animals can significantly reduce the number of animals needed to study a particular biological problem. At a time when the general public is increasingly questioning the extent of animal use in research, the ability of imaging to diminish these numbers is important. This reduction is particularly evident in longitudinal studies, where an imaging assay repeated at sequential time points requires a small fraction of the number of animals that would be required if cohorts were sacrificed at each time point. Furthermore, the statistical evaluation of time-course data is more powerful if individuals are tracked over time and hence serve as their own precedent controls. This lessens biological heterogeneity in averaging across different subjects, and also allows for the identification of outliers with deviant historical time courses.

Imaging can also provide exquisite anatomical details in mice as will be demonstrated later. Mouse imaging at a resolution of 65 mm is much closer to histological visualization than is human imaging at a typical resolution of 1 mm. Furthermore, the feasibility of whole body imaging in the mouse facilitates survey evaluation where the organ or organs affected by a drug, genetic change or disease process may not be known. Beyond just anatomical structure, imaging has growing capabilities to provide functional readouts. These readouts may be physiological, such as those obtained in dynamic motion studies or Doppler measurements of flow, or they may be molecular, reporting on the spatial patterns of drug concentration, metabolic processes and even signaling molecules and specific products of gene expression.

Finally, evaluative assays that are developed based on imaging in animal research can frequently be translated back into clinical imaging, providing a bridge between preclinical and late phase human studies facilitating interpretation.

2 Requirements of imaging for animal studies

The advantages of animal imaging for drug research discussed above will not be realized if one simply puts a mouse into a clinical imaging system. Instead, the technology and know how of human clinical imaging needs to be adapted and re-engineered for imaging the mouse. There are a number of aspects of imaging that need to be reconsidered in adapting clinical radiology to mouse biology. Five specific aspects are identified, and these are used in the rest of the chapter as a framework for describing the adaptation of imaging to the mouse, and for illustrating some of the aspects of disease phenotyping.

The first major aspect in adapting imaging from the human to the mouse is a matter of scale. In linear terms, the mouse is about 15 times smaller than the human (11 cm long as compared with 168 cm for the human). In terms of mass, the mouse is about $15^3 = 3375$ times smaller (20 g as compared with 69 kg for the human). If we are accustomed to seeing clinical imaging at about 1 mm resolution, to maintain "comparable anatomical" resolution, we need to image the mouse at 65 μm resolution. This concept of "comparable anatomy" is a useful guide for determining if we have appropriate resolution for imaging mice. However, it is important to realize that some microscopic anatomical structures (e.g., cell diameters, capillary diameters) do not scale with animal size. Thus, comparable anatomical resolution in the mouse gets us much closer to histological scale than does imaging in the human. On the other hand, major vessels and organs tend to scale with the animal size. If we expect to see the structures in the mouse that we are used to seeing in human imaging, we will need to achieve comparable anatomical resolution. This resolution can be achieved for some imaging modalities and not for others.

Secondly, small-animal imaging will need to achieve both high throughput and operator efficiency if it is going to realize its advantages for drug research. It is in this aspect that biological imaging differs most from clinical imaging. Clinical imaging is piece work by necessity. In the course of several hours, a clinical MR system may study a brain with unknown pathology using several pulse sequence contrasts, look for liver metastases using gadolinium, and do a tagged cardiac motion study, all in one afternoon. In this context, it is worthwhile to have individualized patient setup, carefully selected slice positions and a large repertoire of scan protocols tailored to the anticipated pathologies. In contrast, a mouse biology experiment is likely to consist of five to ten mice in a disease or treatment arm and an equivalent number of controls. These will all require the same imaging technique and the derived assay measurements will need to come from equivalent regions of anatomy. This difference in strategy for mouse imaging favors parallel acquisitions using a general purpose three-dimensional imaging protocol requiring minimal setup time. In both clinical and mouse imaging, the labor costs can become the major cost of the study. Realizing the potential of mouse imaging for drug research requires that staff be deployed efficiently.

Thirdly, beyond simple anatomical structures, mouse imaging will need to provide physiological assessments. This is a requirement that is shared with clinical imaging. However, the adaptation of clinical physiological measures to the mouse is made more difficult by the faster physiological motions in the mouse (respiratory rates of 60 breaths per minute and cardiac rates of 300–500 beats per minute, bpm). Not all human imaging techniques can be adapted to these faster rates.

Fourthly, imaging for the mouse will need to provide as much molecular specificity as possible to enable drug research. Again, this requirement is shared with human imaging where there is now a major research effort in "molecular imaging." Many of the methods being developed translate readily across species. In clinical imaging, improvements in "molecular sensitivity" have generally been offset by poorer spatial resolution with the most sensitive techniques often requiring complementary anatomical imaging to assist interpretation. This trend is exacerbated in the mouse where the spatial resolution is so much more demanding. However, mouse molecular imaging has some advantage in that there are more opportunities for optical techniques than in the human.

Finally, there is a requirement and opportunity for more automated analysis techniques in mouse imaging. Information extraction from human imaging requires highly skilled radiologists and usually results in a narrative report. In contrast, information extracted from mouse images usually can be minimal, unqualified, quantitative, and low cost. Thus, mouse imaging requires a significant development in computer image analysis and quantitative data extraction. It is, therefore, fortuitous that images of mice from an inbred strain are more amenable to computer-based comparison than are images of the genetically heterogeneous human population. Also, unsupervised computer interpretation of mouse images does not suffer from the extreme consequences of false negatives and other errors that plague computer-aided diagnosis in clinical imaging.

This chapter discusses how imaging is being adapted to meet the requirements of animal research in drug discovery. Different modalities are discussed in terms of their abilities to provide these requirements for mouse imaging. Examples of applications are presented to illustrate the promise of structural and functional readouts.

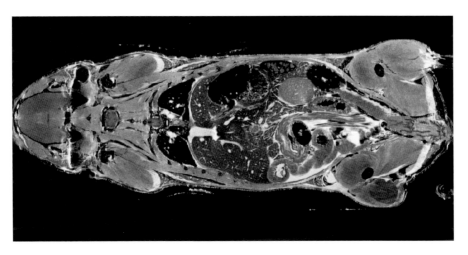

Figure 1.
A 3D anatomical image of a perfusion fixed mouse with Gd contrast. The image is acquired at 7 T with a simple spin echo sequence TR/TE = 600/19 ms and isotropic resolution of 75 µm in an imaging time of 20 h [image provided by R. Behin at the Mouse Imaging Centre (MICe), Toronto].

3   Anatomical resolution

In adapting human imaging to the mouse, some modalities readily achieve the 15-fold increase in resolution required and others do not.

Magnetic resonance (MR) imaging is capable of very high spatial resolution (on the order of 10 µm [4]) provided there is adequate signal-to-noise ratio (SNR). In adapting from the human to the mouse, the signal in a voxel decreases by 3375-fold. This is recovered in three ways: increasing the strength of the magnetic field, using smaller radiofrequency coils that just fit the mouse and for the remainder, increasing the imaging time enabling more signal averaging. Figure 1 shows that these three adaptations can produce "comparable anatomy" [5].

Computed tomography (CT) can also be adapted well to provide excellent spatial resolution in the mouse. Figure 2 shows microCT images with spatial resolutions of about 20 µm isotropic. However, if one wants resolution of soft tissue contrast equivalent to that seen in clinical imaging, the number of X-rays and hence the radiation dose needs to be increased by a factor of > 3375, exceeding the lethal dose to the mouse. Thus, live mouse CT can only be used with lower than anatomically comparable resolution and with poorer soft tis-

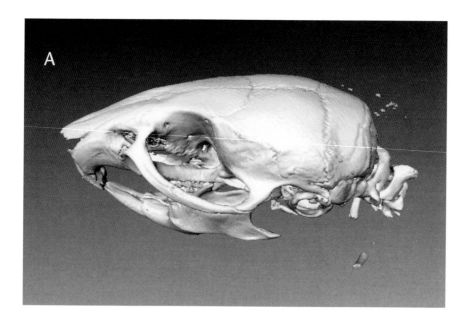

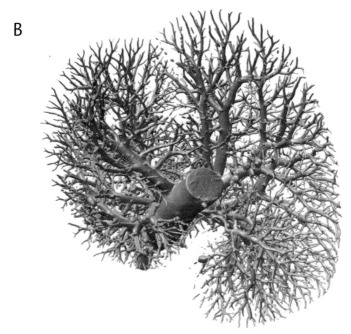

Figure 2.
MicroCT images at an isotropic resolution of 22 μm of (A) a mouse skull and (B) a mouse kidney vascular tree filled with Microfil (images provided by X.L. Yu at the MICe).

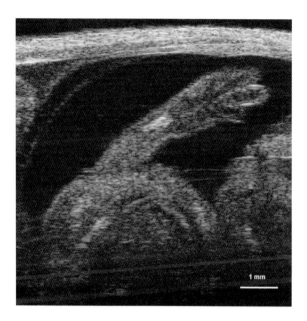

Figure 3.
UBM image acquired at 30 MHz of a live mouse embryo at E16.5 days showing high resolution detail of the developing paw (image provided by YQ. Zhou at the MICe).

sue contrast [6, 7]. Excellent resolution can be obtained for high contrast objects in fixed specimens where dose is of no concern.

Ultrasound (US) can also be adapted to achieve appropriate resolution for mouse imaging [8]. Since the resolution in US is determined by the wavelength, increasing the frequency to 30–50 MHz takes the resolution to the 50-μm range. These higher frequencies are not used in clinical US because the depth of penetration of the ultrasound beam is decreased proportionally, but for smaller patients such as mice, this is in fact desirable. High-frequency US imaging is frequently designated as ultrasound biomicroscopy (UBM) [9], and is illustrated for a live mouse embryo in Figure 3.

The molecularly sensitive human imaging modalities of positron emission tomography (PET) and single photon emission computed tomography (SPECT) cannot be adapted to the mouse achieving comparable anatomical resolution. PET is limited by physics to a resolution of about 1 mm [10]. SPECT can achieve slightly better resolution, but by using a pin hole camera with very low signal efficiency.

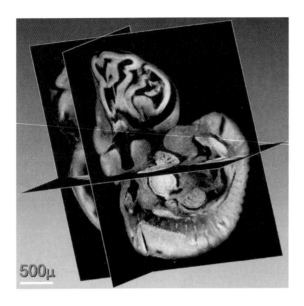

Figure 4.
An OPT image of a fixed mouse embryo clarified in BABB using autofluorescence. The image resolution is approximately 10 μm isotropic (image provided by J.R. Walls at the MICe).

Optical imaging methods represent a new opportunity in mouse imaging that is not adapted from human imaging. They are discussed further under molecular sensitivity. Because of multiple scattering of optical photons, the three-dimensional (3D) spatial resolution of optical techniques is generally worse that 1 mm. One exception is the new technology of optical projection tomography (OPT) [11, 12]; a technique limited to small (< 1 cm) fixed specimens, but allowing spatial resolution down to 10 μm as shown in Figure 4.

4 Throughput and efficiency

Because biological imaging for the mouse usually involves moderately large numbers of animals for both experiments and controls, and because the time to image a mouse may even be longer than for a comparable human study, issues of throughput are paramount. On a related theme, the efficiency of personnel involved in imaging is also critical. A clinical MR scanner will on aver-

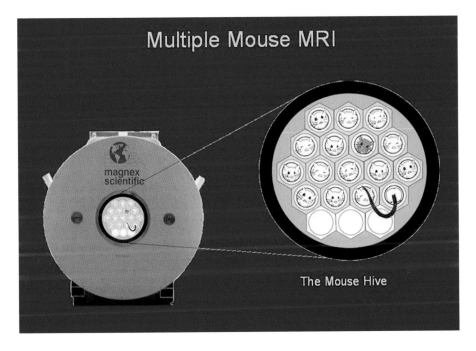

Figure 5.
An MMMRI system for high-throughput mouse imaging. Nineteen independent transmit and receive coils share a common gradient and a 7 T magnetic field.

age have three individuals involved as staff: an MR technologist, a nurse/receptionist, and a radiologist or fellow. It is unlikely that animal imaging can afford such an entourage.

To address the issue of throughput in mouse MR imaging, we have designed [13] a system that can accommodate 19 mice in individual transmit and receive coils that are all shielded from each other as shown in Figure 5. The mice all share the same gradient and the static magnetic field from a 40-cm-diameter, 7-Tesla magnet produced by MAGNEX (Abington, UK). The clear bore inside the shared gradient is 27 cm; sufficient to accommodate individual RF Millipede coils [14] of 32-mm diameter within cylindrical shields of 50-mm diameter. The details and operations of multiple mouse MR imaging (MMMRI) are described in the literature [13]. This system currently images 16 mice in parallel. In the time that it takes to image one mouse, equivalent quality images can be acquired from 16 mice. At the time of writing, live MMMRI is limited to 7 mice due to lack of monitoring

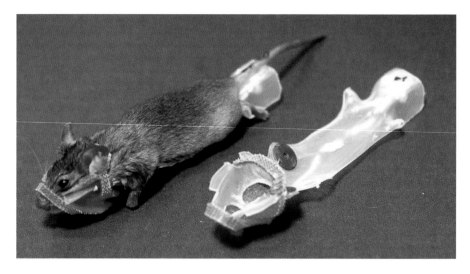

Figure 6.
A mouse handling system for MMMRI that provides individualized cardiac, respiratory and tempera-ture monitoring along with gas anesthesia and scavenging for each mouse. Multiple mice can all be prepared in an induction chamber and mounted onto the mouse holding array. After preparation, they can be inserted as a unit into the coil array of the MR imager. A second group of mice can be prepared while the first set is being imaged (design, fabrication [15] and photograph provided by J. Dazai at the MICe).

channels and independent receivers, but there are no difficulties expected in going to 19 live mice. Handling multiple anesthetized mice with a sin-gle technician requires carefully designed mouse handling equipment [15] as shown in Figure 6. With this system, it is possible to prepare and load 19 mice in 1 h. Figure 7 shows live brain images using an optimized fast spin echo (FSE) pulse sequence with approximately 100 μm isotropic resolution taken in 2 h 45 min [16]. This is somewhat poorer resolution than the tar-get of 65 μm. To achieve this target would require higher magnetic fields and longer scan times [17]. The efficiency of MMMRI is further increased by overlapping scan time with preparation time for subsequent batches of mice.

Several other reports of parallel MRI for mouse phenotyping are in the lit-erature [18]. Methods that use a separate receiver for each mouse preserve the high anatomical resolution of MR. However, simpler methods that put mul-tiple animals in a large receiver coil suffer significant degradation in image quality [19, 20]. One application that benefits considerably from the

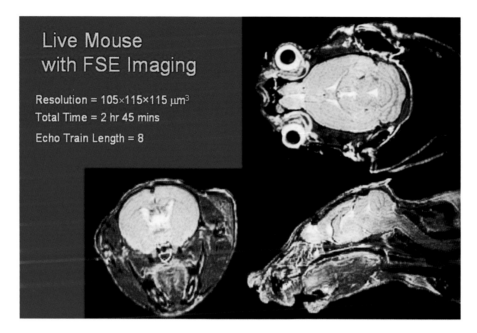

Figure 7.
Live mouse brain images acquired with an FSE (or RARE) imaging sequence with an isotropic resolution of 100 μm and an imaging time of 165 min. Echo train length was 8, TR/TE = 900/12 ms and the center of k-space was acquired from the fourth echo giving some T_2-weighted contrast (image provided by B. Nieman at the MICe).

throughput of MMMRI is the longitudinal study of cancer growth and its response to treatment. Historically, many cancer studies in mice have used subcutaneously implanted tumors as models. This allows for direct estimation of tumor size using calipers. There is now, however, a growing realization that a brain tumor growing under the skin of the flank is not a very realistic model, particularly with respect to routes and prevalence of metastatic spread. Brain tumors growing in the brain are much more relevant, but monitoring the growth curves of tumors in the brain in a single mouse can only be done using imaging, best with MR imaging. We have found MMMRI to be particularly effective for tumor growth monitoring [21]. Even with the limitation of 7 live mice in parallel, we are currently doing a four-arm study: two treatment arms, one control arm with only the carrier, and one additional untreated control arm with 7 mice in each arm imaged every week (up to 10 weeks) following stereotaxic injection of a human xenograft. Imaging

a. Transgene Expression	b. Bacterial Infection	c. Gene Transfer	d. Lymphocyte Trafficking

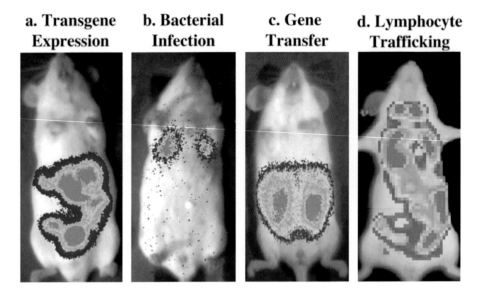

Figure 8.
In vivo applications of bioluminescent imaging. This imaging modality has broad applications in biomedical research that include (a) assessing the levels of transgene expression, (b) the location and extent of bacterial infection, (c) the efficiency of gene transfer and expression, and (d) the trafficking patterns of lymphocytes.

includes three different contrasts: T_1-weighted, diffusion-weighted and T_2-weighted. The whole experiment occupies only 1 day a week of scanner time. Without MMMRI, this single experiment would use the MR scanner full time for 2.5 months.

Another imaging method that can achieve high throughput, again particularly for cancer studies [22], is optical imaging, either using luciferase bioluminescence [23] or fluorescence imaging [24]. These optical techniques are efficient because imaging times are short (10–30 min) and 3–5 mice can be imaged simultaneously side by side. Examples of luciferase imaging are shown in Figure 8.

CT can also be adapted to achieve high throughput. Cone-beam CT acquires data for a full volume reconstruction in a single rotation of the gantry, which can be accomplished in as short a time as 1 s. Such systems have been designed primarily for dynamic studies and have only moderate spatial resolution and throughput. Automated mechanisms for inserting mice into a CT scanner have been reported.

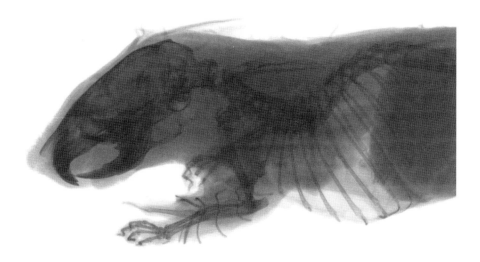

Figure 9.
Digital projection X-ray images are a relatively rapid method for qualitative phenotyping of mouse skeleton. However, because they are projection images, they are significantly less comprehensive than 3D microCT images (image provided by N. Kassam at the Centre for Models of Human Disease).

Two other X-ray imaging technologies are well adapted for high throughput. Faxitron (Wheeling, IL) produces a high-resolution 2D digital image of the mouse skeleton as seen in Figure 9. PIXImus (G.E. Healthcare, Waukesha, WI) is a dual energy X-ray absorption projection that gives estimates of body composition. Although both of these techniques achieve high throughput (limited in time only by the need to anesthetize the mouse), they are projection imaging and do not reveal 3D anatomy. Hence, they are not discussed further.

The throughput and method of operation for PET [25] and SPECT is very similar in mice and human imaging with a single study taking about 1 h. No attempts to significantly increase the throughput have yet been reported.

Finally, US imaging is the most labor intensive of the mouse imaging modalities with studies taking 30–90 minutes per mouse and requiring the involvement of highly skilled individuals [26]. Because US scanning is particularly operator dependent, it is less amenable to automatic scanning and subsequent computer-aided image analysis.

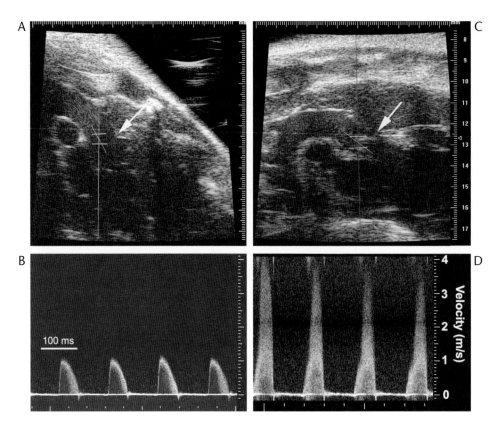

Figure 10.
US imaging and evaluation of flow through the aortic orifice. (A) 2D UBM image with the Doppler sample volume located at the level of aortic orifice of a normal mouse; (B) Doppler flow spectrum obtained from the aortic orifice; (C) 2D UBM image with the Doppler sample volume located at the level of aortic orifice of a mouse with aortic stenosis; (D) Doppler flow spectrum of the aortic jet at the level of aortic orifice, with the peak velocity up to 4 m/s (arrow indicates the aortic orifice) (image provided by YQ. Zhou at the MICe).

5   Physiological phenotyping

Although it is difficult to achieve high throughput for mouse imaging with US, US is probably the best modality for physiological measurements since a single imaging frame is produced in nearly real time. Thus, US is the tool of choice for the evaluation of heart function in the mouse [26]. Not only does US provide excellent visualization of the structural anatomy of the heart, it does so in real time and produces movies of the cardiac dynamics even

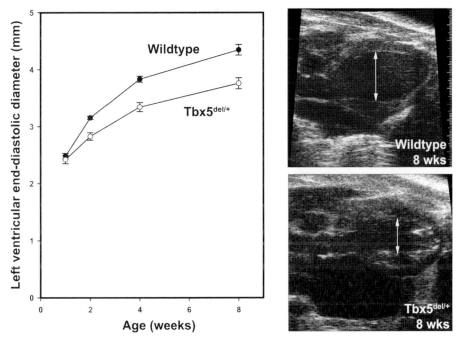

Figure 11.
Cardiac physiological phenotype measured by ultrasound in 12 wild-type and 12 TBx5[del/+] mutants. In the mutant, the left ventricular end-diastolic diameter increases more slowly than in the wild type over the first 8 weeks after birth, and the ventricular wall is thicker) (image provided by YQ. Zhou at the MICe).

though the mouse heart rate is 500 bpm (eight to ten times the human heart rate). These dynamic images can be used to measure ejection fraction and monitor the motion of the heart wall. Mouse US can also measure the Doppler waveform of blood flow in major vessels and flow patterns throughout the heart (Fig. 10). This kind of physiological phenotyping in the mouse is difficult to achieve with any other imaging modality.

As an application example of physiological phenotyping in the mouse using US, Figure 11 shows the average end diastolic diameter of the left ventricle averaged over 12 wild-type mice and 12 heterozygotes with a Tbx5 knockout. This mutant mouse is a model for human Holt Orom's syndrome, which often exhibits an arterial septal defect [27]. Although the ventricular diameters in the mice are similar immediately after birth, over 4–8 weeks the mutant shows wall thickening and significantly decreased left ventricular diameter.

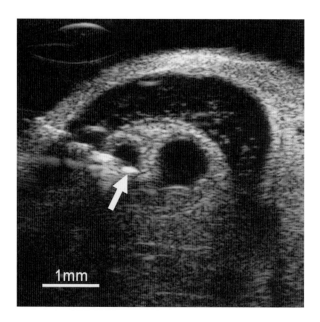

Figure 12.
The use of UBM to guide a needle (arrow) into the neural crest of an E13.5 embryo in utero (image provided by V. Bonn at the MICe).

Another application for real-time mouse US is interventions, image guided. We use US guidance for the introduction of genetic material into specific locations in the embryo in the form of stem cells or adeno virus constructs (Fig. 12). In a more simple application, we use US to guide a needle into the heart without opening the chest for perfusion fixation [28]. Ultrasound is the only mouse imaging modality that presently provides such real-time capability.

As mentioned in the previous section, cone-beam CT for mouse imaging can acquire data for volume images in approximately 1 s (Explore RS MicroCT, G.E. Healthcare, London, Canada). Because of the speed, the resolution is limited to $150 \times 150 \times 450$ µm. This system has been designed and built to enable perfusion time-course studies in stroke models, tumors, and other tissue. An example of a blood flow map in a rat brain is shown in Figure 13 [29]. The technology is not yet widely available and mouse studies have not been completed. The future evolution of dynamic microCT for physiological phenotyping in the mouse will be interesting to watch.

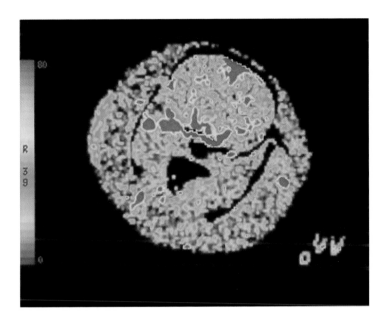

Figure 13.
Blood flow map of a 0.45-mm thick slice of a rat brain measured with dynamic microCT (image provided by T. Lee at the University of Western Ontario, London).

MR is also being adapted as a tool for physiological phenotyping in the mouse. The challenges to this arise from two factors: the intrinsically lower SNR achievable in the comparable anatomical voxel in the mouse, and the tenfold shorter cycle time for cardiac and respiratory processes. However, remarkable cardiac MR images and movies have been made using prospective gating and data acquired over multiple heart beats. These provide assessments of cardiac function in terms of ejection fractions and wall motion [30]. Flow-sensitized images of the coronary vasculature have also been made, although with a perfuse heart preparation at very high magnetic field strengths (17.6 Tesla).

Prospective gating clearly will not work for multiple mouse imaging. However, retrospective gating methods have been adapted from human imaging and provide high-quality dynamic information (Fig. 14) albeit with four- to sixfold oversampling.

MR angiography has been demonstrated in the mouse [31]. As further techniques are developed, we can expect to see arterial spin labeling, blood

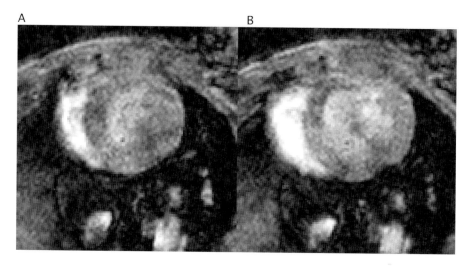

Figure 14.
Retrospectively gated cardiac images acquired in a mode that can be used with MMMRI. A, end dias-tole; B, end systole (image provided by J. Bishop at the MICe).

volume, blood flow, mean transit time vascular permeability, oxygen tension, and perfusion measures for the mouse using MR.

Another vascular-related physiological measure is functional magnetic resonance imaging (fMRI), a major research and clinical tool in the human. fMRI measurements have been demonstrated in the rat [32, 33] (Fig. 15). fMRI in the animal is made more difficult because the light anesthesia needed to overcome motion shuts down some of the neurological processes that one might wish to measure. However, the unique information that fMRI yields means we can expect to see much more fMRI in rats and mice, particularly in the context of development of drugs for mental health.

Finally, there are some physiological measures that can be undertaken in the animal which cannot be done in the human. One example is the use of $MnCl_2$ as a contrast agent [34]. The Mn^{2+} is taken up as a Ca^{2+} analogue by active neurons, and the resulting T_1 contrast highlights active fiber tracks and active regions of the brain. $MnCl_2$ can not be used in this way in humans because of its known neurotoxicity [35]. As the mechanism of action of $MnCl_2$ becomes better understood, we can expect to see it and pos-sibly other animal specific contrast agents being used for physiological phe-notyping.

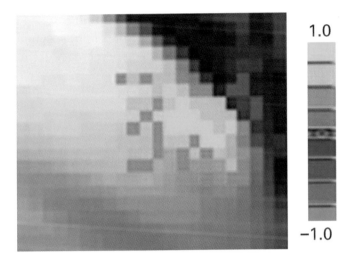

Figure 15.
High-resolution cross-correlation blood-oxygen-level-dependent fMRI activation maps in the whisker barrel cortex (images courtesy of J. Hyde, Milwaukee, WI)

PET and SPECT have about the same application for physiological measurement in the mouse as they exhibit in the human. The minimum temporal resolution is limited to about 10 min (or greater in the mouse due to the lower count rates). Flurodeoxyglucose (FDG) is ideal for measurement of spatial distributions of metabolic activity.

Overall, imaging methods for physiological phenotyping in the mouse are just beginning to be developed. Many more measures can be directly adapted from those in use clinically. Other novel measures specific to animals can also be anticipated. We can expect significant growth in the use of image-based physiological measurements in animal research in the future.

6   Molecular specificity

The spatial mapping of specific molecules using imaging methods could be considered as just another aspect of physiological phenotyping. However, given the intense research and development effort that is currently underway into molecular imaging in both humans and animals, it warrants a separate section. Since a comprehensive discussion of molecular imaging and areas of application have been provided in the previous chapter, this section summarizes the dominant themes and provide some complimentary examples to those provided previously.

The enthusiasm for molecular imaging is easy to appreciate. The ability to map the spatial distribution within the body of specific endogenous biological molecules such as products of individual gene expression, genetic promoters and repressors, cell signaling molecules, neuro transmitters, to name just a few, would be immensely valuable for understanding differentiations, regulation, homeostasis and diseases. Even more important than knowing where these molecules are, is knowing where they act. It is far more valuable to know where antibodies are conjugating, hormones are triggering receptors, metabolites are being used, and drugs are binding, than it is to know that all of them are distributed relatively uniformly by the blood stream. Thus "molecular imaging" really wants to know the spatial distribution within the body of specific molecules at their locations of significant or functional interaction.

The challenge to imaging posed by "molecular imaging" is therefore twofold. First is to find ways to make the molecule report at the time and location of the biologically important interaction. Various approaches are being explored and used: differential uptake, preferential retention, irreversible binding, downstream reporters of transcribed genes, enzymatic activation of MR relaxation agents [36]. The second challenge is amplification. Most imaging techniques have sensitivities only down to the millimolar or micromolar range. However, the biological molecules of interest often are present in the nanomolar range. Thus, there is a need for significant "amplification" for imaging to detect the molecular interaction of interest. Two kinds of amplification are being explored: (1) conjugate linking of the molecular interaction of interest to a much larger reporter as is done with antibody-conjugated bubbles in US, Gd-decorated dendrimers in MR, conjugated iron particles in MR, and fluorescently labeled liposomes in optical imaging; and alternatively (2) using temporal amplification where the reporter is rapidly recycled and able to report millions of times during the image acquisition as is done using fluorophores with nanosecond lifetimes. Molecular imaging will certainly benefit from more and better ways to achieve this required amplification. However, there are already some impressive examples of "molecular imaging" at work.

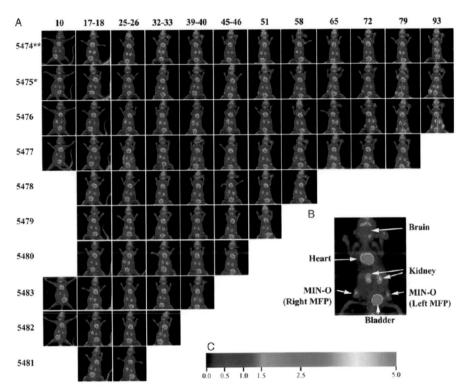

Figure 16.
Longitudinal imaging with PET. (A) Layout of experimental data. Each row of images corresponds to a given animal followed in the study (identified by number at left), and each column corresponds to a time point for imaging. Animals were followed longitudinally from as early as 10 days to as late as 93 days post transplantation of MIN-O tissue. Four animals were not imaged at the earliest time point because of the lack of a visible sign in the other six animals. At the last time point in each row, animals were killed and the mammary fat pads were prepared for *ex vivo* imaging and histology. (B) Example image. An enlarged view of a maximum-intensity projection of a study mouse showing uptake in various tissues, including the MIN-O tissue in the left and right no. 4 mammary fat pads. The mouse is displayed in a supine orientation. (C) Intensity scale. The color scale representing uptake relative to brain. This color scale is used for all PET images. (Figure courtesy of Simon Cherry, UC Davis [37]).

Nuclear imaging (PET and SPECT) has historically been the most effective method for molecular imaging. The fact that the sensor can detect a single molecule at the instant when the nuclear isotope emits gives nuclear imaging a tremendous advantage over other methods. However, nuclear decay is certainly not a recyclable reporter, nor is the timing of the emission in any way related to the biologically important interaction of the molecule that carries the radioisotope. A good application example is shown in Figure 16 [37].

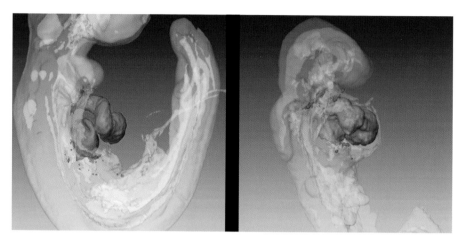

Figure 17.
OPT images comparing heart development in a wild-type embryo with a 90% siRNA knockdown of the gene product Smarcd 3. The heart structures are identified using an anti-PECAM monoclonal antibody that was revealed with an Alexa 488-conjugated secondary antibody (images provided by J.R. Walls at the MICe).

Imaging in the mouse has generated renewed interest in optical imaging. Here, the requisite amplification is mainly provided by the rapid cycle time of fluorescent chromophores and bioluminescent reporters. There is a very large collection of specific optical markers inherited from a century of microscopy. However, to be effective in live animals, the photon window needs to be in the 700–900 nm range to avoid the severe absorption by hemoglobin. New chromophores that operate in this range are being rapidly developed. As an application example of molecular specificity, in OPT where light absorption is much less of a problem because the specimen is clarified, Figure 17 shows an embryonic heart deformation as a result of 90% siRNA knockdown of the gene product Smarcd 3 [38].

Another approach to obtaining molecular specificity in mouse phenotyping by imaging is with chemical shift spectroscopy (Fig. 18) [39]. Chemical shift imaging (CSI) does not need contrast agents and achieves its molecular specificity from the intrinsic NMR frequency shift of the metabolite of interest [40]. Because it has no amplification, CSI is restricted to millimolar concentrations of specific molecules and achieves only moderate spatial resolution of several millimeters.

In summary, molecular imaging in animals holds tremendous promise for drug research. Many of the challenges are being met by intensive research.

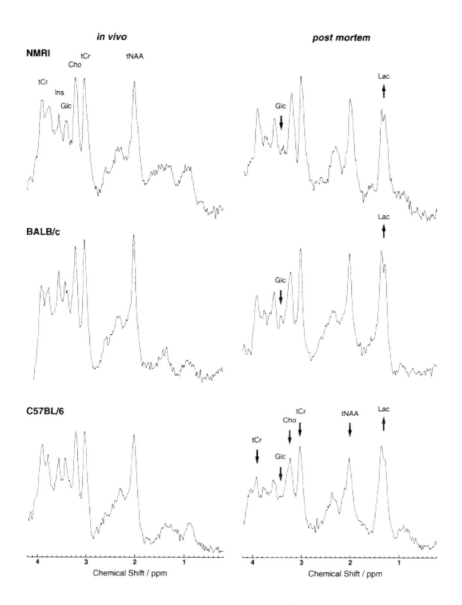

Figure 18.

In vivo (left) and 1 h post mortem (right) proton MR spectra of the same animal for different mouse strains (STEAM, TR/TE/TM = 6000/20/10 ms, 4×3×4 mm³ VOI, corrected for CSF and scaled with respect to brain water content). Metabolite resonances include *N*-acetylaspartate (tNAA), creatine and phosphocreatine (tCr), choline-containing compounds (Cho), *myo*-inositol (Ins), glucose (Glc), and lactate (Lac). Apart from decrease Glc and increased Lac post mortem, the specific vulnerability of the C57BL/6 strain to ischemia is demonstrated by the reduction of tNAA, tCr, and Cho in contrast to NMRI and BALB/c mice. (Figure courtesy of Jens Frohm, Göttingen [39])

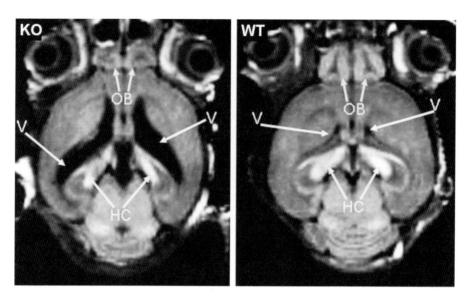

Figure 19.
Comparison of MR images of the live brain of a knockout in the sonic hedgehog pathway compared with a wild-type mouse. The knockout has a reduced hippocampus as was known from histology, but the degree of hydrocephalus is only well appreciated by *in vivo* imaging. The olfactory bulbs are also diminished and the nasal passage is misformed (mouse provided by C.C. Hui, Hospital for Sick Children, Toronto and image provided by N. Lipshitz at the MICe).

6 Automated readouts

The readouts in clinical imaging are predominantly visual. The films, or increasingly, direct digital images, are viewed by a highly trained expert observer and the salient features are dictated into a verbal report. Visual readout is sometimes appropriate for animal imaging. Figure 19 is an example of a comparison between a wild-type and knockout mouse brain in which a number of differences can be visually identified. However, more often in biological imaging, the readout needs to be quantified and the investigator is interested in knowing statistically significant differences between groups of mice. Such assessments are better done by a computer than by visual observation. Moreover, the amount of data that can be generated by high-throughput mouse imaging can exceed that which can be analyzed by a human observer.

There are numerous computer algorithms developed for image readout in human imaging. Computer-aided diagnosis (CAD) for assisting mammo-

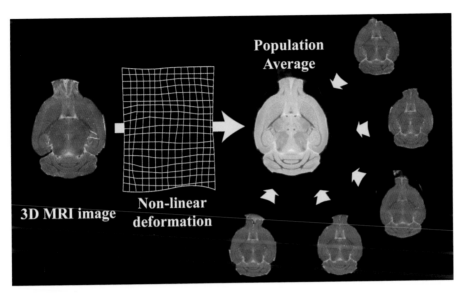

Figure 20.
3D isotropic volume images of the brain from genetically identical mice are registered together to produce an inbred average and a set of deformation fields that are a map of the displacements from each individual to the average.

gram reading has been well developed. The neuroscience community has a long history of quantitative methods for assessment of brain images. In general, however, unassisted computer readouts of mouse images are an active research area that needs more development.

We have been working on registration algorithms for the mouse brain [41]. Figure 20 shows data from 3D high-resolution (~60 μm isotropic) images of genetically identical mice. Nine such datasets are co-registered through multi-scale non-linear deformations based on both intensity comparisons and edge alignment [42, 43]. The image synthesized by averaging the individual aligned datasets provides an unbiased estimator of the average structural anatomy of the brain of this mouse strain. The average image shows greater detail than any of the component images. Note that neuroanatomical structures that are under tight genetic control are enhanced, while structures that vary among individuals such as small blood vessels are averaged out. Since the average differs from the individual images by a known deformation at every point, an estimate of the population variance for the normal anatomy of this strain can be calculated as shown in Figure 21. It is remark-

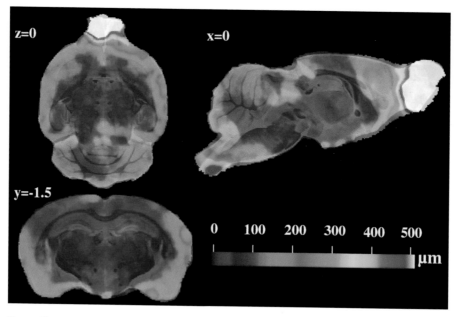

Figure 21.
An average brain overlaid with a color map of the average displacement of the individual voxels to register them to the average. There are some regions of large displacement: the brain stem which has been arbitrarily severed, the olfactory bulbs which even in a fixed specimen are floppy, and small compression at the lateral sides of the brain where the walls of the test tube compress the sample. But over most of the brain volume, the mean square displacement is 100–200 μm. This shows the anatomic reproducibility among genetically identical individuals. This measure also defines the variance of normal, against which any genetic variation needs to be defined (analysis provided by N. Kovacevic at MICe). (Printed with permission of Cerebral Cortex [44].)

able that the root mean square displacement over most of the brain is limited to 100–200 μm [44]. Knowledge of normal variance is essential if one wishes to identify significance differences in anatomy due to mutations, diseases or even environmental perturbations. As an illustration of the sensitivity of this kind of computer automated image readout, Figure 22 shows an average brain image synthesized from a mix of three strains. Looking closely at an arbitrary voxel of this grand average, one can see that the contributing voxels cluster together by strain and that the differences between strains is significantly greater that the variance within the strain. Another use for these registration techniques is to track growth patterns from images of different mice at different points in development. An excellent example of this has

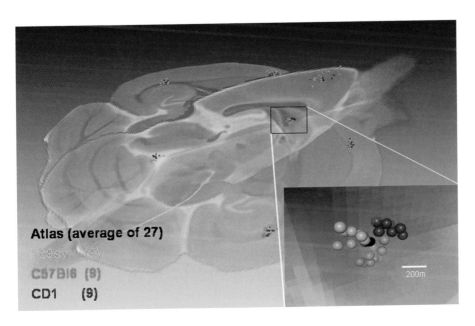

Figure 22.
A brain average constructed from 27 isotropic images (9 individuals each from 3 strains). If we pick a voxel at random from this average and look at the locations of the individual mouse voxels that contributed to this average, we see that the individual strains cluster together, showing that the variation within strains is much less than the differences between strains (image provided by N. Kovacevic at the MICe).

been reported by Mori et al. [45]. We believe that this kind of automated readout will be essential for optimal use of mouse imaging.

In contrast to the brain where structures are highly detailed and very similar, automated readout will be much more difficult in the abdomen and probably impossible for organs like intestines. In the body, registration attempts will need to be supplemented and assisted by segmentation of individual organ structures. Figure 23 shows the segmentation of kidneys from abdominal 3D images of mouse using adaptive shape models. Approaches such as these will help to define average normal anatomy and its variance allowing for the identification of anatomical abnormalities.

Beyond just comparative measures of anatomy, computer automated readout will, in the future, assist in understanding function. One example is the use of trabecular architecture obtained from 3D microCT imaging to biomechanically calculate bone strength and risk of fracture. Another example

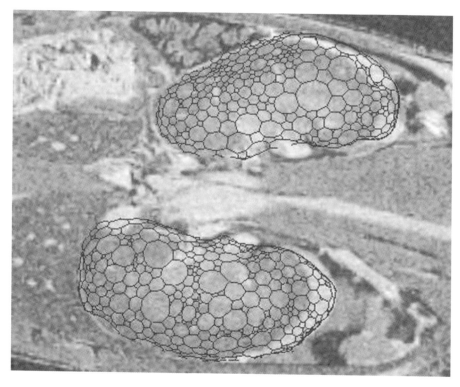

Figure 23.
Computer-aided analysis of mouse imaging in the body is more difficult than in the brain. Because of the relative freedom of motion of the organs, simple registration will not be feasible. However, adaptive shape models can be used to segment out individual organs. This figure shows kidney volumes obtained by automated shape recognition compared with manual segmentation. Automated computer analysis is promising for abdominal phenotyping (image provided by L. Baghdadi at the MICe).

is the use of vascular trees to calculate perfusion from flow models. As biological imaging is used more and more for quantitative analysis of disease and response to treatment, we will see more use of sophisticated computer algorithms to provide automated readouts.

7   Conclusions

As we have seen in this chapter, small-animal imaging, with a major focus on mouse as a genetically controllable model, already plays a major role in disease phenotyping. Clinical imaging techniques are being successfully adapted to the study of small animals. Just as different imaging modalities have complementary roles to play in clinical imaging, mouse imaging also requires complementary and even new modalities such as optical techniques to provide a full evaluation of disease phenotype. The complementary measurements of high-definition anatomy and molecular sensitivity seem to be even more divergent at the scale of small animals, and will probably find more need to be used in concert and even integrated into hybrid imaging equipment (e.g., SPECT-CT, MR-PET, etc.). Throughput and efficiency are particularly critical in animal imaging and need more development. So also does automated computer readout, but the existence of inbred strains and known genetic substrates makes this exciting area of development easier than the analysis of human data.

Already, we are seeing cancer studies in mice with time course and response to treatment using MR and CT. Cardiac function is being analyzed with UBM and MR, and can provide quantitative readouts. Normal and abnormal vascular development and its modulation with drugs can be well characterized with microCT and MR angiography. Drug uptake and bio-distributions over the whole body can be done with PET and SPECT.

As the imaging technology and methods advance, we can expect to see exponential growth in the use of imaging in drug discovery and development.

Acknowledgements

The authors acknowledge funding from the Canada Foundation for Innovation and the Ontario Innovation Trust for providing facilities along with The Hospital for Sick Children. Operating funds from the National Cancer Institute of Canada – Terry Fox Program Projects, Canadian Institutes of Health Research, the National Institutes of Health and the Ontario Research and Challenge Fund are gratefully acknowledged. This work could not have been done without the creativity and perseverance of the members of the Mouse Imaging Centre (MICe) in Toronto and the many biological collaborators who provide mice and ideas. Many colleagues, who are acknowledged in the captions, have provided figures for this chapter.

References

1 The International Human Genome Mapping Consortium (2001) A physical map of the human genome. *Nature* 409: 934–941

2 Mouse Genome Sequencing Consortium (2002) Initial sequencing and comparative analysis of the mouse genome. *Nature* 420: 520–562

3 Balaban RS, Hampshire VA (2001) Challenges in small animal noninvasive imaging. *ILAR J* 42: 248–262

4 Ciobanu L, Pennington CH (2004) 3D micron-scale MRI of single biological cells. *Solid State Nucl Magn Reson* 25: 138–141

5 Johnson GA, Cofer GP, Gewalt SL, Hedlund LW (2002) Morphologic phenotyping with MR microscopy: the visible mouse. *Radiology* 222: 789–793

6 Ford NL, Thornton MM, Holdsworth DW (2003) Fundamental image quality limits for microcomputed tomography in small animals. *Med Phys* 30: 2869–2877

7 Boone JM, Velazquez O, Cherry SR (2004) Small-animal X-ray dose from micro-CT. *Mol Imaging* 3: 149–158

8 Foster FS, Zhang MY, Duckett A, Zhou YQ, Henkelman RM, Chen J, Adamson SL (2002) Ultrasound micro-imaging of the mouse. *Med Phys* 29: 1329–1329

9 Zhou YQ, Foster FS, Qu DW, Zhang M, Harasiewicz KA, Adamson SL (2002) Applications for multifrequency ultrasound biomicroscopy in mouse from implantation to adulthood. *Physiol Genomics* 10: 113–126

10 Yang Y, Tai YC, Siegel S, Newport DF, Bai B, Li Q, Leahy RM, Cherry SR (2004) Optimization and performance evaluation of the microPET II scanner for *in vivo* small-animal imaging. *Phys Med Biol* 49: 2527–2545

11 Sharpe J, Ahlgren U, Perry P, Hill B, Ross A, Hecksher-Sorensen J, Baldock R, Davidson D (2002) Optical projection tomography as a tool for 3D microscopy and gene expression studies. *Science* 296: 541–545

12 Sharpe J (2004) Optical projection tomography. *Annu Rev Biomed Eng* 6: 209–228

13 Bock NA, Konyer NB, Henkelman RM (2003) Multiple-mouse MRI. *Magn Reson Med* 49: 158–167

14 Wong WH, Sukumar S (2000) *"Millipede" imaging coil design for high field micro imaging applications.* Proc 8th Annual Meeting ISMRM, Denver, 1399

15 Dazai J, Bock NA, Nieman BJ, Davidson LM, Henkelman RM, Chen XJ (2004) Multiple mouse biological loading and monitoring system for MRI. *Magn Reson Med* 52: 709–715

16 Nieman BJ, Bock NA, Bishop J, Sled JG, Chen XJ, Henkelman RM (2005) Fast spin-echo for multiple mouse MR phenotyping. *Magn Reson Med* 54: 532–537

17 Aoki I, Wu YJ, Silva AC, Lynch RM, Koretsky AP (2004) *In vivo* detection of neuroarchitecture in the rodent brain using manganese-enhanced MRI. *Neuroimage* 22: 1046–1059

18 Matsuda Y, Utsuzawa S, Kirimoto T, Haishi T, Yamazaki Y, Kose K, Anno I, Marutani M (2003) Super-parallel MR microscope. *Magn Reson Med* 50: 183–189

19 Xu S, Gade TP, Matei C, Zakian K, Alfieri AA, Hu X, Holland EC, Soghomonian S, Tjuvajev J, Ballon D et al. (2003) In vivo multiple-mouse imaging at 1.5 T. *Magn Reson Med* 49: 551–557

20 Schneider JE, Bhattacharya S (2004) Making the mouse embryo transparent: identifying developmental malformations using magnetic resonance imaging. *Birth Defects Res Part C Embryo Today* 72: 241–249

21 Bock NA, Zadeh G, Davidson LM, Qian B, Sled JG, Guha A, Henkelman RM (2003) High-

resolution longitudinal screening with magnetic resonance imaging in a murine brain cancer model. *Neoplasia* 5: 546–554

22   Choy G, Choyke R, Libutti SK (2003) Current advances in molecular imaging: noninvasive in vivo bioluminescent and fluorescent optical imaging in cancer research. *Mol Imaging* 2: 303–312

23   McCaffrey A, Kay MA, Contag CH (2003) Advancing molecular therapies through in vivo bioluminescent imaging. *Mol Imaging* 2: 75–86

24   Yang M, Raynoso J, Jiang P, Li L, Moossa AR, Hoffman RM (2004) Transgenic nude mouse with ubiquitous green fluorescent protein expression as a host for human *tumors. Cancer Res* 64: 8651–8656

25   Serganova I, Doubrovin M, Vide J, Ponomarev V, Soghomonyan S, Beresten T, Ageyeve L, Seganov A, Cai S, Balatoni J et al (2004) Molecular imaging of temporal dynamics and spatial heterogeneity of hypoxia-inducible factor-1 signal transduction activity in tumors in living mice. *Cancer Res* 64: 6101–6108

26   Zhou YQ, Foster FS, Nieman BJ, Davidson LM, Chen XJ, Henkelman RM (2004) Comprehensive transthoracic cardiac imaging in mice using ultrasound biomicroscopy with anatomical confirmation by magnetic resonance imaging. *Physiol Genomics* 18: 232–244

27   Mori AD, Bruneau BG (2004) TBX5 mutations and congenital heart disease: Holt-Orom syndrome revealed. *Curr Opin Cardiol* 19: 211–215

28   Zhou YQ, Davidson LM, Henkelman RM, Nieman BJ, Foster FS, Yu LX, Chen XJ (2004) Ultrasound-guided left ventricular catheterization: a novel method of whole mouse perfusion for microimaging. *Lab Invest* 84: 385–389

29   Purdie TG, Lee TY (2003) Carbon dioxide reactivity of computer tomography functional parameters in rabbit VX2 soft tissue tumour. *Phys Med Biol* 48: 849–860

30   Wiesman F, Ruff J, Engelhardt S, Hein L, Dienesch C, Leupold A, Illinger R, Frydychowicz A, Hiller KH, Rommel E et al (2001) Dobutamine-stress magnetic resonance microimaging in mice. *Circ Res* 88: 563–569

31   Kobayashi H, Shirakawa K, Kawamoto S, Saga T, Sato N, Hiraga A, Watanabe I, Heike Y, Togashi K, Konishi J et al (2002) Rapid accumulation and internalization of radiolabeled herceptin in an inflammatory breast cancer xenograft with vasculogenic mimicry predicted by the contrast-enhanced dynamic MRI with the macromolecular contrast agent G6-(1B4M-Gd)(256). *Cancer Res* 62: 860–866

32   Lu H, Patel S, Luo F, Li SJ, Hillard CJ, Ward BD, Hyde JS (2004) Spatial correlations of laminar BOLD and CBV responses to rat whisker stimulation with neuronal activity localized by Fos expression. *Magn Reson Med* 52: 1060–1068

33   Keilhotz SD, Silva AC, Raman M, Merkle H, Koretsky AP (2004) Functional MRI of the rodent somatosensory pathway using multislice echo planar imaging. *Magn Reson Med* 52: 89–99

34   Pautler RG, Koretsky AP (2002) Tracing odor-induced activation in the olfactory bulbs of mice using manganese-enhanced magnetic resonance imaging. *Neuroimaging* 16: 441–448

35   Aschner M, Aschner JL (1991) Manganese neurotoxicity: cellular effects and blood-brain barrier transport. *Neurosci Biobehav Rev* 15: 333–340

36   Meade TJ, Taylor Ak, Bull SR (2003) New magnetic resonance contrast agents as biochemical reporters. *Curr Opin Neurobiol* 13: 597–602

37   Abbey CK, Borowski AD, McGoldrick ET, Gregg JP, Maglione JE, Cardiff RD, Cherry SR (2004) In vivo positron-emission tomography imaging of progression and transformation in a mouse model of mammary neoplasia. *Proc Natl Acad Sci USA* 101: 11438–11443

38   Lickert H, Takeuchi JK, Von Both I, Walls JR, McAuliffe F, Adamson SL, Henkelman RM, Wrana JL, Rossant J, Bruneau BG (2004) Baf60c is essential for function of BAF chromatin remodeling complexes in heart development. *Nature* 432: 107–112

39   Schwarcz A, Natt O, Watanabe T, Boretius S, Frahm J, Michaelis T (2003) Localized proton MRS of cerebral metabolite profiles in different mouse strains. *Magn Reson Med* 49: 822–827

40   Naumova AV, Weiss RG, Chacko VP (2003) Regulation of murine myocardial energy metabolism during adrenergic stress studied by in vivo 31P NMR spectroscopy. *Am J Physiol Heart Circ Physiol* 285: H1976–H1979

41   Kovacevic N, Henderson J, Chen J, Henkelman M (2004) Deformation based representation of groupwise average and variability. *Lecture Notes in Computer Science* 3217: 616–622

42   Collins DL, Evans AC (1997) Animal: validation and applications of nonlinear registration-based segmentation. *Int J Pattern Recogn* 11: 1271–1294

43   Woods, RP, Grafton ST, Watson JDG, Sicotte NL, Mazziotta JC (1998) Automated image registration: II. Intersubject validation of linear and nonlinear models. *J Comput Assist Tomogr* 22: 163–165

44   Kovacevic N, Henderson JT, Chan E, Lifshitz N, Bishop J, Evans AC, Henkelman RM, Chen XJ (2005) 3D atlas of average and variability for an inbred mouse brain. *Cerebral Cortex* 15: 639–645

45   Zhang J, Miller MI, Yarowsky P, Van Zijl P, Mori S (2005) Mapping postnatal mouse brain development with diffusion tensor microimaging. *Neuroimage* 26: 1042–1051

Progress in Drug Research, Vol. 62
(Markus Rudin, Ed.)
©2005 Birkhäuser Verlag, Basel (Switzerland)

Evaluation of drug candidates: Efficacy readouts during lead optimization

By Markus Rudin[1],
Nicolau Beckmann[2]
and Martin Rausch[2]

[1]Institute for Biomedical Engineering
University of Zurich/ETH Zurich
Switzerland
<rudin@biomed.ee.ethz.com>
[2]Novartis Institute for Biomedical
Research
CH-4002 Basel
Switzerland

Glossary of abbreviations

ADC, apparent water diffusion coefficient; APP, amyloid precursor protein; BBB, blood-brain barrier; BAL, bronchoalveolar lavage; CA, contrast agents; CBF, cerebral blood flow; CBV, cerebral blood volume; CNR, contrast-to-noise ratio; COPD, chronic obstructive pulmonary disease; FDG, fluoro-dexoyglucose; FLT, 3'-fluoro-3'-deoxythymidine; fMRI, functional magnetic resonance imaging; HEP, high-energy phosphates; HIF-1, hypoxia-inducible factor-1; IHC, immunohistochemistry; MCAO, middle cerebral artery occlusion; MRS, magnetic resonance spectroscopy; MTC, magnetization transfer contrast; MTR, magnetization transfer ratios; OA, osteoarthritis; PCr, phosphocreatine; PET, positron-emission tomography; PG, proteoglycans; PK, pharmacokinetic; RA, rheumatoid arthritis; ROI, region-of-interest; rtPA, recombinant tissue plasminogen activator; SPECT, single-photon computerized tomography; TK, thymidine kinase 1; USPIO, ultrasmall particles of iron oxide.

1   The objective: Evaluation of drug efficacy and safety during lead optimization

The purpose of screening large compound libraries in high-throughput biochemical or cellular assays is the identification of chemical lead structures, which, once validated for efficacy in secondary assays, have to be optimized in several regards during the so-called lead optimization phase. Criterion for a lead compound is its 'drugability', i.e., is the structure amenable to modification that might enhance the target interaction?; is it likely to be delivered to the target site?; does the structure contain elements that might be associated to known toxicological effects? Aspects to be addressed in the lead optimization process are:

a. The binding affinity: the binding affinity to the drug target, which has to be optimized to a range of typically nanomolar activity. Different approaches are being pursued. If the structure of its molecular target is known, structure-based drug design allows defining optimal derivatization strategies of the basic molecular scaffold. Alternatively, a series of derivatives is synthesized to establish a structure-activity relationship, enabling the design of optimized drug candidates.

b. The specificity: Does the drug candidate cross-react with other potential drug targets? High specificity is envisaged to minimize the potential side-effect profile.

c. The pharmacokinetic (PK) properties: What are the rate and efficiency of absorption, the plasma half-life of the compound? Is it metabolized and how? What are the predominant routes of elimination? These parameters are commonly determined from analysis of plasma samples collected at different time points following drug administration. Knowledge of PK parameters in humans allows optimizing the dosing regimen and to reach the trough level required for pharmacological efficacy. In addition, whole-body autoradiographic analysis in rodents using radiolabeled (^{14}C or ^{3}H) compound yields information on the drug's biodistribution, enabling the estimation of drug levels in the target tissue. Similar studies can be carried out *in vivo* both in animals and humans using positron-emission tomography (PET) in combination with compounds labeled with short-lived positron-emitting nuclei (^{11}C or ^{18}F). PET biodistribution and receptor occupancy analyses have been extensively carried out for drugs acting on the central nervous system (CNS). Such application of PET are discussed in detail in by Bergström and Langström (Chapter 8 of this volume).

d. The safety profile: Any pharmacological intervention will potentially evoke side effects or even cause toxicity. It is important to detect such an undesired profile as early as possible in both *in vitro* and *in vivo* (whole animal) studies.

Many of these aspects are today handled using sophisticated *in vitro* assays, e.g., absorption from the gastrointestinal tract or penetration of other cellular membranes may be studied using an artificial membrane assay [1]. Similar, metabolic activity can be derived from a CaCO-2 cell assay. Many analogous test batteries have been developed that allow for testing potential drug candidates. Nevertheless, all these system are artificial and are at best approximations of the *in vivo* situation. There is currently no way avoiding the combined evaluation of all these aspects and the interplay thereof in the intact organism, i.e., in the animal and in animal models of human disease. The latter are indispensable tools for the identification of potential indications.

Evaluation of drug biodistribution, efficacy and safety in animals requires readout modalities that are preferentially non-invasive to be translatable to clinical phases. Imaging technologies providing structural, physiological, metabolic and more recently also molecular readouts have evolved into indispensable tools in this regard. In this chapter we illustrate the role of imaging during preclinical lead optimization. We first describe the qualitative and quantitative readouts provided by modern imaging techniques that can be used to characterize drug effects, illustrate the approaches with application from various indication areas, and finally discuss the position of imaging with regard to alternative analysis methods and potential improvements required to enhance the value of imaging for drug research and development.

2   The tools: Imaging methods for qualitative and quantitative assessment of therapy response

2.1   Mechanisms determining image contrast

Classical imaging methods allow the characterization of tissue based on morphological and morphometric readouts. The sensitivity of detecting an anatomical or pathological structure, and hence, the diagnostic value of an imaging approach, depends critically on the contrast-to-noise ratio (CNR), i.e. the ratio of the intensity difference between a specific structure and its environment divided by the average noise figure in the image.

For non-contrast-enhanced imaging techniques the signal intensity is governed by microstructural properties of the tissue, which are characteristic for the imaging modality applied: For X-ray computerized tomography (CT), X-rays are scattered at electrons in the tissue leading to an attenuation of the beam intensity, which depends on the tissue density and composition, and on the X-ray energy. Signal intensity in magnetic resonance imaging (MRI) is governed by a variety of tissue-specific parameters: the density ρ of water protons in tissue, the longitudinal and transverse relaxation rates R_1 and R_2, which relate the magnetic nuclei investigated to their magnetic environment, spin exchange processes (e.g., due to chemical reaction or due to transfer of magnetic coherence), and the microscopic (diffusion, microcirculation) and macroscopic motion (e.g., blood flow) of water in the tissue. Light propagation in tissue is diffusive, hence in diffuse optical tomography (DOT) the signal intensity, i.e., the photon flux at the detector, is determined by the scattering and absorption properties of tissue.

In many cases, this endogenous contrast is not sufficient to unambiguously identify a specific tissue structure or pathology. Contrast agents (CA) are administered to increase the CNR. Contrast enhancement is specific for the methodology applied. CT-CAs are electron-dense materials with a high X-ray scattering cross-section, leading to significant beam attenuation, while MRI-CA affect the signal intensity indirectly by increasing the water proton relaxation rates. In both cases contrast enhancement is related to the local concentration of the CA.

Both for nuclear and fluorescence/bioluminescence imaging the 'CA' administered is the only source of signal. Hence, one would expect contrast to be intrinsically high. Yet, CNR between a target tissue and its environment might still be low as the CA may accumulate in both structures. In fact, the development of probes that yield high signal-to-background ratio, i.e. a high CNR between the tissue-of-interest and its environment is a major objective of modern imaging approaches.

Nuclear imaging detects γ-rays that are emitted from a metastable radionuclide using a detector array that is arranged around the imaging object (see Chapter 2 of this volume). Spatial resolution is obtained either by geometric collimation as in the case of single-photon computerized tomography (SPECT), or by electronic collimation based on coincidence detection for PET. The intensity in the reconstructed image is in first order proportional to the local amount of the radionuclide, provided that the appropriate corrections for confounding physical events and instrumental imperfections are being made [2, 3]. Analogous to DOT, image reconstruction in fluorescence molecular tomography (FMT) has to deal with the diffusive light propagation in tissue, which corresponds to solving the inverse problem in electrodynamics. Assuming successful reconstruction, the image intensity is governed by several parameters, the attenuation and scattering of the light both at the excitation and the emission frequency, and the fluorescent properties of the probe, i.e., its concentration, fluorescence yield and lifetime. Proper image reconstruction considering these aspects should yield accurate estimates of the local dye concentration.

2.2   Deriving quantitative data from image datasets

Comparative evaluation of drug candidates requires objective quantitative or semi-quantitative readouts of treatment effects on structural, physiological, metabolic or molecular tissue parameters. In the following section we discuss methods to derive such information from imaging datasets.

2.2.1 Structural parameters

Pathologies lead to microscopic and macroscopic alteration of tissue structure, which may be reflected by and altered appearance in images, i.e., the pathological transformation of the tissue leads to changes in the respective imaging parameters. Hence, measurement of the value of the imaging parameter in a specific region-of-interest (ROI) allows staging of tissue and also the evaluation of therapy response. Typical examples are the stroke signature of ischemic tissue following cerebral infarction, or the characterization of cartilage quality in models of osteoarthritis. The stroke signature is a multi-parametric characterization of a tissue region, i.e., a tissue voxel v is described by a time-dependent parameter profile $v(T_1,T_2,ADC,CBF,...;t)$, which is of prognostic value [4, 5]. Cartilage quality is assessed by determining the magnetization transfer ratio, which reflects the integrity of the macromolecular structure (in particular collagen) [6], and contrast enhancement following administration of a charged paramagnetic CA. The amount of CA uptake by cartilage is indicative of the integrity of the proteoglycan network [7, 8].

Alternatively, a scoring system can be applied to translate an altered appearance of tissue in images into a quantitative readout, analogous to scoring methods used for histopathological analysis. Important prerequisites to minimize operator bias of such types of semi-quantitative image analysis are (1) that the interpreter is not aware of the respective treatments, and (2) that the data are analyzed by more than one interpreter. This approach has been applied, e.g., to assess the efficacy of immunosuppressive treatment in rat models of chronic rejection of kidney allografts [9].

Yet, readouts based on the morphological appearance that are of primordial importance for diagnostic imaging, are rarely used for assessment of therapy response. Far more common is the evaluation of drug efficacy based on morphometric measures such as tissue volumes, cross-sectional areas, distances, etc. The actual geometrical measurement is preceded by an image segmentation step, which allows identifying the structure-of-interest from the surrounding tissue. Segmentation can be carried out operator interactively by defining the perimeter of the structure. This approach is appropriate when CNR is not sufficient to allow for automated segmentation. High CNR values on the other hand allow for automated procedures based on intensity thresholds or more sophisticated algorithms exploiting the intensity difference between target and surrounding tissue. Alternatively, the ROI can be selected by choosing a seed point and applying of a region-growing algorithm. Once the ROI is segmented, morphometric measures can be made, e.g., the area is determined by counting the pixel in the segmented structure and multiplying by the pixel dimensions. Volumes are derived by repeating the procedures for multiple cross-sectional slices comprising the structure-of-interest and multiplying by the slice distance. Such procedures have been widely applied to determine volumes of normal and pathological organs or tissue structures [10, 11]. Other morphometric measures are distances to assess the thickness of tissue structures, e.g., of myocardial wall [12, 13] or articular cartilage [14].

2.2.2 Measurement of physiological processes and tissue metabolism

Alterations in tissue contrast due to either an endogenous contrast mechanism or to the administration of an exogenous MRI CA, fluorescent dye or radionuclide tracer reflect underlying physiological processes. The analysis of the dynamic signal enhancement yields the local concentration-time curve of the CA/tracer, which has to be interpreted within the framework of a tissue model to derive quantitative physiological parameters such as tissue perfusion rates, vascular permeability, or changes in local cerebral blood oxygenation. Physiological readouts have turned out to be sensitive indicators of the tissue state. Similarly changes in tissue metabolic activity frequently precedes structural pathology. Non-invasive measurements of glucose utilization [15], turnover of energy phosphates such as ATP [16], or studies of phospholipid metabolism [17] have been shown to be of value both for disease phenotyping and to evaluate therapy efficacy.

We illustrate here approaches to derive quantitative physiological parameters with a few selected examples. Let us consider first the case of contrast enhancement by administration of an exogenous CA, which distributes into various tissue compartments. MRI CA are paramagnetic or superparamagnetic compounds, which exhibit strong local effects on the relaxation of nearby water protons. Quantitative determination of tissue relaxivities $R_i(t)$ (= $1/T_i(t)$) as a function of time allows the estimation of the local CA concentration according to

$$R_i(t) = R_{i,0} + \sum_k r_{i,k} \cdot c_k(t) \cdot v_k \tag{1}$$

where $R_{i,0}$ with $i = 1,2$ is the tissue relaxivity prior to the administration of the CA, $r_{i,k}$ the molar relaxivity of the k-th tissue compartment, $c_k(t)$ the concentration of the CA and v_k the volume of the respective compartment. If the molar relaxivities are $r_{i,k} = r_i$ assumed to be identical for all tissue compartments, i.e., $r_{i,k} = r_i$ for all k, the average tissue concentration is obtained as

$$c(t) = v^{-1} \cdot \sum_k c_k(t) \cdot v_k = \frac{(R_i(t) - R_{i,0})}{v \cdot r_i}, \tag{2}$$

with the voxel volume $v = \sum_k v_k$. Similarly, time-activity curves recorded with PET yields local tracer concentrations when corrected for the decay properties of the radionuclide.

Quantitative physiological information is obtained from tissue models. These models commonly comprise several tissue compartments characterized by a homogenous CA/tracer concentration c_k, i.e., rapid equilibration within a compartment is assumed, and a tracer distribution volume v_k (Fig. 1). CA/tracer exchange between compartments is governed by first-order rate constants. Mathematically, these tissue models are described by a set of coupled differential equations

$$\frac{d}{dt} \mathbf{c}(t) = \mathbf{K} \cdot \mathbf{c}(t) + \mathbf{c}_{input} \tag{3}$$

where $\mathbf{c}(t)$ is the vector composed of the concentrations in the individual compartments, $\mathbf{K}$ the kinetic matrix accounting both for tracer exchange between and for chemical reactions within a compartment, while the vector $\mathbf{c}_{input}$ describes the CA/tracer input function. The CA/tracer concentration in an individual voxel is obtained as a weighted sum of the contributions $c_k(t)$ of the individual compartments contained in the voxel (eq. 2). Fitting to the experimental observations, e.g., to tissue activity-time curves and the arterial input function, yields the individual rate constants and distribution volumes, which reflect the underlying physiological processes. For instance, in the framework of the models shown in Fig. 1b, k_1^* and k_2^* describe [18F]fluoro-dexoyglucose (FDG) uptake and metabolic conversion (hexokinase activity) to [18F]FDG-6-phosphate, respectively, as a measure of metabolic activity [15]. Similarly, the rate constant k_1 in Fig. 1c accounts for the vascular leakage of a CA into the extracellular space and is a measure for the vascular permeability*surface product [18]. It has to be kept in mind that the data inter-

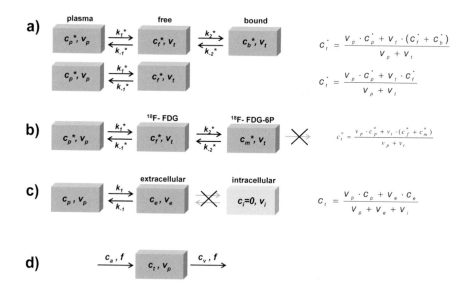

Figure 1.
Multi-compartment tissue models for assessment of receptor binding (a), uptake and metabolism of ^{18}F-FDG (b), extravasation of a contrast agent (c), and local tissue perfusion (d). In (a) the upper scheme describes, e.g., a brain region expressing the receptor, while the lower case is a reference region not expressing the target. Assuming blood-tissue exchange to be identical for the various brain regions, the combined analysis of the two cases will increase the robustness of the fitting procedure. b) ^{18}F-FDG is taken up by tissue and phosphorylated to ^{18}F-FDG-6-phosphate (^{18}F-FDG-6P) by hexokinase. ^{18}F-FDG-6P is not further processed and is trapped in tissue as an indicator of glucose utilization. (c) MR CA such as Gd-DTPA leak out of the vascular bed into the extracellular space; however, it does not penetrate into the cells. Signal enhancement is proportional to the extravasated CA and thus an indicator for the vascular permeability. (d) Intravascular markers enter tissue through an artery, are distributed through the capillary system and collected by draining veins. Analysis of the tracer concentration in tissue yields information on local perfusion values according to the tracer dilution model.

pretation is only as good as the underlying tissue models. Models are commonly chosen to be as simple as possible to minimize the number of independent model parameters, yet to still give a reasonable description of the experimental data. For instance, when deriving glucose utilization data using the FDG techniques, the two substrates are competing for the glucose transporter and hexokinase. This implies that reactions of the unlabeled substrate have to be considered when analyzing FDG results. In addition, it has to be considered that the kinetic constants for the FDG reactions (k_i^*, eq. 5) are not identical to those for the glucose reaction (k_i, eq. 5). When computing the glucose utilization rate vGluMR using the model shown in Figure 1b, this can be accounted for by correcting the values derived from the FDG experiment using a so-called lumped constant LC, yielding

$$v_{GluMR} = \frac{k_1 \cdot k_2}{k_{-1} + k_2} \cdot c_p(t) = \frac{1}{LC} \cdot \frac{k_1^* \cdot k_2^*}{k_{-1}^* + k_2^*} \cdot c_p(t) \qquad (4)$$

$c_p(t)$ being the glucose concentration in plasma [19].

Tissue perfusion is a critical parameter for proper tissue function; therefore, methods to quantitatively assess local blood flow values have been developed quite early. Perfusion values are commonly derived from so-called indicator dilution experiments using tracers that are confined to the vascular compartment [20]: The intravascular CA enters the tissue-of-interest via a feeding artery, distributes through the capillary network and is collected by a draining vein. Comparing the tracer concentration profiles in both artery and vein allows the estimation of the mean transit time $\bar{t}$, from which the perfusion rate f can be estimated according to

$$f = \frac{v_p}{\bar{t}} \ . \qquad (5)$$

Estimation of perfusion rates requires knowledge of the tissue blood volume v_p. MR bolus tracking experiments are based on this principle, the measurement of local contrast enhancement being proportional to the capillary concentration of the CA. Quantitative perfusion rates f can be derived from the measured concentration-time curve in tissue $c_t(t)$ provided the arterial input function $c_a(t)$ is known [21],

$$f = \frac{1}{\rho} \cdot \left(\frac{1 - H_{artery}}{1 - H_{capillary}} \right) \cdot \left(\int_0^\infty c_t(t) \cdot dt \right) \cdot \left(\int_0^\infty c_a(t) \cdot dt \right)^{-1} , \qquad (6)$$

ρ being the density of the tissue, and H_{artery} and $H_{capillary}$ the respective hematocrit values. Quantitative perfusion values are of high diagnostic values and have also been used to evaluate therapy efficacy.

Administration of exogenous compound may potentially cause adverse reactions and hence influence the physiological parameters to be measured. This is less an issue for nuclear imaging approaches that use radioligands at tracer concentration. In contrast to nuclear and fluorescent imaging, MRI allows the use of labeling strategies that do not involve the administration of a exogenous CA, thereby eliminating any potential disturbance of the physiology. This is achieved by either applying magnetic labeling techniques or

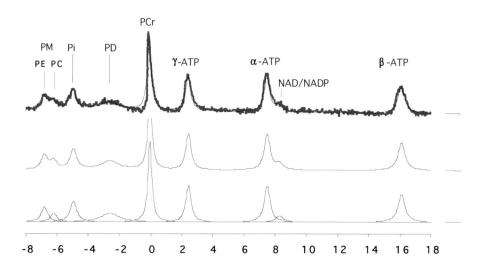

Figure 2.
Phosphorus (^{31}P) MR spectrum of rat brain displaying resonances of phosphomonoesters (PM), phos-phorylethanolamine (PE), and phosphorylcholine (PC), pyrophosphate (Pi), phosphodiesters (PD), phosphocreatine (PCr) and α-, β-, and γ-resonances of nucleoside triphosphates including ATP. Curve fitting using Lorentzian line shapes has been applied to determine signal intensities. The fine line in the upper spectrum and the middle trace show the fitted spectrum, the bottom trace the individual signals.

by exploiting endogenous contrast mechanisms due to paramagnetic com-pounds such as deoxy-hemoglobin. Magnetic labeling involves generation of non-equilibrium longitudinal magnetization: the lifetime of the labeled state is governed by longitudinal relaxation R_1, i.e., processes to be studies are char-acterized by time constants τ in the range $0.1 = \tau \cdot R_1 = 10$. The most common example using this concept are perfusion measurements based on the so-called arterial spin labeling method. Briefly, arterial water proton spins are magnetically labeled in a plane proximal to the actual imaging plane by applying either a saturation or inversion pulse. The labeled spins enter the imaging plane after a delay $\Delta (\propto \tau)$, causing an attenuation of the observed sig-nal, which is proportional to the local perfusion rate f. The signal in the imag-ing plane is governed by R_1 relaxation and tissue perfusion according to [22]

$$\frac{M_{steady-state}}{M_o} = (R_1 + \frac{f}{\lambda}) \cdot \left[R_1 + \frac{f}{\lambda} \cdot (1 - \exp\{-R_1 \cdot \Delta\}) \right] \qquad (7)$$

with λ being the blood-tissue distribution coefficient of water. Knowledge of R_1 values and of λ allows the determination of tissue perfusion in a completely non-invasive manner. In a refined analysis, cross-relaxation between bulk and macromolecular-bound water within the tissue compartment also has to be included [23].

Changes in local MRI signal intensity might also be caused by endogenous paramagnetic compounds, which change concentration due to alterations in the physiological state of the tissue. The best known example is blood oxygenation level-dependent (BOLD) contrast [24]. While oxygenated hemoglobin (HbO_2) is diagmagnetic, its deoxygenated form (Hb) is paramagnetic. The effect of deoxy-hemoglobin on the R_2 relaxivity of tissue water is given by [25]

$$R_2(t) = R_{20} + \alpha \cdot \gamma \cdot v_p \cdot (1 - Y(t)) \cdot \Delta\chi \cdot B_0 \qquad (8)$$

with α being a proportionality constant, γ the gyromagnetic ratio of the proton, v_p the blood volume fraction, (1-Y) the fraction of intravascular deoxy-hemoglobin, $\Delta\chi$ the susceptibility difference between fully oxygenated and deoxygenated blood, and B_0 the static magnetic field. Increasing the ratio $[HbO_2]/[Hb] = Y/(1-Y)$ leads to a decrease in water relaxivity R_2 (and R_2^*) and hence to a signal increase in T_2-weighted MRI experiments. This is the basis of functional MRI (fMRI) methods to assess brain activity: Increased neuronal activity prompts an increase in local perfusion rates via the neuro-vascular coupling. The increased oxygen supply exceeds the oxygen extraction by activated brain parenchyma, leading to an increase of the ratio $Y/(1-Y)$ and to a decrease of R_2. fMRI studies have, e.g., been applied to assess the functional plasticity of the brain [26] and to study functional recovery in cytoprotected cerebral tissue following focal cerebral ischemia [27].

Similar to physiological changes, metabolic responses have been shown to be a sensitive indicator of pathology and of therapy response. We have briefly discussed the non-invasive assessment of tissue glucose utilization as a measure of energy turnover using PET in combination with the glucose substrate ^{18}F-FDG. Deoxyglucose and its fluorinated analogue FDG are taken up by tissue via the glucose transporter and phosphorylated by hexokinase; however, it is not further processed along the glycolytic cascade [28]. FDG accumulation in tissue is therefore considered an indicator of glucose utilization, and frequently used to assess neuronal activity or glycolytic activity in highly proliferating tissue. Energy consumption can be directly studied by measuring levels and fluxes of high-energy phosphates (HEP) using phosphorus (^{31}P) magnetic resonance spectroscopy (MRS). Tissue levels of the HEP adenosine triphosphate (ATP) and phosphocreatine (PCr) and the degradation product pyrophosphate are obtained by determining the intensity of the corresponding spectral signals (Fig. 2). Due to the relatively poor spectral resolution, i.e., overlapping signals, spectral deconvolution procedures are required for accurate intensity measurements. Deconvolution algorithms have been developed both for the spectral [29] and in the time domain [30]. In addition, signal intensities have to be corrected for relaxation effects unless spectra are recorded under fully relaxed conditions. ^{31}P MRS has been extensively applied in drug research, in particular at the preclinical level [11, 31]. Steady-state levels of HEP turned out to be poor indicators of the tissue metabolic state: energy metabolism is highly regulated with production matching energy consumption, and drastic challenges are required to induce alteration in ATP levels. Direct measurement of energy turnover rates has been shown to provide superior sensitivity. This can be achieved using the magnetic labeling techniques described, measuring the exchange of longitudinal non-equilibrium magnetization between two compounds coupled by a chemical reaction, e.g., the transfer of a phosphate group between ATP and PCr via the creatine kinase reaction. Such magnetization transfer techniques allow the determination of reaction rates and substrate fluxes [16] and have been applied to assess the effect of drugs on the energy metabolism in heart [32] and brain [33, 34].

Alterations in cell metabolic activity such as abnormal cell proliferation or lipid metabolism have also been probed by measuring either DNA or protein synthesis rates or membrane turnover. PET-based approaches use radio-labeled precursor molecules such as thymidine analogues [35], fluorinated amino acids [36], and ^{11}C- [37] or ^{18}F-labeled choline [38]. These readouts of proliferative activity have been shown to provide valuable prognostic information in oncological indications, and have been used to evaluate tumor therapies. Alternatively, membrane turnover can be assessed using MRS techniques [17].

The most recent addition to the arsenal of imaging technologies are molecular imaging methods that allow the study of molecular processes in the intact organism, i.e., the annotation of structural data with molecular signatures. Molecular imaging approaches are characterized by high demands on sensitivity, as the molecular targets are present in low concentration, on specificity to distinguish the targeted interaction from non-specific background signals, and spatial resolution, in particular when considering applications in small rodents. As no imaging methods meets all these criteria, a molecular imaging facility has to comprise multiple imaging modalities The combined use of these technologies provides unique information on the expression of a potential drug target (e.g., a receptor or an enzyme), on the PK properties and receptor interaction of potential drug candidates, on the target activation due to the drug-target interaction (e.g., the activation of a signaling cascade), and on the migratory properties of labeled cells. These methods are extensively discussed in Chapters 3, 4 and 8, and we only briefly describe some examples in the context of the applications mentioned.

3 Imaging applications during lead optimization: Selected examples

In discussing imaging applications during lead optimization, we focus on pre-clinical drug evaluations since the results of such studies contributes the basis for decision making on further development of potential drug candidates in man. In the last decade this field has grown tremendously and it is beyond the scope of this chapter to provide a comprehensive review. Instead we select a few examples to illustrate the application of imaging technologies to document therapy efficacy in animal models of human disease and to assist translation of drug candidates into clinical development.

3.1 CNS disorders

Brain is not accessible to biopsies, therefore, the diagnosis and characterization of cerebral disorders using traditional techniques is based in secondary readouts such as neurological deficits or behavioral abnormalities, and ultimately on post-mortem histological analysis of brain specimens. It is not surprising that non-invasive imaging methods providing structural, functional and molecular information have become important tools both for disease phenotyping, i.e. diagnosis of CNS pathologies, and for the evaluation of therapeutic interventions. In fact, the number of imaging studies referring to the brain outnumbers those to any other organ. In the subsequent sections we describe the use of imaging for the development of drugs addressing neurovascular, neurodegenerative and neuroinflammatory disorders.

3.1.1 Evaluation of anti-ischemic drug in models of cerebral ischemia

Stroke is a leading cause of death in industrialized nations. Today, the only clinically approved treatment is thrombolysis using recombinant tissue plasminogen activator (rtPA) [39, 40]. Only a very small fraction of stroke patients (~5%) is amenable to rtPA treatment. This illustrates the high medical need to develop novel pharmacological therapies to alleviate the severe consequences of a cerebral ischemic insult for the patients. While the pathophysiological cascade leading to reversible tissue necrosis in human embolic stroke is quite well understood [41, 42], translation of this knowledge into efficacious clinical therapy concepts has not been successful up to now, despite many promising preclinical results. The reason for these failures are manifold, the discussion of which is beyond the scope of this article.

Focal cerebral ischemia is caused by transient or permanent occlusion of a major cerebral artery. Cessation of local perfusion and thereby supply of oxygen and nutrients initiates a cascade of detrimental effects, which lead to loss of function and ultimately to necrosis of affected brain areas [41, 42]. Lack of oxygen and glucose lead to energy failure within minutes due to the shut-down of aerobic ATP synthesis. Energy depletion affects all energy-dependent processes of the cell, including membrane pumps required to maintain ion homeostasis, and intracellular signaling cascades via ATP-dependent protein kinases. A consequence of failing ATP-dependent membrane pumps is the accumulation of intracellular Ca^{2+}, prompting a cascade of disastrous downstream events for the cell: loss of $[Ca^{2+}]_i$ regulation ultimately leads to cell death. Failure of membrane pumps causes the concentration gradients of Na^+ and K^+ to break down, leading to membrane depolarization. The altered ion distribution changes the cellular osmolality, prompting a massive inflow of water into the cells (cytotoxic edema). Additional relevant factors ultimately leading to tissue necrosis are excitatory neurotransmitters such as glutamate. Inactivation of glutamate via glial and neuronal uptake is energy dependent; hence, during energy failure glutamate accumulates leading to exhaustive neuronal stimulation. Elevated glutamate levels cause opening of receptor-operated Ca^{2+} channels (NMDA receptors), and correspondingly contribute to the increased $[Ca^{2+}]_i$ levels with the consequences already mentioned. In addition, glutamate interaction with metabotropic glutamate receptors (mGluR) activates second-messenger-mediated signal transduction processes via GTP binding proteins. Glutamate-induced spreading depressions are believed to play a relevant role with regard to infarct growth [43, 44]. In models of focal cerebral ischemia the transient changes in the apparent water diffusion coefficient (ADC) observed during spreading depression does not fully recover, leading to an overall growth of the ischemic lesion [44]. In addition to these acute effects, delayed infarct growth due to recruitment of penumbral regions has been observed at time points beyond 48 h after infarction. This delayed loss of neurons is due to apoptosis [45], which is commonly associated with neuroinflammation due to the proximity of apoptotic neurons and immune-competent cells [46].

Potential therapeutic interventions target the individual processes of the pathophysiological cascade and the molecular targets involved. It is obvious that long-term tissue survival is only be achieved following restoration of blood supply to the ischemic lesion, i.e., either be recanalization of the occluded vessel by thrombolysis or by enhancing collateral blood supply. As already stated, recanalization by administration of rtPA is currently the only approved treatment for acute stroke, provided it can be applied within 3 h following stroke onset [39, 40, 47]. A second therapeutic strategy is to reduce Ca^{2+} influx via voltage-gated channels by administration of Ca^{2+} channel blockers. Such treatments have shown remarkable efficacy in animal models of focal cerebral ischemia [48, 49]. Control of $[Ca^{2+}]_i$ levels can also been achieved via inhibition of receptor-operated channels such as the N-methyl-D-aspartate (NMDA) channel. Neuroprotective efficacy in rat stroke models has been demonstrated for a number of non-competitive [50] and competitive NMDA antagonists [51, 52]. Other compound classes evaluated were glycine antagonists [53, 54], glycine being a NMDA receptor co-agonist, prevention of excitotoxicity using antagonists of the α-amino-3-hydroxy-5-methyl-isoxazole-4-propionate (AMPA) receptor [55, 56], free radical scavengers such as the so-called lazaroids [57], death protease inhibitors preventing apoptotic cell loss [58, 59] or anti-inflammatory treatment [60–63]. More recently, tissue repair strategies using neuronal stem or progenitor cells have been proposed: treatment with either stem cells [64] or fetal neural grafts

[65] in a rat stroke model resulted in a significantly improved neurological outcome.

Today, imaging techniques, and in particular MRI based methods, have been developed to visualize individual aspects of the pathophysiological cascade both in humans and in animals, which are the focus of our discussion. High resolution MR angiography detects the initial event, the occlusion of a cerebral artery [66]. The ensuing perfusion deficit in the ischemic area is identified by applying perfusion-sensitive imaging methods such as MRI [22, 67, 68]. Ischemia-associated hypoxia leads to increased levels of deoxy-hemoglobin and correspondingly to increase R_2^* relaxivity. Areas of decreased oxygen tension can be detected using susceptibility-weighted MRI [69]. Energy depletion leads to the failure of membrane pumps, altered cellular osmolality, and as a consequence to the formation of a cytotoxic edema in the ischemic tissue region. Redistribution of water between the extracellular and intracellular tissue compartment affects the ADC, which is the weighted average of the two contributions. Areas with altered ADC can be detected acutely following infarction by applying diffusion-sensitive imaging methods [70]. It has been shown that diffusion-weighted MRI provides an early reliable readout of cerebral infarction [71, 72], even at a stage, where tissue damage is still reversible [73]. Breakdown of the blood-brain barrier (BBB) is revealed by contrast-enhanced MRI following the administration of extracellular CA that do not cross the intact BBB such as Gd-DTPA. The formation of a vasogenic edema leads to an increase of tissue water, which is reflected by altered MRI tissue parameters, most characteristically by an increase in the T_2 relaxation time. In fact, infarct volume derived from T_2-weighted MR images are commonly used to evaluate treatment efficacy [11, 48]. More recently, imaging strategies to visualize inflammatory events during the post-acute phase have been developed. Inflammatory processes are characterized by recruitment of immune-competent cells, such as lymphocytes and monocytes, to the lesion site. These cells of the monocyte phagocytotic system (MPS) are often found at the border of ischemic/necrotic tissue. Ultrasmall particles of iron oxide (USPIO) have been developed as CA for visualization of structures with phagocytotic function such as the spleen or lymph nodes [74], these nanoparticles are efficiently internalized by monocytes/ macrophages via absorptive endocytosis and can be applied to track such cells. Application of the approach to models of permanent [75] and transient middle cerebral artery occlusion (MCAO) [76] in rats displayed massive infiltration of blood-borne monocytes to areas of focal ischemia revealing ongoing inflammatory activity.

Imaging methods have been widely applied to characterize the efficacy of anti-ischemic drugs targeting various phenotypic readouts of cerebral ischemia.

3.1.1.1 Metabolic readouts of efficacy

Due to the vital role of energy metabolism for proper tissue function, non-invasive ^{31}P MRS has been applied to monitor levels of HEP such as ATP and PCr. Cerebral HEP synthesis not matching HEP consumption ultimately leads to energy failure, brain dysfunction, and ultimately to tissue necrosis. During global cerebral ischemia PCr levels disappear within 2 min following cessation of blood flow, while ATP reservoirs are depleted within typically 4 min [77]. Intracellular pH values drop from a normal value of pH 7.15 to values around pH 6.5, depending on the resting blood glucose levels [77–79]. Pretreatment with cytoprotective compounds delays ATP depletion and acidosis significantly [77]. Yet, HEP levels are of limited value as an indicator of tissue state, in particular when studying milder forms of ischemia/hypoxia: as long as their synthesis rate is capable of accounting for the energy consumption, HEP levels remain unchanged. HEP turnover, on the other hand, has to match the demands due to tissue function; therefore, assessment of turnover rates should provide superior sensitivity to metabolic stress. This has been demonstrated in normal rat brain that was exposed to varying 'workloads': cerebral steady-state ATP levels were not responsive to alterations in energy consumption; however, there was a high correlation between the forward rate constant for the creatine kinase reaction (as measure for ATP turnover) and the integrated cerebral electrical activity [34]. A similar correlation has been observed for the glucose perfused rat heart [32]. Kinetic information has been derived from magnetization transfer experiments monitoring the transfer of a magnetic label between to reaction partners [16, 32, 80, 81]. Applying this concept, it could be demonstrated that calcium antagonists reduce HEP turnover both in the normoxic and ischemic brain [33].

MRS studies, while providing valuable mechanistic information, are limited by lack of sensitivity, small dynamic range, and poor spatial resolution, Therefore, MRS has played a minor role in the management of stroke patients and for the development of novel anti-ischemic therapies. In contrast, MRI methods have emerged as an indispensable tool to identify and stage cerebral ischemic tissue. Today, MRI can be applied to visualize different phases of the pathophysiological cascade of stroke, from the initial vascular occlusion visualized by MR angiography [66] to the chronic phase involving neuroinflammatory [75, 76] and apoptotic processes. Application of functional MRI methods allows this comprehensive structural and physiological characterization to be complemented by readouts of CNS function [3, 82].

3.1.1.2 Structural readouts of efficacy

Most of the preclinical studies evaluating drug efficacy are based on morphometric readouts in focal cerebral ischemia models. The underlying assumption is that reduction of the structural damage, i.e., reduction of the infarct volume, will necessarily translate into an improved behavioral or correspondingly clinical outcome. In other words, infarct volume serves as efficacy biomarker. The classical MRI method for assessment of cerebral infarct volume is based on T_2 contrast: formation of a vasogenic edema leads to significantly elevated T_2 values, providing a good demarcation between ischemic and intact tissue [11, 48, 83]. An excellent correlation between infarct volumes determined *in vivo* using T_2-weigthed MRI and lesion volume derived from histology has been demonstrated [84].

From a patient management point-of-view T_2-weighted MRI is of limited value as cerebral tissue displaying an increased T_2 value is already irreversibly damaged. Earlier indicators that provide a significant contrast for tissue that is still salvageable would be highly relevant for evaluation of drug efficacy. Readouts proposed are the ADC in brain parenchyma and local perfusion rates. Assessment of cerebral blood flow (CBF) identifies hypo-perfused brain regions immediately. In rat focal cerebral ischemia models perfusion deficits have been visualized within seconds after occlusion of a major brain artery such as the MCA [72]. Similarly, the formation of a cytotoxic edema is an early event in the pathophysiological cascade. Cytotxic edema is reflected by a redistribution of water between the intra- and extracellular compartments. As the extracellular diffusibility exceeds the intracellular one ($D_{ex} < D_{in}$), an increase in the intracellular volume fraction due to cytotoxic edema causes a decrease of the ADC, which constitutes the weighted average of the two contributions. Decreases in cerebral ADC values occur within minutes after onset of ischemia [85], i.e., diffusion-weighted MRI detects early microstructural changes following an ischemic insult. More importantly even, it has been demonstrated at least in animal models of global [86] and focal ischemia

[87] that ADC changes are reversible: in both cases reperfusion led to normalization of ADC values that were decreased during the ischemic episode.

These early ischemia markers (ADC, CBF) are potentially of predictive value with regard to the final infarct volume. For instance, in the rat unilateral permanent MCAO model, the extent of the lesion as derived from CBF maps recorded 1 h post infarction (based on relative CBF values in the ischemic region that were significantly smaller than contralateral values) predicted the outcome at 48 h with good accuracy for untreated animals [5]. In contrast, the ischemic regions as derived from maps of ADC and T_2 significantly grew between 1 h and 48 h post infarction. This has been also reported in clinical stroke: a significant perfusion/diffusion mismatch, with the 'perfusion lesion' being larger than that derived from ADC maps, implied significant growth of the ADC lesion [88].

Pathological brain regions are characterized by deviations of MRI parameters from 'normality' (Fig. 3). Needless to say, that this procedure is to some extent arbitrary. How much must T_2 values deviate from normality to be identified as abnormal? This depends on a variety of factors such as the general signal-to-noise ratio of the image and the morphological heterogeneity of the corresponding brain area. Moreover, clinical stroke is highly heterogeneous, and spontaneous re-canalization may occur with profound influence on the evolution of the MRI parameters and thus their prognostic quality, while in animal models rather homogeneous conditions can be achieved. Accurate volume determinations depend on a high CNR between infarcted and healthy brain parenchyma: this is commonly provided by T_2-weighted images recorded 24 or 48 h following infarction. A considerable number of drug candidates have been evaluated using this approach [11]. Alternatively, contrast based on other MRI parameters (ADC, CBF) has been used for the identification of the ischemic territory. This enables the estimation of the final infarct volume in the absence of treatment, prior to the onset of drug treatment.

3.1.1.3 Assessment of drug efficacy using functional readouts

It should not be forgotten that the objective of stroke therapy is not to reduce infract volume but to improve the clinical outcome for the patient, i.e., to preserve/restore brain functionality. Cytoprotective therapy using a variety of pharmacological strategies has been demonstrated to reduce the volume of infarction in animal models of focal cerebral ischemia. Demonstration that

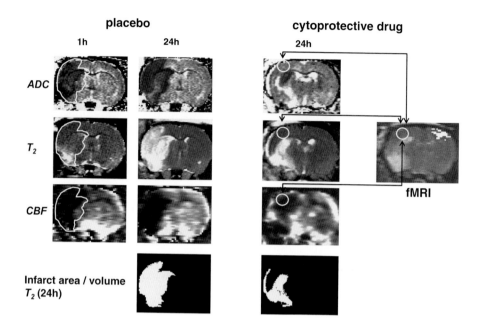

Figure 3.
Multi-parametric characterization of focal cerebral infarction in the rat due to MCAO. Shown are maps of the ADC, transverse relaxation time (T_2), and regional CBF. The images of a placebo-treated animal display the evolution of the 'MRI lesion' between 1 and 24 h following the MCAO. While ADC and CBF maps recorded after 1 h predict the lesion size measured at 24 h (white contour), the T_2 lesion is hardly observable at this early time point. Treatment with the dihydropyridine calcium antagonist isradipine significantly reduced the infarct volume as revealed by the segmented images shown in the bottom row. Analysis of the functional responsiveness of the cytoprotected somato-sensory cortex using fMRI in combination with a forepaw stimulation paradigm displayed compromised fMRI activity for this animal, despite structural integrity of the brain area (ADC, T_2). This is probably due to reduced CBF values in corresponding cortical area as compared to the contralateral side, which displays a normal fMRI response.

these regions are functional would be evidence that the assessment of the infarct volume is a valid efficacy biomarker for anti-ischemic therapy. Studies in rats that had undergone permanent MCAO and treatment with calcium antagonists confirmed the hypothesis only in part: at days 5–12 following MCAO some recovery of the function was observed; however, only a fraction of the animals showed a fully recovered fMRI response, while the remaining animals of the drug-treated group displayed no cerebral blood volume (CBV) response at all. In all animals, significant reduction of the infarct volume was found as compared to placebo-treated animals, in particular the somato-sensory cortex was spared from becoming necrotic [27, 89]. Obviously, structural integrity is a necessary, yet not sufficient, prerequisite for functional integrity (Fig. 3). The different responses have been attributed to differences in the CBF values in the cytoprotected territory [27]: CBF is sufficient to ensure survival of cells but not sufficient in all cases to ensure proper functionality.

3.1.1.4 Cell tracking to assess efficacy of cell-based therapies

Two factors contribute to the attractiveness of using MRI techniques for cell tracking studies: (1) the high temporo-spatial resolution provided by MRI, and (2) the potentially high payloads of labels that can be achieved for a cell without affecting its vital functions. Cell trafficking studies can be applied to qualitatively monitor the migration of cells within the intact organism. Quantitative analysis is feasible by either measuring the volume occupied by the labeled cells [90] or by estimation of local cell densities via quantitative analysis of relaxation effects or fluorescence intensity. Such readout will become relevant for assessing the efficacy of both inflammatory or (stem) cell-based therapies [91, 92].

3.1.2 Evaluation of therapy concepts for targeting neurodegeneration: Alzheimer's disease

Diagnosis of Alzheimer's disease (AD) is based on test batteries evaluating the cognitive performance of a patient. Reliable diagnosis is currently only possible post mortem, by identification of the pathological hallmarks of AD, the deposits consisting of β-amyloid peptides (Aβ plaques) and neurofibrillary tangles composed of tau protein. Visualization of these deposits under *in vivo* conditions would therefore be of high diagnostic relevance.

Attempts to visualize plaques by exploiting the intrinsic contrast to the surrounding parenchyma both in tissue specimen from humans [93] and from transgenic mice [94, 95] have turned out to be problematic due to unrealistic measurement times as a result of the high demands on spatial resolution. In a recent study in amyloid precursor protein (APP)-presenilin (PS) double-transgenic mice carrying both the mutant genes for APP and PS, Aβ plaques could be visualized using both spin-echo and gradient-echo pulse sequences at 9.4 T. Typical data acquisition times were 1–1.5 h [96]. All these studies demonstrated that high spatial resolution with voxel volumes of less than ($100\ \mu m^3$) is required to visualize plaques in brain parenchyma, rendering translation into a clinical setting difficult due to constraints in measurement time and sensitivity.

An alternative concept is to amplify plaque-related signals by administering Aβ-specific CA. Several MRI approaches have been reported. However, they suffer from a principal problem: they require breaking of the BBB, e.g., with mannitol, to allow the bulky reporter molecules to penetrate the brain parenchyma [97]. In this regard, approaches that use plaque-specific PET ligands [98] or fluorescent dyes [99] seem more promising. These tracers have been shown to readily cross the intact BBB and specifically label Aβ plaques. While the fluorescent dye has yielded promising results in transgenic mice, it is of limited value for clinical applications due to insufficient light penetration through the human skull. From a clinical perspective, plaque-selective PET ligands seem to be the most promising imaging agent for visualization and quantification of the plaque load in humans.

Quantification of the plaque load is considered highly attractive for diagnosis, disease staging, and therapy evaluation. Nevertheless, it has been reported that the correlation between Aβ plaque load and clinical status in AD patients is rather weak, i.e., significant plaque deposition was observed in completely unsymptomatic elderly people [100]. To what extent quantitative assessment of plaque load constitutes a reliable biomarker of therapy efficacy in AD remains to be shown.

In view of the difficulty of direct visualization of the primary morphological hallmarks of AD, a number of methods that probe secondary structural changes have been developed. Advanced disease is characterized by substantial loss of neurons reflected by massive cerebral atrophy. APP23 mice, a transgenic AD model in which the APP precursor protein is overexpressed, develop characteristic neuropathological features of AD such as Aβ deposits [101, 102]. These pathomorphological alterations occur in an age-dependent manner and are associated with behavioral and learning deficits [103, 104]. In these animals cerebral atrophy became obvious only in old animals during advanced disease, and was found to be of little prognostic value for evaluating pharmacological interventions. Alternative approaches are based on the quantitative assessment of MRI parameters susceptible to micro-structural changes in brain parenchyma due to plaque and tangle formation. Changes in regional brain MR relaxation times have been observed in two murine models of AD: transgenic APP-PS mice, which express high levels of Aβ in several brain regions, displayed decreased T_2 values in these areas. On the other hand, cerebral T_2 values in mice carrying only a mutant gene for PS, which show subtly elevated levels of Aβ without Aβ deposition were not significantly different from those observed in control animals [105]. These results indicate that T_2 might constitute a sensitive marker of parenchymal abnormalities due to massive deposition of insoluble Aβ. Similarly, the ADC in brain parenchyma should reflect the extracellular deposition of Aβ plaques: restrictions to interstitial fluid diffusion should translate into a reduction of the tissue ADC. Significantly decreased ADC values were observed in cortical regions of APP23 mice that displayed high numbers of insoluble Aβ plaques as compared to wild-type animals [106]. A final example of a secondary readout: it has been described that AD-related vasculopathies also affects lager vessels, including the principal feeding arteries of the brain. Studies in 24-month-old APP23 mice using MR angiography revealed significant flow abnormalities in vessels such as the circle of Willis or the MCA of transgenic animals, findings that were confirmed by post-mortem analysis using vessel casting techniques [107].

A common feature of these various morphological phenotyping approaches, except for the target-specific imaging methods probing the plaque load of the mice, is their lack of sensitivity. Reliable deviations from normal values (brain atrophy, ADC, T_2, vascular defects) are only observed in advanced disease states, i.e., in old animals.

In AD, early symptoms comprise functional (cognitive) deficits, which appear prior to gross-morphological alterations of associated brain regions [96]. Hence, functional neuroimaging might detect alterations of neuronal function before anatomical abnormalities become detectable in structural images. fMRI was applied to APP23 mice of various ages to evaluate the response to standardized challenges in comparison to age-matched wild-type animals. The stimuli comprised pharmacological stimulation using the $GABA_A$ receptor antagonist bicuculline, physiological stimulation by inducing hypercapnia, and electrical stimulation of the hind paws. All three stimulation paradigms evoked CBV responses in 15- and 24-month-old APP23 mice that were significantly smaller when compared to age-matched wild-type mice [108, 109]. In young animals of 6–8 months, there was no difference between the transgenic and wild-type group. Data analysis revealed that the impaired response in transgenic mice might be due to a compromised vascular reserve capacity caused by the severe cerebral amyloid angiopathy

(CAA) found in this model – and in AD patients [110, 111]: perivascular Aβ deposits impair the ability of the cerebral arteriolar and/or capillary compartment to effectively regulate CBF. In fact, the age dependence of the fMRI response correlated rather with the time course of CAA than with the increase parenchymal Aβ plaque load.

Currently, imaging techniques have hardly been used for preclinical drug evaluation in models of AD. This is due to the fact that the commonly used structural methods showed limited sensitivity, changes becoming only detectable during advanced disease stages. It is to be anticipated that molecular readouts providing selective information on the plaque load will change the picture. In particular, the fluorescent oxazine dye that selectively binds to Aβ plaques is of high interest, providing a rapid semi-quantitative readout using planar reflectance imaging [99] or potentially quantitative information when using fluorescence molecular imaging methods [112].

3.1.3 Assessing the efficacy of drugs for treatment of neuroinflammatory processes or diseases

Inflammatory processes can be triggered by several diseases of the CNS. In general, inflammation is not just the response to viral or bacterial infection, but also to antigens that have been presented or released by an organ as a consequence of a pathological event. Antigens may be degradation products produced by affected tissue following, e.g., stroke, hemorrhage or tissue loss due to neurodegeneration. Autoimmunity will prompt an immune-response aiming at the elimination of the source of the antigen. In the majority of CNS diseases, inflammation is regarded as a factor that aggravates tissue damage. One representative example is stroke, where cell necrosis within the core of the lesion might extent to adjacent tissue regions due to inflammatory factors (cytokines, chemokines) released by the injured tissue [113–115]. These factors induce the accumulation of lymphocytes, which by triggering a cascade of deleterious events may lead to delayed tissue damage despite the restoration of cerebral perfusion. However, since the main tissue damage is clearly due to metabolic stress, and since the role of inflammation could not be entirely elucidated, the development of anti-inflammatory drugs has always played a subordinated role in the treatment of ischemic or neurodegenerative CNS disorders.

In autoimmune diseases, however, inflammatory processes represent the major cause of tissue damage, and hence they are the main target for the development of treatment regimes. Multiple sclerosis (MS) represents the most relevant example for this class of diseases, and so far drug development was strongly focused on this disease [116].

In MS, the myelin sheath, which covers the axons of neurons and which is important for the fast transmission of action potentials from the soma to the synapses, is recognized as antigen by T lymphocytes (T cells). The T cells initiate an immune response, which attracts and activates macrophages and leads to a destruction of the myelin, and in later stages to axonal degradation. Since the capacity of remyelination is limited, this process cannot be reversed, which results in an aggravation of tissue damage over months and years, and finally leads to motor and cognitive impairment in MS patients. Several avenues have been pursued to prevent the immune attack on the myelin sheath, ranging from limiting the access of T cells to CNS to the modulation of T cell function.

Imaging techniques used so far for studying the burden of disease, or the effect of treatment in MS patients, have been focused on the indirect visualization of inflammation and tissue damage rather than monitoring the accumulation or function of T cells directly. MRI offers some opportunities to measure secondary effects of T cell infiltration, such as increased BBB permeability, sclerosis, scare formation or atrophy [117–119]. These parameters have been studied extensively in the clinics for the evaluation of potential drug candidates and for staging of patients.

Preclinical research and drug development in MS relies on animal models of experimental autoimmune encephalomyelitis (EAE), which mimic several pathological aspects of the human disease [120]. These models have been established for several different species including mice, rats and non-human primates. In these models the disease develops much faster than in humans. Typically, symptoms appear some days after immunization (acute phase), which, depending on the model, is followed by a chronic phase (symptom aggravation over some weeks) or complete remission. The effect of drugs on the disease can, in principle, be studied by a neurological score assessing the functional deficit in these animals or measurement of body weight as a non-specific readout of the animal status. Histology of CNS specimen yields a detailed analysis of the pathological events. Most importantly, immunohistochemistry (IHC) provides highly specific information on which type of T cells or blood-borne monocytes have infiltrated brain tissue, or whether brain residing microglia or astrocytes have been activated in response to the inflammatory stimulus. Specific staining techniques allow visualizing apoptotic processes and neurodegeneration and studying the dynamics of chemokine receptor presentation on or internalization by immune cells.

Analogous to clinical studies in MS patients, imaging strategies for preclinical drug evaluation were mostly based on the assessment of acute inflammation by measuring damage of the BBB using contrast-enhanced MRI or demyelination using magnetization transfer contrast (MTC). These parameters can be routinely assessed with high sensitivity and robustness. In particular, BBB damage is regarded as one important hallmark of acute inflammation, and seems to be correlated with infiltration of immune cells into the CNS [121]. BBB damage can be visualized by intravenous administration of paramagnetic CA such as Gd-DOTA (Laboratoire Guerbet, France) or Gd-DTPA (Schering AG, Germany) [122]. These low molecular weight CA are administered intravenously and diffuse across the impaired vascular lineage into the tissue, where they induce an increase of the longitudinal relaxation rate of water protons, and hence a signal increase in T_1-weighted MR images. While in animals the same readout could be derived from histology (e.g., by measuring plasma protein extravasation), *in vivo* imaging BBB damage allows longitudinal measurements and thereby the dynamic studies of BBB permeability over time, including phases of opening and repair. Moreover, Gd-enhanced MRI provides a faster and more efficient readout: it does not involve complex processing of tissue and allows quick whole-brain scans.

This technique has been used for studying the effects of various potential drug candidates for treatment of MS or EAE, irrespective of the mechanisms of action or of the molecular target of the compound. One example is beta-interferon, which interacts with the function of the BBB by down-regulating several inflammatory factors, thereby abolishing inflammatory events in the CNS [123]. In a couple of preclinical imaging studies it could be shown that treatment with beta-interferon reduces BBB permeability, which correlated with a reduction of neurological symptoms. Nevertheless, this Gd-enhanced imaging provides only a very unspecific readout of the disease processes and does not yield any direct evidence on the underlying mechanism, e.g., demonstrating reduced cell infiltration or tissue damage. Secondly, studying BBB damage is of limited value for the assessment of late-stage neurodegenerative processes observed in progressive MS. For these patients, lesion development is often not accompanied by opening of the BBB, and Gd-enhanced MRI does not provide any information on disease progression and treatment efficacy.

In addition to imaging of primary inflammatory events, the consequences of neurodegenerative processes can be visualized on the basis of MTC. Magnetization transfer ratios (MTR) measure the loss of myelin by assessing the amount of protons bound to white matter structures [124, 125]. While MTR can be determined within a reasonable period of time under *in vivo* conditions, quantitative assessment of MT rates (quantitative MT imaging, qMTI) requires long measuring times, rendering its application impractical. However, qMTI offers several important advantages: parameters determined are tissue properties such as the transversal relaxation times of bound protons, water/proton exchange rates and the concentration of bound water protons, and do not depend on the measurement parameters chosen such as MTR.

The application of MTI for the assessment of drugs efficacy has been of limited success as the animal models currently used in preclinical research rather reflect aspects of neuroinflammation than of neurodegeneration; hence, demyelination is not playing a major role. New models using new mice models or employing adoptive transfer EAE in non-human primates open a new avenue to study neurodegenerative aspects under preclinical conditions. Using these models, MTR imaging has been used to demonstrate the modulation of neurodegenerative events in response to drug treatment [126].

While Gd-enhanced and MTR imaging have already become established tools in clinical and preclinical research and drug development, recent developments in the area of CA development have allowed inflammatory processes to be studied at a mechanistic level.

In particular the use of superparamagnetic nanoparticles has proven useful for labeling and tracking of phagocytotic cells such as blood-borne macrophages entering brain tissue during inflammation (Fig. 4) [75, 76, 127–130]. In addition, target-specific CA labeling cell adhesion molecules such E-selectin or inter-cellular adhesion molecule 1 (ICAM-1) have been developed and tested in animal models of CNS inflammation [131, 132]. However, due to the low tissue concentration of these molecular targets, the effect of such specific CA on the proton relaxation rate and, therefore, on the contrast in MR images is limited, compromising the sensitivity of these target-specific imaging approaches. Furthermore, issues with regard to the delivery of bulky CA limit their use to endovascular targets such as adhesion mol-

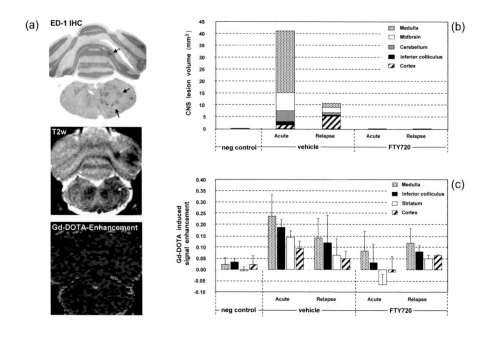

Figure 4.
(a) Imaging data from an EAE rat acquired during the chronic phase of the disease. The ED-1 IHC stain shows macrophages in the medulla and brain stem of a rat as brown spots. USPIO-labeled macrophages can be visualized by T_2-weighted MRI as hypointense areas. The spatial distribution of these areas corresponds to the histological findings. In this animal no clear-cut BBB damage could be observed by Gd-DOTA-enhanced MRI during this phase of the disease. FTY720 abolishes the infiltration of macrophages during the acute and chronic phase of the disease as indicted by USPIO-enhanced MRI and reflected by the lesion volumes (b). However, residual BBB can be observed during the chronic phase of the disease in particular in the medulla (c). It cannot be excluded that this pathology is related to the damage, which emerged during the acute inflammatory episode and which was not repaired during the remitting period.

ecules. Currently, target-specific imaging techniques are not mature enough to be widely used for preclinical drug evaluations.

3.2 Oncology

Imaging has evolved to an indispensable tool for management of cancer patients; in fact, the need for diagnostic methods enabling the early detection of proliferating tissue was a major stimulus for the development of imaging techniques, in particular of MRI. In 1971, Damadian reported significantly prolonged T_1 relaxation time in various types of neoplastic tissues, and suggested the application of such measurements for tumor detection [133].

For cancer diagnostics, the primary objective of non-invasive imaging is the early detection of tissue that has undergone malignant transformation, the characterization and staging of tumors, and the identification of metastatic lesions. From a drug discovery and development point of view, a non-invasive imaging method should provide a rapid, quantitative and reliable readout of the efficacy of treatment with an oncological drug candidate.

The classic readout when assessing tumor proliferation and treatment efficacy is tumor volume using structural imaging methods such as CT, MRI or ultrasound. The same methods have been applied to study animal tumor models. For example, the somatostatin analogues octreotide [134] and bicalutamide [135] have been shown to significantly reduce the growth of Dunning prostate R3327 tumors in the rat. Somatostatin analogues have also been used in other neuroendocrine tumor models, e.g., octreotide to evaluate beneficial effects on established estrogen-induced pituitary hyperplasia [136], or RC 160 for the treatment of liver metastases of a colon tumor line [137]. Such evaluations are dependent on a high CNR allowing an accurate segmentation of neoplastic tissue from its host environment. Animal models frequently involve subcutaneously implanted tumor xenografts; therefore, imaging might not be required for tumor volume determination, calipers can be used instead. The application of non-invasive imaging approaches for volumetric measurements is justified mainly for orthotopic deep-lying neoplastic lesions not accessible to caliper measurements. Moreover, imaging methods should be used to complement morphometric information by providing additional information on tumor morphology (heterogeneity), physiology and most recently on tumor-specific molecular constituents.

While clinically established, structural readouts are commonly late indicators. It may take several weeks until a therapeutic intervention can translate into a measurable effect on the proliferation rate or on the tumor volume. This is undesirable from several perspectives: from a drug developer's perspective an early readout is desired to optimize the dosing regimen. More important, however, is the fact that in the case of a patient who is not responsive to therapy precious time might be lost with potentially severe consequences for the patient.

Morphological manifestation of pharmacological interventions must be preceded by physiological, metabolic and/or molecular responses. Hence, visualization and quantification of these parameters should provide earlier evidence of drug efficacy than the classical structural readouts. Such study paradigms target various tumor hallmarks, i.e., physiological and molecular processes associated with tissue proliferation, tumor metabolism (in particular glucose utilization), neoangiogenesis, i.e., the formation of novel tumor vasculature, or apoptotic processes.

3.2.1 Proliferation

Potential indicators of excessive proliferation are increased synthesis rates for DNA, proteins and other cell constituents such as lipid/phospholipids membrane building blocks. Not surprisingly, imaging approaches, and in particular PET methods, have been developed to probe each of these processes. PET-based approaches use radiolabeled precursor molecules such as labeled thymidine analogues [35], amino acids [36], or choline [37, 38] (see Section 2.2). These readouts of proliferative activity have been shown to provide valuable prognostic information in oncological indications and have been used to evaluate tumor therapies.

Thymidine kinase 1 (TK) is a key enzyme in DNA synthesis. It phosphorylates thymidine, a prerequisite for DNA incorporation. TK activity increases approximately tenfold as cells enter the S-phase of the cell cycle, during which DNA is synthesized [138]. TK activity can be monitored by administration of radiolabeled substrates. An obvious choice is [2-^{11}C]thymidine, which is currently being evaluated both clinically and in animal research [139, 140]. Yet, the short half-life of the radionuclide and the rapid *in vivo* degradation constitute severe limitations [141]. Thus, increased metabolic stability of the tracer and the of radioisotopes with longer half-life such as ^{18}F would offer significant advantages for PET imaging. [^{18}F]-3'-Fluoro-3'-deoxythymidine (FLT) fulfills these requirements and has been thoroughly evaluated as potential indicator of DNA synthesis. Analogous to thymidine, FLT is taken up by cells, phosphorylated by TK, leading to intracellular trapping within the cell [35, 142]. Hence, the PET signal represents the integrated TK activity over the exposure period assuming that substrate delivery is not the rate-limiting step. Tumor levels of radiolabeled nucleotides (thymidine analogues) then reflect DNA synthesis and, correspondingly, cell proliferation. It has been shown that cellular uptake rates of labeled nucleotides by neoplastic tissue can serve as early indicator of therapy efficacy [143, 144]. Nevertheless, further validation of the approach is required.

Rapid cell proliferation is associated with high protein synthesis rates with high demands on resupply of amino acids. There is experimental evidence that amino acid transport is up-regulated in experimental tumors [145]. Two strategies can be pursued for amino acid-based PET tumor imaging: (1) the measurement of amino acid transport into the cells, and (2) the measurement of amino acid transport into the cells followed by protein incorporation rate (protein synthesis rate) using radiolabeled amino acid analogues. The second readout is a combination of several processes and a detailed quantitative analysis is not straightforward. A large number of ^{11}C- and ^{18}F-labeled amino acid tracers is currently being evaluated as potential tracers for detection, delineation and staging of proliferating tumors [36]. The obvious advantage of using isotopic substitution by ^{11}C, leaving all the properties of the unlabeled amino acid unchanged, is counterbalanced by the disadvantage of the short half-life of the radio-isotope, too short for the process to be measured, i.e., the protein synthesis, so that by using ^{11}C-labeled amino acids, one essentially measures amino acid transport. While the half-life of ^{18}F-labeled amino acids allows the assessment of protein synthesis rates in principle, pre-clinical and clinical PET studies indicate that also for these tracers the tissue uptake rates are clearly dominated by amino acid transport across the cell membrane [146]. Coenen et al. [147] observed significant [^{18}F]fluorotyrosine (^{18}F-FTyr) incorporation into brain proteins only in preclinical studies in mouse cerebral tissue. Despite this limitation, the use of radiolabeled amino acids both as diagnostic tools for tumor/metastasis detection and as potential indicators of treatment response is highly attractive. Dynamic assessment of uptake rates in combination with multi- (two-) compartment tissue modeling will provide reliable parameters for the amino acid transport rate, allowing the quantitative evaluation of changes induced by a therapeutic intervention.

Increased proliferation rates are associated with increased rates of membranes synthesis. Hence, substrates required for membrane synthesis bear the potential to serve as proliferation markers. In fact, early observations in MRS studies of tumors revealed some characteristic common spectral features: (1) elevated signal intensities of endogenous phsophomonoester (PME) and -diester (PDE) signals have been observed in most non-brain tumors, (2) elevated signal intensity of the 'choline' signal in brain tumors, and (3) early decreases in the PME signal or in the PME/PDE ratio were found to be good predictors of therapy response [148]. These data highlight a critical role of PME and PDE in the biosynthetic and degradative pathways of proliferative, as compared to normal, tissue. *In vivo* MRS is currently being evaluated by several groups for its potential as prognostic tool and as potential biomarker for treatment efficacy. As compared to MRS, which measures endogenous metabolites, PET provides superior sensitivity and spatial resolution. However, PET applications require the development of a radio-labeled precursors such as choline. Substitution of one of the methyl-groups by $^{11}CH_3$ yielded [^{11}C]choline, which has been first evaluated for imaging of brain tumors [37]. [^{11}C]Choline turned out to be superior to FDG PET imaging, as the latter gives rise to the high background signal caused by the high metabolic rate of normal brain tissue. Excellent tumor-to-background contrast was also observed in primary prostate cancer and its lymph node and bone metastases, and demonstrated the potential of the approach to detect small tumor foci [149]. The already-described limitations of ^{11}C-labeled tracers prompted the development of [^{18}F]fluorocholine (^{18}F-FCho), which was first evaluated in prostate tumor cell lines [38, 150]. ^{18}F-FCho is rapidly phosphorylated by choline kinase and trapped by the cell.

3.2.2 Metabolism

Proliferating tissue is commonly associated with high metabolic rates, in particular with high glycolytic activity, as compared to normal tissue [151]. A critical mediator in this regard is hypoxia-inducible factor-1 (HIF-1), a transcription factor that is up-regulated under hypoxic conditions [152] and by oncogenes [153], which induces glycolysis and angiogenesis. Measurement of glucose utilization rates has evolved as a sensitive tool for the characterization of primary tumors and for the detection of metastases. Systemically administered ^{18}F-FDG is taken up by cells via the glucose transporter and phosphorylated at the 6-position by hexokinase. The lack of a hydroxyl group at the 2-position prevents further processing and the metabolite is trapped in the cell. Hence, the total amount of activity measured at a given location represents the integrated glycolytic activity in the interval between tracer administration and PET measurement (typically 40 min) [15]. The method is clinically established in the management of cancer patients.

There is convincing evidence in multiple clinical drug trials that changes in glycolytic rate precede any effects on the overall tumor volume. This has been demonstrated breast cancer patients undergoing hormone therapy [154] or who were treated with a combination of chemotherapeutics [155]. A spectacular report concerns patients suffering from gastrointestinal stromal tumors (GIST) treated with the Abelson kinase inhibitor imatinib (Gleevec®). Within 24 h after onset of treatment glucose utilization was significantly reduced to a level hardly detectable over background activity, while there was no effect on tumor volume for several weeks [156]. A significant reduction of the tumor load was observed in these patients after 24 weeks only. These studies indicate that assessment of glucose utilization bears a high potential for the early characterization of a therapy response, at least in favorable cases. The availability of micro-PET systems allows for similar studies in animal models. This close correspondence of study designs will facilitate the translation from preclinical to clinical compound evaluations.

3.2.3 Angiogenesis

Neo-vascularization is a critical factor promoting the tumor growth. The assessment of tumor vascularity, or more accurately vascular permeability, using extravascular MR CA, has been proposed as a qualitative indicator for tumor malignancy [157]. Dynamic contrast-enhanced (DCE) MRI methods using low-molecular-weight CA such as Gd-DTPA or Gd-DOTA that leak into the extracellular space are currently widely used for tumor diagnostics, and are being evaluated by several research groups as potential biomarker for therapy efficacy. The signal enhancement caused by an increase in the relaxation rate R_1 is due to CA extravasation, which by itself depends on the tracer PK, tumor perfusion, vascular transfer constant (permeability*surface area product), and interstitial leakage space [18, 158]. Alterations in CA uptake by the tumor may, therefore, reflect changes in any of these factors or of a combination thereof. In animal studies, additional information can be obtained using intravascular macromolecular CA, such as magnetite nanoparticles [74], which have, for example, been used to assess CBF and CBV [159] or for labeling of macrophages [75, 76]. The steady-state signal attenuation caused by the nanoparticles reflects the total amount of tracer in the tissue and, assuming equilibrated blood concentrations, tissue blood volume, which might be considered a non-invasive surrogate of the microvascular density. It has to be kept in mind though that changes in the mean vessel diameter will also influence tissue blood volume without altering microvascular density [160].

Vascular endothelial growth factor (VEGF, also known as vascular permeability factor) is an angiogenic factor produced by most solid tumors [161], and is involved in the induction of vascular permeability as well as in the promotion of new vessel formation [162]. The expression of VEGF and that of its receptors on the endothelial cells is strongly regulated by hypoxia and is thought to play a crucial role in tumor neo-vascularization and tumor growth. Therefore, inhibition of VEGF constitutes an attractive concept for control of tumor proliferation. Efficacy of VEGF receptor inhibition should be reflected by a decreased vascular permeability (vascular transfer constant) and potentially also in tumor blood volume. This has been demonstrated for human breast carcinoma xenografts in rats (MDA-MB-345), which when treated with an anti-VEGF antibody showed significantly reduced vascular leakage of the macromolecular CA albumin-(Gd-DTPA30) [163]. In an orthotopic kidney tumor model in mice, the VEGF-R tyrosine kinase inhibitor, PTK787, also significantly reduced vascular transfer constant as determined by MRI using the CA Gd-DOTA [162]. The same compound was shown to decrease vascular leakage and extracellular volume in B16 melanoma in BL6 mice both in primary tumors and cervical lymph node metastases. CA extravasation in lymph node metastases decreased significantly within 48 h after onset of therapy [164]. Clinical studies in patients suffering from liver metastases have yielded corresponding results, indicating that, in fact, vascular permeability measures may serve as biomarkers of efficacy [165].

3.2.4 Apoptosis

Programmed cell death or apoptosis is an essential process for normal development and function of tissue. Down-regulation of apoptosis is associated with excessive cell proliferation associated with malignancies. Correspondingly, induction of apoptosis is an attractive therapy concept in oncology and many of the well-known cytostatics in fact display an apoptotic component. Several imaging strategies for visualizing activation of the apoptotic pathway are conceivable, two of which targeting molecular players in the apoptotic cascade are discussed briefly below.

Cells undergoing apoptosis redistribute aminophospholipids that are normally localized at the cytoplasmic leaflet to the outer (extracellular) leaflet of the cell membrane [166]. These extracellular aminophospholipids, primarily phosphatidylserine, are recognized by phagocytotic cells prompting a signal for cell removal [167]. Hence, the occurrence of apoptotic cells is a transient event, i.e., detection is only feasible in a limited time window between the induction of the apoptotic cascade and cell death/removal. Externalized phosphatidylserine moieties are recognized by annexin-V [168], which binds to its target with high affinity and specificity. Specific imaging probes are designed by coupling reporter groups such as radioligands [169], MRI CA [170] or fluorescent dyes [171, 172] to annexin-V or related targeting moieties, such as the C2 domain of synaptotagmin I. Using such approaches, the induction of apoptosis using cytostatic such as cyclophosphamide could be demonstrated within hours after drug administration [173, 174]. Externalization of aminophospholipids provides an attractive imaging target. Phosphatidylserines are sensitive indicators of the process to be studied, which can be easily assessed using macromolecular reporter constructs. Essentially any imaging modality can be used for detection of the target-specific interaction, each one having advantages and disadvantages. Nevertheless, a word of caution has to be added: transient externalization of phosphatidylserine is not necessarily associated with apoptosis; it can also occur during traumatic or physiological stress [174]. Therefore, accumulation of labeled annexin-V type ligands at the target organ does not uniquely reflect the occurrence of apoptotic processes.

Cytosolic caspases play a central role in the apoptotic cascade and the assessment of caspase activities would provide direct evidence of the activation of an apoptotic pathway. A critical issue when targeting caspases is their intracellular location: any reporter substrate to be processed would have to cross the intact cell membrane. An alternative imaging strategy, at least for imaging apoptosis in animal models, is the use of reporter gene assays using fluorescent proteins or luciferases as reporter proteins. Laxman et al. [175] have designed a corresponding reporter construct, in which the reporter (firefly luciferase) was silenced until activated by cleavage of a DEVD peptide sequence by caspase-3. Apoptosis was induced in a murine xenograft model (human glioma) by administration of TNF-α-related apoptosis-inducing ligand (TRAIL).

Indirect imaging approaches sensitive to microstructural or metabolic changes associated with apoptosis have also been proposed. Metabolic changes involve increased levels of fructose-1,6-bisphosphate (FBP) and cytidine-diphosphocholine (CDPC), which can be monitored using ^{31}P MRS [176] The most prominent spectral changes observed in ^{1}H MRS spectra are decreased choline and increased signals arising from intracellular lipids [177]. The decreased choline signal is attributed to the reduced proliferation rate (see above). Microstructural changes that affect the relative volumes of the intra- and extracellular compartments will be reflected in altered values of the water ADC. In fact, following apoptosis-induced therapy increases in water ADC values have been observed early after treatment onset, i.e., before any effects on tumor volume have been detected [178, 179]. An issue with both structural and metabolic markers is their lack of specificity: any mechanism that affects proliferation may influence choline levels, and microstructural changes might be imposed by other processes than apoptosis. Nevertheless, they seem to indicate an early response to therapeutic interventions and, therefore, are currently being evaluated as potential biomarkers for anti-proliferative, apoptosis-inducing efficacy of tumor therapies.

To conclude this section, some remarks concerning molecular imaging approaches that are discussed in some detail in Chapters 3 and 4 of this volume need to be made. Mechanistic information can be derived from using target-specific or target-activated probes. Well-known examples are the polymer-based quenched fluorescence reporters that are activated by the targeted protease [180, 181]. This assays allows the visualization and quantification (if tomographic procedures are used) of the protease activity *in vivo*, which can be used to evaluate potential enzyme inhibitors [182]. Comparison of the fluorescent intensity in drug-treated and control animals yields a direct proof of mechanism of the therapeutic concept.

As an alternative to morphometric measurements, reporter gene approaches can be applied to measure the tumor burden in preclinical cancer models. Tumor cell lines are genetically modified to stably express a reporter gene such as green fluorescent protein [183], firefly luciferase [184] or herpes simplex virus-1 thymidine kinase (HSV1-TK) [185]. The intensity of fluorescence or bioluminescence signal, or correspondingly the HSV1-TK activity are considered a surrogate for the tumor volume. The strength of the approach is high sensitivity, which allows the detection of micro-metastases, and the rapid readout, in particular when multiple lesions are present. The principal disadvantage is poor spatial resolution.

3.3 Inflammatory and degenerative joint diseases

Imaging has been extensively applied to study inflammatory and degenerative diseases of the joints. The analysis originally focused on pathological changes affecting bony structures. Modern imaging approaches, however, provide detailed insight into soft-tissue structures involved, which are earlier indicators of joint disease. Most recently, molecular imaging methods have been introduced that allow targeting of specific molecular events involved in joint destruction. Today, multimodal imaging approaches offer a powerful tool set for diagnosis, for monitoring disease progression, and for the evaluation of therapy response.

3.3.1 Evaluation of drug efficacy based on structural appearance

Clinically planar X-ray and X-ray CT are probably the most established technologies for the assessment of joint diseases. Similarly, micro-CT provides high resolution morphological and architectural three-dimensional (3D) information allowing characterizing bone and joint-related changes in arthritis models in small animals. For instance, the technique has been used to quantify cortical bone loss and periosteal new bone formation for therapeutic evaluation in a murine model of collagen-induced arthritis (CIA) [186] or to detect disease progression in the subchondral bone of the knee joint of rats in an osteoarthritis (OA) model [187]. Such data demonstrate the potential of *in vivo* micro-CT for routine, high-throughput analysis and screening of new therapies for joint diseases. Nevertheless, micro-CT involves significant radiation dose to achieve the image resolution required, limiting experiments involving repeated imaging the same animal [188] and translation into the clinics.

Structural MRI has also been extensively used in conjunction with animal models of arthritis. In particular, articular structures can be exquisitely imaged due to the fact that 75% of the weight of the cartilage is water; hence, cartilage yields a strong MRI signal. In rheumatoid arthritis (RA) models, the technique provided qualitative and quantitative readouts of analysis of changes in soft tissue and bone structure [189–192]. Because of the complicated joint structures, qualitative image analyses based on a scoring system have been used as a primary readout characterizing the disease process and the effects of compounds. Scores accounted for changes in soft tissue, such as edema formation, joint separation, cyst formation, and structural changes of bone such as cortical erosion or the formation of osteophytes. For instance, Jacobson et al. [194] validated the use of MRI to follow *in vivo* disease progression in an adjuvant arthritis model in the rat: 2D MR images were scored prior and after injection of Gd-containing CA following subcutaneous administration of *Mycobacterium butyricum*. Using this approach, it was shown that the selective COX-2 inhibitor ABT-963 significantly reduced bone loss and soft tissue destruction [193]. Similar protective effects on joint integrity have been found for SB 242235 [194], a potent and selective inhibitor of p38 mitogen-activated protein kinase, and for SB 273005 [195], a potent, orally active nonpeptide antagonist of the integrin $\alpha_v\beta_3$ vibronectin receptor.

Increases in joint space volumes of metatarsophalangeal and proximal interphalangeal joints of the mid toes of the hind paw were observed in the course of CIA in Dark-Agouti rats [189]. These *in vivo* readouts reflecting cartilage and bone erosion correlated well with histological findings [196]. Paw swelling assessed by a micro-caliper was receding before significant changes in the joint architectures have been observed in MR images, indicating the superiority of high-resolution MRI for monitoring disease-modifying drug efficacy. No significant changes in the joint architecture were observed in rats receiving immunosuppressive treatment by cyclosporine A.

While MRI applications in acute RA models focused on assessment of cartilage erosion, such readouts are of limited value for chronic diseases such as OA. In OA, cartilage erosion is a late event that is preceded by progressive changes in the macromolecular network constituting articular cartilage; visualization of such changes should provide early indicators of disease progression, and several MRI techniques have been developed to probe the integrity of the biomolecular structure of the cartilage matrix. In animal studies, spatial resolution is one of the main hurdles to overcome since articular cartilage rarely exceeds 1-mm thickness even in rabbits or dogs. Thus, macroscopic signs of cartilage degeneration may not be visible during pre-clinical investigations in the early stage of OA. Only in rare occasions has *in vivo* MRI been used to quantify the loss of cartilage volume in conjunction with disease progression in animals [197, 198].

Early cartilage lesions in OA are primarily characterized by a loss of proteoglycans (PG) and loosening of the collagen framework [199]. The delayed Gd-enhanced MRI of cartilage technique has been proposed as a method capable of detecting PG loss in the osteoarthritic tissue [7]. This contrast-enhanced imaging method allows measurement of the fixed charge density (FCD) of cartilage, reflecting the negatively charged glycosaminoglycan (GAG) side chain concentration. Following intravenous administration, the negatively charged Gd complex $Gd(DTPA)^{2-}$ penetrates the interstitial fluid of cartilage to reach an equilibrium concentration that is governed (1) by the $Gd(DTPA)^{2-}$ concentration gradient and (2) by the electrostatic interactions, which are related to the FCD. The local $Gd(DTPA)^{2-}$ concentration and, hence, the related FCD, can be derived from T_1 maps as previously described [7], provided the $Gd(DTPA)^{2-}$- relaxivity is tissue independent [200]. The capability of this method to quantitatively assess cartilage degeneration was assessed in a rabbit [201] and in a goat model of OA [8], in which PG depletion was induced by an intra-articular injection of papain. A significant correlation between the $Gd(DTPA)^{2-}$-induced T_1 changes and the PG content has been found. The reproducibility was such that a 20% drug effect on PG levels could be detected with groups sizes of ten animals.

Due to the high content of macromolecules, cartilage exhibits a significant magnetization transfer (MT) effect reflecting the exchange process between bulk and matrix-bound water. MT contrast can be exploited for improved contrast and consequently better delineation of articular structures [202, 203]. More importantly, MT imaging may provide information on the chemical/structural status of cartilage. In fact several *in vitro* studies have demonstrated that the MT effect in cartilage is dominated by the contribution of collagen, while the influence of PG is significantly smaller [6, 204]. The observed changes in MT ratios are likely to reflect changes in collagen structure rather than changes in collagen concentration [6].

3.3.2 Assessment of inflammatory processes/cellular and molecular imaging

Inflammation is characterized by vascular changes such as increased tissue perfusion and capillary permeability, and possibly angiogenesis, secretion of chemokines and cytokines, as well as the infiltration of immunocompetent cells such as lymphocytes and blood-borne monocytes. Analogous to the situation described for tumors, leakage of extracellular CA into the interstitial space depends on local tissue perfusion and microvascular permeability. In RA, the uptake of CA such Gd-DTPA in the synovium has been demonstrated to significantly correlate with histopathological features of synovitis such as polymorphonuclear leucocyte infiltration, hyperemia and fibrin deposition [205].

Macrophages possess widespread pro-inflammatory, destructive, and remodeling capabilities that critically contribute to the acute and chronic phases of RA [206]. The feasibility of MRI techniques to assess macrophage infiltration into sites of inflammation as disease readout has been explored in mouse [207], rat [208] and rabbit [209] models of RA. Small particles of iron oxide (SPIO) or USPIO particles have been applied for *in situ* macrophage labeling, exploiting their phagocytotic activity (see Section 3.1.1). In a rat antigen-induced arthritis model, significant negative correlation was found between the MRI signal intensity in the knee and the histologically determined iron content in macrophages located in the same region of animals that had received SPIO (Endorem®) 24 h before image acquisition [185]. Starting 4 days following the antigen injection, images from arthritic knees exhibited distinctive signal attenuation in the synovium. This signal attenuation was significantly smaller in knees from animals treated with dexamethasone (0.3 mg/kg/day by gavage) and completely absent in contralateral knees that had been challenged with vehicle.

Alternatively, macrophages can be visualized by targeting surface molecules such as the F4/80 antigen. Using this concept, early signs of experimental arthritis have been detected in a mouse model of antigen-induced arthritis. By targeting the antigen with intravenously administered anti-F4/80 monoclonal antibodies (mAb) labeled with the indocyanine dye Cy5.5, macrophages infiltration into the inflamed synovial membrane could be monitored. Significant accumulation of the fluorochrome probes was observed in inflamed knee joints and, to a lesser extent, in contralateral non-arthritic knee joints [210].

Another characteristic of inflammation is high protease activity, which contributes significantly to joint destruction; hence, targeting of proteases using protease-activatable imaging probes constitutes an attractive strategy for visualization and possible quantification of inflammatory events [183,

184]. For example, by intravenous administration of a cathepsin B-activatable near-infrared fluorescent probe, activity of this protease could be detected at an early stage in a murine model of OA involving intra-articular injection of collagenase I [211]. The probe consisted of a poly-lysine backbone to which fluorescent groups were covalently bound. Due to the proximity of the fluorophores, fluorescence is effectively quenched. Proteases that target the Lys-Lys cleavage site, including cathepsin B, activate the probe, leading to an increase in fluorescence yield by typically two orders of magnitude. Measurement of the fluorescence signal intensity due to protease activity has been used to semi-quantitatively assess the response to antirheumatic therapy [212].

3.4   Pulmonary disease

Today, imaging methods are not commonly used for evaluation of drugs targeting pulmonary diseases as established clinical and preclinical testing procedures allowing assessing the efficacy of pulmonary-active compounds exist. Spirometry yields a simple *in vivo* readout of airway resistance. Invasive procedures, such as analysis of bronchoalveolar lavage (BAL) fluid and histopathological analyses are commonly applied in animal studies providing detailed information of drug efficacy. Nevertheless, the use of non-invasive imaging methods for the characterization of pulmonary diseases and analysis of therapeutic interventions is attractive as (1) they provide 3D spatially resolved structural, functional and more recently molecular information, (2) they enable longitudinal studies in a individual, and (3) they may allow a straightforward translation from preclinical to clinical research.

Currently, CT is the imaging modality of choice for diagnosis of lung diseases in a clinical setting. Due to the huge difference in X-ray attenuation of lung parenchyma and water-containing tissue (with attenuation coefficients for air and tissue being −1000 and ±100 Hounsfield units, respectively), lung structures can be imaged with high contrast. The development of micro-CT devices allows translating these techniques to small animals, e.g., rodents; high-resolution thoracic images can be obtained when applying respiratory gated data acquisitions [213, 214]. Radiation dose is approximately 0.15 Gy for a respiratory-gated micro-CT imaging protocol. The combination of high-resolution CT imaging and respiratory-gated acquisitions appears well-suited to serial *in vivo* scanning. Although being an ex vivo study, Langheinrich et al. [215] showed recently that micro-CT is feasible for structural evaluation of the lung fine structure and its alterations during endotoxin-induced lung injury. Systemic application of endotoxin led to a significant increase in the soft-tissue volume of the lungs (i.e., tissue edema) and significant thickening of the alveolar walls at micro-CT. Simultaneously, endotoxin-treated rat lungs showed a significant reduction in total air space.

Significant efforts have been devoted to developing MRI-based lung imaging procedures. Lung is a challenging organ to image by MRI. Signal intensity is low due to the low density of tissue water of approximately 20–30% as compared to other tissues (70–80%), and due to very short T_2 and T_2^* relaxation times. These are caused by differences in magnetic susceptibility between lung tissue and air, which comprises about 80% of the pulmonary volume, leading to significant magnetic field inhomogeneity and thus rapid dephasing of the MR signal. To detect a signal from lung parenchyma, especially at high fields, MR techniques with very short echo time have to be applied [216]. Image quality is further degraded as consequence of artifacts caused by cardiac and respiratory movements. These problems are more evident in small rodents, because of their higher cardiac and respiratory rates. Only recently has the technique been applied to preclinical pharmacological studies in the area of respiratory diseases [217].

Breathing-related motion artifacts can be minimized by applying scan-synchronous ventilation acquisition schemes [218, 219], for which breathing is restricted to the recovery period after data acquisition. In addition, artifacts due to the cardiac motion are reduced by triggering the image acquisition by electrocardiogram recordings. Although the combination of projection reconstruction methods with synchronous ventilation and cardiac gating enables the recording of high-resolution images of the rat lung, the approach is limited by long acquisition times, typically 30–40 min per image [220]. For drug testing *in vivo* in animal models of airways diseases, however, it is important to keep the acquisition conditions as simple as possible so that repeated measurements interfering minimally with the physiology of the animals can be carried out on a routine basis. This consideration has prompted the development of imaging protocols that do not need either involving respiratory or cardiac gating [220, 221].

3.4.1 Assessment of inflammatory lung disease via visualization of edema formation

Inflammatory processes induced in models of airways diseases can be followed non-invasively in rats by monitoring edema formation caused by inflammatory processes. For instance, actively sensitized Brown Norway (BN) rats exposed to allergen (ovalbumin, OVA) develop airway hyperresponsiveness and eosinophilic inflammation together with an increase in activated T cells (CD25[+]) in the airways [222, 223], thus reflecting the key features of asthmatic inflammation. Intense edematous signals detected in the lungs of sensitized rats challenged with OVA [223] were shown to be significantly correlated with inflammatory parameters determined in the BAL fluid collected from the same animals [224]. The strongest correlations were with the number of eosinophils, eosinophil peroxidase activity (a marker of eosinophil activation), and the total protein content (a marker for plasma extravasation). Importantly, the signal detected by MRI correlates significantly with the perivascular edema assessed by histology [225]. Since edema is an integral component of experimental pulmonary inflammation, MRI provides a non-invasive tool for monitoring the course of the inflammatory response and the consequence of anti-inflammatory therapy. This could be demonstrated by administrating drug candidates both before or after the allergen challenge [224–226]. Interestingly, in contrast to conventional post-mortem fluid BAL analysis MRI was able to pick up rapid anti-inflammatory efficacy of compounds applied after OVA [226].

Administration of endotoxin (lipopolysaccharide; LPS) to rodents elicits an inflammatory response similar to that observed in chronic obstructive pulmonary disease (COPD) patients. LPS activates mononuclear phagocytes, leading to the release of a number of cytokines, which increase the adherence of neutrophils to endothelial cells [227, 228], thus facilitating a massive infiltration of neutrophils into the lung [229]. Exposure of BN rats to LPS leads to pulmonary neutrophilia [226, 230] and induces mucus cell metaplasia [231]. Following an LPS challenge of non-sensitized BN, the MR signals in the lungs are heterogeneous and significantly less intense than those detected after OVA administration to actively sensitized animals. They persist for 8 days following dosing [232]. Histology and BAL fluid analysis suggest that the long-lasting MRI signal following LPS is due to secreted mucus.

3.4.2 Regional assessment of lung function

Inflammation in airways leads to pathophysiological changes in the structure of the lung tissue, including thickening of the smooth muscle in the airway wall, which may influence airways responsiveness [233] as well as ventilation. The progressive structural change known as airway remodeling, which is driven by chronic local inflammation, is a fundamental component for development of irreversible airway hyperresponsiveness (for a review, see [234]).

Effects of airway remodeling and hyporesponsiveness following allergen or endotoxin challenges, respectively, can be monitored non-invasively in spontaneously breathing rats using MRI methods [235] as changes in oxygenation levels affect the signal intensity of lung parenchyma. Molecular oxygen is weakly paramagnetic and thereby acts as a CA affecting the relaxivity of nearby water protons in lung tissue. This contrast mechanism has been explored to derive ventilation-related information from the human lung [236, 237]. In the rat lung, a highly significant negative correlation has been found between the parenchymal signal and the partial pressure of oxygen in the blood, for different amounts of oxygen administered [236]: increased parenchymal signal intensity is indicative of reduced oxygen levels and thus potential ventilation deficits.

In actively sensitized rats, increased parenchymal signal intensity (in areas devoid of edematous signals) was detected from 6 h up to 180 h after challenge, at a time when edematous signals reflecting inflammation had completely resolved. Histological analysis revealed airway remodeling in the lungs of OVA-challenged rats characterized as increased bronchial epithelium thickness and smooth muscle area, as well as bronchial goblet cell hyperplasia. The increased parenchymal signal was consistent with a significant reduction of air space determined by histology, showing impaired lung ventilation in these animals [236].

In contrast, significantly decreased parenchymal signal intensity was detected 24 h after intratracheal instillation of LPS [236]. The effect was abolished by pretreatment with N^G-nitro-L-arginine methyl ester (L-NAME), an inhibitor of nitric oxide (NO) synthase (NOS). Potential broncho-dilatory activity of NO in the inflammatory response elicited by endotoxin has been demonstrated by Pauwels et al. [238]. In the same model, LPS-induced airway hypo-responsiveness was eliminated by NOS inhibitor L-NAME [239].

These effects are in line with the observation of marked expression of inducible NOS in rat macrophages recovered from the airways 16 h after local LPS instillation [240].

Instead of indirect assessment of ventilation through oxygen-mediated relaxation effects, ventilation can be visualized directly by administration of hyperpolarized noble gas isotopes ^{3}He and ^{129}Xe (for a review, see [241]). The nuclear spin polarization of these isotopes can be increased by optical pumping by four to five orders of magnitude compared to that of protons. This increase in polarization translates directly into the MRI signal intensity significantly enhancing the sensitivity of MRI approach. Small animal respirators compatible with polarized ^{3}He allow a fine control of the delivered gas volume and of the lung ventilation timing [221, 242]. Synchronization of the imaging sequence with the gas delivery can be used for performing dynamic lung ventilation studies. For instance, cine-type imaging allows imaging of the gas distribution in the lung at very high temporal and spatial resolution [243–245]. An advantage of this approach is that the absence of any background signal: signals detected are exclusively due to the administered hyperpolarized gas.

The potential of ^{3}He MRI for assessing airway constriction has been investigated in methacholine-induced broncho-constriction rat models. Using a Cine-MRI approach comprising the acquisition of a dynamic series of images over 150 gas breaths, Chen and Johnson [246] showed heterogeneously distributed airways constriction, resulting in a partition of the lung between ventilated and non-ventilated regions. Superposition of helium and proton images allowed the detection of airway obstructions that led to air-trapping in the non-ventilated lung regions. The diameter of the principal airways decreased in average by 11% following methacholine administration. Dynamic ventilation image series obtained from a single breath were also used to generate parametric pixel-by-pixel maps of gas arrival time, filling time constant, inflation rate and gas volume in distal areas of the lung [247]. An average 12% inflation rate decrease was measured following the administration of 85 µg methacholine. The inflation rate decreased further after 170 µg methacholine.

Emphysema is a pulmonary disease characterized by alveolar wall destruction, resulting in enlargement of gas exchange spaces without fibrosis, ultimately resulting in severe impairment of gas exchange [248]. This condition is one of the most critical components of COPD. Experimental emphysema can be induced in rats by the application of a single dose of porcine pancreatic elastase [249]. Elastase-treated rats displayed a significantly larger ADC of the hyperpolarized ^{3}He gas as compared to normal animals, indicating alveolar expansion [250, 251].

At present, ^{3}He MRI techniques generate superior functional information of the lung as compared to the indirect methods based on oxygen level-dependent proton relaxation rates. However, it cannot be excluded that besides information on the inflammatory state, proton MRI might also yield relevant information on lung function despite its inherently lower sensitivity.

Ventilation imaging is complemented by regional assessment of lung perfusion; in fact, the ventilation-perfusion mismatch is considered a critical indicator of lung pathology. Blood flow to the lung is commonly assessed using the tracer dilution approaches already described. MRI has been used in combination with a blood-pool magnetic CA, polylysine-Gd-DTPA40 (polylysine-Gd-DTPA40) for detecting pulmonary perfusion defects in a rat pulmonary embolus model [252]. After CA administration, the signal intensity of the well-perfused lung areas increased more than 200%, whereas contrast enhancement in the embolized lung increased by only 25%. Signal intensities of the perfused lung remained stable for 1 h due to the long circulation time of the CA, the signal intensities of the embolized lung gradually increased for 20 min as the air embolus dissolved [253]. MRI assessment of lung perfusion is also feasible by analyzing the first pass of a low molecular weight CA such as Gd-DTPA (Fig. 5).

3.4.3 Visualization of molecular processes in the lung

More recently, molecular imaging approaches have been applied to targeted interaction in lung tissue. As an example, PET imaging has been applied to study the time-dependent expression of mutant HSV1-TK and an enhanced green fluorescent protein in the lungs of transfected rats [253]. Pulmonary gene transfer was performed via intratracheal administration of a replication-deficient adenovirus containing the corresponding fusion gene. Imaging was performed at several time points following the gene transfer, using 9-(4-[^{18}F]fluoro-3-hydroxymethylbutyl)guanine as imaging substrate for the mutant kinase. The substrate is phosphorylated by the thymidine kinase and

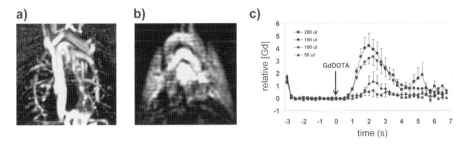

Figure 5.
Perfusion imaging of rat lung. (a) Time-of-flight angiography of major thoracic vessels. High contrast is obtained by saturating the stationary protons, while inflowing proton spins of vascular water yields full signal intensity. (b) Lung perfusion map recorded in the time interval 1.5–3 s following the administration of 200 µl Gd-DOTA (0.1 mM) into the tail vein. At this early time point signal enhancement is predominantly observed in lung arteries, lung parenchyma and ascending and descending aorta. (c) Average CA concentration in lung parenchyma as a function of time and dose of Gd-DOTA. CA-induced signal changes are observed as early as 1 s following tail vein injection and reach a maximum at 2 s. Data represent mean ± SEM of four rats.

trapped in the cell, analogous to FDG. PET signals were already significantly increased 4–6 h after gene transfer, maximal after 4 days, and no longer detectable by 10 days. *In vivo* results were confirmed by *ex vivo* assays of TK activity and green fluorescent protein.

4   Imaging: essential or nice to have

Establishment and operation of a multimodality imaging facility is rather resource intense; therefore an important aspect to be addressed concerns the relevance of the imaging contributions for decision making in drug discovery and development. Could similar information have been generated more economically and/or more efficiently using alternative methods, e.g., the classical established pharmacological techniques or '-omics' technologies? What is the added value of using sophisticated imaging techniques?

Undisputed imaging applications are those which provide unique information or when information can be obtained more efficiently or more economically than with classical analytical methods. The possibility to derived high-resolution structural, functional and meanwhile also cellular and molecular information in a non-invasive manner is highly relevant for pharmacological studies, in particular when studying chronic degenerative disease.

Treatment efficacy can be evaluated in individuals over extended periods of time, allowing analysis of morphological and physiological changes with respect to a pretreatment reference state. Intra-individual variability is thereby significantly reduced and statistically significant data might be obtained with significantly reduced group sizes. Imaging can also be applied for stratification of treatment groups: prior to therapy administration, patients or animals can be classified into 'homogenous' treatment groups, which should translate into data with better statistical relevance. Applications of non-invasive techniques such as imaging allow the correlation of structural and functional imaging data with other 'clinical' readouts characterizing the individual, such as cognitive or behavioral performance when studying, e.g., CNS disorders. Collection of as much comprehensive information as possible enhances the reliability of diagnosis, prognosis and therapy management.

The high temporal resolution (sub-seconds to seconds) of several imaging methods/protocols allows recording of dynamic data that are difficult to assess otherwise. An example is the functional analysis of the heart. Dynamic cardiac MRI imaging provides cardiac functional parameters such as diastolic and systolic ventricular volumes, stroke volume and ejection fraction [254–256]. Analogous information is provided by dynamic CT and ultrasound imaging. In addition, MRI allows the recording of myocardial stress maps, which can be derived when applying so-called myocardial tagging techniques [257, 258]. Another example utilizing the high temporo-spatial resolution of fMRI are functional studies of the brain following cognitive, sensory or pharmacological stimulation (Fig. 6). The functional CNS response can be recorded with a temporal resolution of seconds. Classically, functional information is obtained in preclinical research by applying autoradiographic procedures measuring tissue uptake of [14C]deoxyglucose [28] or [14C]iodoantipyrine [259] or using electrophysiological recordings. While the first approach yields high spatial, yet no temporal resolution, the measured activity corresponding to the time-integral over the exposure period, the second readout yields excellent temporal resolution at predefined fixed locations.

Collection of high-resolution 3D structural and functional information translates into improved quality of information. For instance, full volumetric coverage of a subcutaneous tumor with clear identification of neoplastic versus normal tissue will yield better data than caliper measurements in three

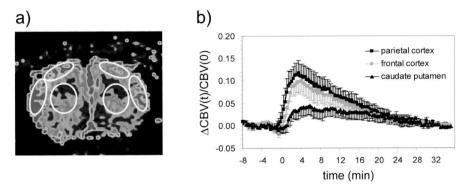

Figure 6.
High temporo-spatial resolution in fMRI studies of rat brain. (a) Transverse cross-section at the level of caudate putamen (8 mm anterior to the intra-aural line) corresponding to the integrated intensity over the period 0–20 min following intravenous administration of amphetamine at a dose of 1 mg/kg. Four slices covering the forebrain of the rat were recorded simultaneously. High activity is observed in cortical structures. This type of image corresponds to autoradiographic data. (b) Changes of CBV as a function of time in ROI indicated in (a). Amphetamine was injected as a bolus at $t = 0$. Time resolution was 15 s per set of images.

directions. Whether this degree of quality is required depends on the specific question asked.

Similarly, 3D imaging of a specific body region reduces the potential problem of sampling errors when collecting tissue specimen, which is of particular relevance when studying heterogeneous tissues. Of course, this has to be balanced against the specificity of histological specimen analysis. In fact, the two readouts are complementary: histological analysis is required for validation of the imaging approaches, while imaging-guided tissue sampling will enhance the specificity of the specimen.

An important advantage of using non-invasive imaging readouts is the fact that tissue is analyzed in its host environment. Any artifacts due to tissue collection and processing (fixation, and histological processing, or extraction) are thereby largely reduced. For instance, tissue collection is invariably linked to a period of global ischemia for a specimen, which will affect the levels of energy metabolites. Similarly, histological processing of tissue will lead to morphological distortions that will affect any morphometric measurements. When analyzing vessel cross-sectional areas in a rat model of carotid artery restenosis (following endothelial denudation using a balloon catheter), significantly reduced vascular perimeters were observed in fixed carotid specimen as compared to the *in vivo* measurement using MR angiographic procedures [260]. Obviously, perfusion fixation led to significant tissue shrinkage affecting the quantitative analysis.

Despite the significant cost associated with the installation and operation of an imaging facility, the use of imaging may still be more economic than conventional analysis tools that might be rather labor intense. As an illustration let us consider drug evaluations using rat focal cerebral ischemia models. Infarct volumes are typically derived from T2-weighted MR images, which yield a high CNR, sufficient for applying intensity-based image segmentation procedures during image analysis. Using standardized image acquisition procedures it is possible to collect data from 10 rats per hour, i.e., data collection and analysis for drug study involving three treated groups and a control group with ten animals each can be completed within 4 h. This has to be compared to the classical post mortem analysis using gross-morphological and/or histological tissue analysis. Brains have to be removed, fixed, sliced, stained and analyzed – a task requiring significant personnel resources, which will take 2–3 days. Needless to say that after the imaging experiments the animals are still alive and can be used for additional experiments, e.g., behavioral tests.

Finally, the use of imaging methods for characterizing animal models of human disease will definitely facilitate the translation between preclinical and clinical drug development. Similar study designs can be applied, potential biomarkers can be identified and validated, and studies in animals can be used to rationalize experimental findings in humans using analogous biomedical readouts.

5   Limitations of current imaging approaches

Despite the success of imaging both as diagnostic tool and for the assessment of therapy evaluation there is significant room for improvement to further enhance their values for biomedical research.

Throughput of imaging is certainly an issue to be addressed. Today, the effective data acquisition time essentially depends on the question to be answered: For morphological or morphometric characterization of an established lesion, the time required to acquire a dataset is the rate-limiting step. Hence the application of fast imaging protocols will have a major impact on the throughput achievable. Modern MRI procedures use parallelization of data acquisition [261], thereby shortening acquisition times, or allow collection of data from several animals simultaneously [262].

Sophisticated tools have been developed for quantification of imaging data. Nevertheless, there is a high need further improvements in this area. The biomedical researcher is not interested in method-specific imaging parameters such as relaxation time, fluorescence intensity or local activity measures. Results should be provided as physiological values such tissue perfusion, oxygenation levels, tracer concentrations. In many cases, absolute values have to be derived. For instance, in cerebral ischemia models, perfusion values in the ischemic territory are frequently expressed as percentage of contralateral 'normal' values, which allows the identification of the affected brain region. As there are threshold CBF values for cell function and cell survival, the relevant information would be: Is the residual perfusion above or below these thresholds [263]? This requires a detailed understanding of the underlying biochemical and biophysical processes and the development of more extensive tissue models than those described in Section 2. Imaging data might be interpreted in the context of system biological models. Multimodal imaging approaches combining structural, functional and molecular information should provide complementary information required to validate such models.

A final point to be mentioned in the context of both preclinical and clinical drug development is standardization. Imaging results, in particular MRI data depend on the specific image acquisition procedure applied. This renders the comparison of data collected at different centers difficult, sometimes even impossible. For multicenter clinical studies the use of standardized measurement procedures in mandatory, across centers and irrespective of the specific equipment at each center.

6 Conclusion

Imaging methods providing quantitative structural, functional and more recently also cellular and molecular information in a non-invasive manner have become valuable tools for the preclinical and clinical evaluation of drug candidates. Imaging enables longitudinal studies in an individual, which is attractive when studying chronic diseases both for monitoring the progression of the untreated disease and for studying long-term efficacy of therapeutic interventions. Obvious advantages of serial data acquisition are a significant elimination of inter-individual variability, thereby enhancing the statistical relevance of the data, the possibility to evaluate therapy response with respect to a pretreatment reference state, and stratification of therapy groups to achieve homogeneous cohorts. *In vivo* imaging results can be correlated with other 'clinical' readouts of a disease allowing a comprehensive characterization of a disease state.

Biomedical applications, and in particular drug development, demand quantitative data and significant efforts have been made to rationalize imaging results in the context of tissue models. Most commonly, models comprising multiple tissue compartments that are linked by exchange processes have been used. Future developments in this respect are required to derive the physiological and molecular tissue parameters of interest for the biomedical researcher.

An important aspect in drug development is the availability of biomarkers of therapeutic efficacy, which should provide a rapid readout of whether a patient is responsive to treatment. This is relevant both for the drug developer and for the patient. Several candidate imaging biomarkers are currently evaluated (see Section 3 of this chapter, and Chapter 9 in this volume), and it is anticipated that they will have a major impact on the design of clinical trials. Of course, biomarkers are not confined to imaging, techniques such as genomics, proteomics and metabonomics [264] will become highly relevant for translational applications.

The field of non-invasive imaging is in rapid development: established modalities such as CT, MRI, and PET are being optimized with respect to efficiency of data acquisition, data analysis, and operating comfort. For all these modalities small animal versions are currently available aimed at facilitating translational applications. Novel techniques such as bioluminescence and fluorescence imaging have emerged and are rapidly becoming an attractive tool for the biologist; they are cheap, use stable reporter systems and are characterized by high sensitivity. They exploit readouts widely used in molecular biology, which can be further developed to *in vivo* application. However, translation to the clinics is not straightforward due to biophysical limitations (penetration of light) and due to the fact that many of the reporter system are difficult or virtually impossible to apply in humans. Yet, for experimental research optical imaging methods will become highly relevant.

Combination of the various imaging techniques currently available either by post-processing (image fusion) or by simultaneous recording will allow a comprehensive characterization of a biological problem. Disease processes might be studied at the receptor level, by monitoring individual signaling cascades, and finally the morphological, physiological and metabolic consequences of these molecular events. As such, multimodal imaging might become an interesting tool for system biology. It will help the drug developer to assess, understand and optimize therapeutic intervention for the individual.

References

1   Wohnsland F, Faller B (2001) High-throughput permeability pH profile and high-throughput alkane/water log P with artificial membranes. J Med Chem 44: 923–930

2   Phelps ME (2004) PET: molecular imaging and its biological applications. Springer, New York

3   Rudin M (2005) Molecular imaging – Basic principles and applications to biomedical research. Imperial College Press (London)

4   Jiang Q, Chopp M, Zhang AG, Knight RA, Jacobs N, Windham JP, Peck D, Ewing JR, Welch KMA (1997) The temporal evolution of MRI tissue signatures after transient middle cerebral artery occlusion in rat. J Neurol Sci 145: 15–23

5   Rudin M, Baumann D, Ekatodramis D, Stirnimann R, McAllister KH, Sauter A (2001) MRI analysis of the changes in apparanet water diffusion coefficient, T2 relaxation time, and cerebral blood flow and volume in the temporal evolution o cerebral infarction following permanent middle cerebral artery occlusion in rats. *Exp Neurol* 169: 56–63

6   Laurent D, Wasvary J, Yin J, Rudin M, Pellas TC, O'Byrne E (2001) Quantitative and qualitative assessment of articular cartilage in the goat knee with magnetization transfer imaging. *Magn Reson Imag* 19:1279–1286

7   Bashir A, Gray ML, Hartke J, Burstein D (1999) Nondestructive imaging of human cartilage glycosaminoglycan concentration depletion in articular cartilage. *Magn Reson Med* 41: 857–865

8   Laurent D, Wasvary J, Rudin M, O'Byrne E, Pellas T (2003) *In vivo* assessment of proteoglycan content in articular cartilage of the goat knee. *Magn Reson Med* 49: 1037–1046

9   Beckmann N, Bruttel K, Joergensen J, Rudin M, Schuurman H (1996) Magnetic resonance imaging for the evaluation of rejection of a kidney allograft in the rat. *Transpl Int* 9: 175–183

10   Rudin M, Sauter A (1992) *In vivo* NMR in pharmaceutical research. *Magn Reson Imag* 10: 723–731

11   Rudin M, Beckmann N, Porszasz R, Reese T, Sauter A (1999) *In vivo* magnetic resonance in pharmaceutical research: current status and perspectives . *NMR Biomed* 12: 69–97

12   Manning,WJ, Wei JY, Fossel ET, Burstein D (1990) Measurement of left ventricular mass in rats using electrocardiogramm-gated magnetic resonance imaging. *Am J Physiol* 258: H1181–1186

13   Rudin M, Pedersen B, Umemura K, Zierhut W (1991) Determination of rat heart morphology and function *in vivo* in two models of cardiac hypertrophy by means of magnetic resonance imaging. *Bas Res Cardiol* 86: 165–174

14   Watson PJ, Carpenter TA, Hall LD, Tyler JA (1996) Cartilage swelling and loss in a spontaneous model of osteoarthritis visualized by magnetic resonance imaging. *Osteoarthritis Cartilage* 4: 197–207

15   Phelps ME, Huang SC, Hoffman EJ, Selin C, Sokoloff L, Kuhl DE (1979) Tomographic measurement of local cerebral glucose metabolic rate in humans with (F-18)2-fluoro-2-deoxy-D-glucose: validation of method. *Ann Neurol* 6: 371–388

16   Rudin M, Sauter A (1992) Measurement of reaction rates *in vivo* using magnetization transfer techniques. In: M Rudin, J Seelig (eds): *NMR Basic Principles and Progress*, Vol 27: *In vivo Magnetic Resonance Spectroscopy II.*). Springer-Verlag, Berlin, Heidelberg, 257–293

17   Podo F (1999) Tumour phospholipids metabolism. *NMR Biomed* 12: 413–439

18   Tofts PS (1997) Modeling tracer kinetcis in dynamic GdDTPA MR imaging. *J Magn Reson Imag* 7: 91–101

19   Reivich M, Alavi A, Wolf A, FowlerJ, Russel J, Arnett C, MacGregor RR, Shiue CY, Atkins H, Anand A et al (1985) Glucose metabolic kinetic model parameter determination in humans: the lumoed constants and rate constants for [18F]fluorodeoxyglucose and [11C]deoxyglucose. J *Cerebr Blood Flow Metab* 5: 179.192

20   Meier P, Zierler KL (1954) On the theory of the indicator-dilution method for measurement of blood flow and volume. *J Appl Physiol* 6: 731–744

21   Rausch M, Scheffler K, Rudin, M, Radü E (2000) Analysis of input functions from different arterial branches with gamma variate functions and cluster analysis for quantitative blood volume measurements. *Magn Reson Imag* 18: 1235–1243

22   Detre JA, Leigh JS, Williams DS, Koretsky AP (1992) Perfusion imaging. *Magn Reson Med* 23: 37–45

23   Zhang W, Silva AC, Williams DS, Koretsky AP (1992) Measurement of brain perfusion by volume-localized NMR spectroscopy using inversion of arterial water spins: accounting for transit time and cross-relaxation. *Magn Reson Med* 25: 362–371

24   Ogawa S, Lee TM, Kay AR, Tank DW. (1990) Brain magnetic resonance imaging with contrast dependent on blood oxygenation. *Proc Nat Acad Sci USA* 87: 9868–9872

25   Scheffler K, Seifritz E, Haselhorst R, Bilecen D (1999) Titration of the BOLD effect: separation and quantitation of blood volume and oxygenation changes in the human cerebral cortex during neuronal activation and ferumoxide infusion. *Magn Reson Med* 42: 829–836

26   Dijkhuizen RM, Singhal AB, Mandeville JB, Wu O, Halpern EF, Finklestein SP, Rosen BR, Lo EH (2003) Correlation between brain reorganization, ischemic damage, and neurologic status after transient focal cerebral ischemia in rats: a functional magnetic resonance imaging study. *J Neurosci* 23: 510–517

27   Sauter A, Reese T, Pórszász R, Baumann D, Rausch M, Rudin M (2002) Recovery of function in cytoprotected cerebral cortex in rat stroke model assessed by functional MRI. *Magn Reson Med* 47: 759–765

28   Sokoloff L, Reivich M, Kennedy C, Des Rosiers MH, Patlak CS, Pettigrew KD, Sakurada O, Shinohara M (1977) The [14C]deoxyglucose method for the measurement of local cerebral glucose utilization: theory, procedure, and normal values in the conscious and anesthetized albino rat. *J Neurochem* 28: 897–916

29   Mierisova S, Ala-Korpela M (2001) MR spectroscopy quantitation: a review of frequency domain methods. *NMR Biomed* 14: 247–259

30   d eBeer R, van Ormondt D (1992) Analysis of NMR data using time domain fitting procedures. In: M Rudin, J Seelig (eds): *NMR Basic Principles and Progress*, Vol 27: *In vivo Magnetic Resonance Spectroscopy II*. Springer-Verlag Berlin Heidelberg, 201–248

31   Rudin M, Sauter A (1992) *In vivo* phosphorus-31 NMR: Potential and limitations. In: M Rudin, J Seelig (eds): *NMR Basic Principles and Progress*, Vol 28: *In vivo Magnetic Resonance Spectroscopy III*. Springer-Verlag, Berlin Heidelberg, 161–188

32   Bittl JA, Ingwall JS (1985) Reaction rates of creatine kinases and ATP synthesis in the isolated rat heart. *J Biol Chem* 26: 3512–2517

33   Rudin M, Sauter A (1989) Dihydropyridine calcium antagonists reduce the consumption of high-energy phosphates in the rat brain. A study using combine 31P/1H magnetic resonance spectroscopy and 31P saturation transfer. *J Pharm Exp Ther* 251: 700–706

34   Sauter A, Rudin M (1993) Determination of creatine kinase kinetic parameters in rat brain by NMR magnetization transfer: Correlation with brain function. *J Biol Chem* 268: 13166–13171

35   Shields AF, Grierson JR, Kozawa SM, Zheng M (1996) Development of labelled thymidine analogues for imaging tumor proliferation. *Nucl Med Biol* 23: 17–22

36   Laverman P, Boerman OC, Corstens FHM, Oyen WJG (2002) Fluorinated amino acids for tumour imaging with positron emission tomography. *Eur J Nucl Med* 29: 681–690

37   Hara T, Kosaka N, Shinoura N, Kondo T (1998) PET imaging of prostate cancer using carbon-11-choline. *J Nucl Med* 39: 990–995

38   DeGrado TR, Coleman RE, Wang S, Baldwin SW, Orr MD, Robertson CN, Polascik TJ, Price DT (2000) Synthesis and evaluation of 18F labeled choline as an oncologic tracer for positron emission tomography: initial findings with prostate cancer. *Cancer Res* 61: 110–117

39   Hacke W, Brott T, Caplan L, Meier D, Fieschi C, von Kummer R, Donnan G, Heiss WD, Wahlgren NG, Spranger M et al (1999) Thrombolysis in acute ischemic stroke: controlled trials and clinical experience. *Neurology* 53 Suppl 4: S3-14

40   Leira EC, Adams HP (1999) Management of acute ischemic stroke. *Clin Geriatr Med* 15: 701–720

41   Siesjö BK (1978) *Brain energy metabolism*. John Wiley & Sons, New York

42   Hossman KA (1982) Treatment of experimental cerebral ischemia. *J Cerebr Blood Flow Metabl* 2: 275–297

43   Rother J, deCrespigny AJ, D'Arcueil H, Moseley ME (1996) MR detection of cortical spreading depression immediately after focal ischemia in the rat. *J Cerebr Blood Flow Metab* 16: 214–220

44   Busch E, Gyngell ML, Eis M, Hoehn-Berlage M, Hossman KA (1996) Potassium-induced spreading depressions during focal cerebral ischemia in rats: contribution to lesion growth assessed by diffusion – weighted NMR and biochemical imaging. *J Cerebr Blood Flow Metab* 16: 1090–1099

45   Banasiak KJ, Xia Y, Haddad GG (2000) Mechanisms underlying hypoxia-induced neuronal apoptosis. *Progr Neurobiol* 16: 202–213

46   Del Zoppo GJ, Ginis I, Hallenbrck JM, Iadecola C, Wang X, Feuerstein GZ (2000) Inflammation in stroke: putative role of cytokines, adhesion molecules and iNOS in brain response to ischemia. *Brain Pathol* 10: 95–112

47   Schellinger PD, Warrach S (2004) Therapeutic time window of thrombolytic therapy fol-
      lowing stroke. *Curr Atheroscler Rep* 6: 288–294

48   Sauter A, Rudin M (1986) Calcium antagonists reduce the extent of infarction in rat mid-
      dle cerebral artery occlusion model as determined by quantitative magnetic resonance
      imaging. *Stroke* 17: 1228–1234

49   Germano IM, Bartkowsky HM, Berry I, Moseley M, Brant-Zawadski M,Pitts LH (1986)
      Magnetic resonance imaging in the evaluation of nimodipine-treated acute experimen-
      tal focal cerebral ischemia. *Acta Radiol Suppl Stockh* 369: 49–52

50   Sauter A, Rudin M (1995) Strain-dependent drug effects in rat middle cerebral artery
      occlusion model of stroke. *J Pharm Exp Ther* 274: 1008–1013

51   Sauer D, Martin P, Allegrini PR, Bernasconi R, Amacker H, Fagg GE (1992) Differing effects
      of alpha-difluormethylornithin and CGP40116 on polyamine levels and infarct volume
      in a rat model of focal cerebral ischemia. *Neurosci Lett* 141: 131–135

52   Urwyler S, Campbell E, Fricker G, Jenner P, Lemaire M, McAllister K, Neijt HC, Park CK,
      Perkins M, Rudin M et al (1996) Biphenyl-derivatives of 2-amino-7-phophono-heptanoic
      acid, a novel class of potent competitive N-methyl-D-aspartate receptor antagonists. II.
      Pharmacological characterization *in vivo*. *Neuropharmacol* 35: 655–669

53   Qiu H, Hedlund LW, Gewalt SL, Benveniste H, Bare TM, Johnson GA (1997) Progression
      of a focal ischemic lesion in rat brain during treatment with a novel glycine/NMDA
      antagonist: an *in vivo* three-dimensional diffusion-weighted MR microscopy study. *J
      Magn Reson Imag*ing 7: 739–744

54   Petty MA, Neumann-Haefelin C, Kalisch J, Sarhan S, Wettstein JG, Juretschke HP (2003)
      in vivo neuroprotective effects of ACEA 1021 confirmed by magnetic resonance imaging
      in ischemic stroke. *Eur J Pharmacol* 474: 53–62

55   Buchan AM, Li HS, Cho S, Pulsinelli WA (1991) Blockade of AMPA receptors prevents
      CA1 hippocampal injury following severe but transient forebrain ischemia in adult rats.
      Neurosci Lett 132: 1358–1362

56   Nellgard B, Wieloch T (1992) Postischemic blockade of AMPA but not NMDA receptors
      mitigates neuronal damage in the rat brain following transient severe cerebral ischemia.
      J Cereb Blood Flow Metab 12: 2–11

57   Muller TB, Haraldseth O, Jones RA, Sebastiani G, Lindboe CF, Unsgard G, Oksendal AN
      (1995) Perfusion and diffusion-weighted MR imaging for *in vivo* evaluation of treatment
      with U74389G in a rat stroke model. *Stroke* 26: 1453–1458

58   Wiessner C, Sauer D, Alaimo D, Allegrini PR (2000) Protective effects of casapase
      inhibitors in models for cerebral ischemia *in vitro* and *in vivo*. *Cell Mol Biol* 46: 53–62

59   Deckwerth TL, Adams LM, Wiessner C, Allegrini PR, Rudin M, Sauter A, Hengerer B, Say-
      ers RO, Rovelli G, Aja T et al (2001) Longterm protection of brain tissue from cerebral
      ischemia by peripherally administered peptidomimetic caspase inhibitors. Drug Dev Res
      52: 579–586

60   Li PA, Uchino H, Elmer E, Siesjö BK (1997) Amelioration by cyclosorine A of brain dam-
      age following 5 or 10 min of ischemia in rats subjected to preischemic hyperglycemia.
      Brain Res 753: 133–140

61   Sharkey J, Crawford JH, Butcher SP, Marston HG (1996) Tacrolimus (FK506) ameliorates
      skilled motor deficits produced by middle cerebral artery occlusion in trats. *Stroke* 27:
      2282–2286

62   Bochelen D, Rudin M, Sauter A (1999) Calcineurin inhibitors FK506 and SDZ ASM 981

alleviate the outcome of focal cerebral ischemic/reperfusion injury. *J Pharm Exp Ther* 288: 653–659

63   Hughes PM, Allegrini PR, Rudin M, Perry VH, Mir AK, Wiessner C (2002) Monocyte chemoattractant protein-1 deficiency is protective in a murine stroke model. *J Cereb Blood Flow Metab* 22: 308–317

64   Modo M, Stroemer RP, Tang E, Patel S, Hodges H (2002) Effects of implantation site of stem cell grafts on behavioral recovery from stroke damage. *Stroke* 33: 2270–2278

65   Mattsson B, Sorensen JC, Zimmer J, Johansson BB (1997) Neuronal grafting to experimental neocortical infracts improves behavioral outcome and reduces thalamic atrophy in rats housed in enriched but not in standard environments. *Stroke* 28: 1225–1231

66   Reese T, Bochelen D, Sauter A, Beckmann N, Rudin M (1999) Magnetic resonance angiography of the rat cerebrovascular system without the use of contrast agents. *NMR Biomed* 12: 189–196

67   Villringer A, Rosen BR, Belliveau JW, Ackerman JR, Lauffer RB, Buxton RD, Chao YS, Wedeen VJ, Brady TJ (1988) Dynamic imaging with lanthanide chelates in normal brain: contrast due to magnetic susceptibility effects. *Magn Reson Med* 6: 164–174

68   Rudin M, Sauter A (1991) Noninvasive determination of regional cerebral blood flow in rats using dynamic imaging with Gd(DTPA). *Magn Reson Med* 22: 32–46

69   Roussel SA, van Bruggen N, King MD, Houseman J, Williams SR, Gadian DG (1994) Monitoring the initial expansion of focal ischaemic changes by diffusion-weighted MRI using a remote controlled method of occlusion. *NMR Biomed* 7: 21–28

70   Moseley ME, Vendland MF, Kucharczyk J.(1991) Magnetic resonance imaging of diffusion and perfusion. *Top Mag Reson Imag* 3: 50–67

71   Mintorovitch J, Moseley ME, Chileuitt L, Shimizu H,Cohen Y, Weinstein,PR (1991) Comparison of diffusion-and T2-weighted MRI for the early detection of cerebral ischemia and reperfusion in rats. *Magn Reson Med* 18: 39–50

72   van Dorsten FA, Hata R, Maeda K, Franke C, Eis M, Hossmann KA, Hoehn M (1999) Diffusion- and perfusion-weighted MR imaging of transient focal cerebral ischaemia in mice. *NMR Biomed* 12: 525–534

73   van Lookeren Campagne M, Verheul JB, Nicolay K, Balazs R. (1994) Early evolution and recovery from excitotoxic injury in the neonatal rat brain: a study combining magnetic resonance imaging, electrical impedance, and histology. *J Cereb Blood Flow Metab* 14: 1011–1023

74   Weissleder R, Elizondo G, Wittenberg J, Lee AS, Josephson L, Brady TJ (1990) Ultrasmall superparamagnetic iron oxide: an intravenous contrast agent for assessing lymph nodes with MR imaging. *Radiology* 175: 494–498

75   Rausch M, Sauter A, Fröhlich J, Neubacher U, Radü EW, Rudin M (2001) Dynamic pattern of USPIO enhancement can be observed in macrophages after ischemic brain damage. *Magn Reson Med* 46: 1018–1022

76   Rausch M, Baumann D, Neubacher U, Rudin M (2002) *In-vivo* visualization of phagocytotic cells in rat brains after transient ischemia by USPIO. *NMR Biomed* 15: 278–283

77   Sauter A, Rudin M (1987) Effects of calcium antagonists on high-energy phosphates in ischemic rat brain measured by 31P NMR spectroscopy. *Magn Reson Med* 4: 1–8

78   Delpy DT, Gordon RE, Hope PL, Parker D, Reynolds EOR, Shaw D, Whitehead MD (1982) Noninvasive investigation of cerebral ischemia by phosphorus magnetic resonance. *Pediatrics* 70: 310–313

79   Prichard JW, Alger JR, Behar KL, Petroff OAC, Shulman RG (1983) Cerebral metabolic studies *in vivo* by 31P NMR. *Proc Natl Acad Sci USA* 80: 2748–2751

80   Forsen S, Hoffman RA (1963) Study of moderately rapid chemical exchange reaction by means of nuclear magnetic double resonance. *J Chem Phys* 40: 1189–1196

81   Koretsky AP, Wang S, Klein MP, James TL, Weiner MW (1986) 31P NMR saturation transfer measurements of phosphorus exchange reactions in rat heart and kidney *in situ*. *Biochemistry* 25: 77–84

82   Rudin M, Weissleder R (2003) Molecular imaging in drug discovery and development. *Nat Rev Drug Discov* 3: 123–131

83   Buonanno FS, Pykett IL, Brady TJ, Vielma J, Burt CT, Goldman MR, Hinshaw WS, Pohost GM, Kistler JP (1983) Proton NMR imaging in experimental ischemic infarction. *Stroke* 14: 173–177

84   Allegrini PR, Sauer D (1992) Application of magnetic resonance imaging to the measurement of neurodegeneration in rat brain: MRI data correlate strongly with histology and enzymatic analysis. *Magn Reson Imag* 10: 773–778

85   van der Toorn A, Sykova E, Dijkhurzen RM, Vorisek I, Vargova L, Skobisova E, van Lookeren-Campagne M, Reese T, Nicolay K (1996) Dynamic changes in water ADC, energy metabolism *Magn Reson Med* 36: 52–60

86   Davis D, Ulatowski J, Eleff S, Izuta M, Mori S, Shungu D, van Zijl PC (1994) Rapid monitoring of changes in water diffusion coefficients during reversible ischemia in cat and rat brain. *Magn Reson Med* 31: 454–460

87   Hasegawa Y, Fisher M, Latour LL, Dardzinski BJ, Sotak CH (1994) MRI diffusion mapping of reversible and irreversible ischemic injury in focal brain ischemia. *Neurology* 44: 1484–1490

88   Neumann-Haefelin T, Wittsack HJ, Wenserski F, Siebler M, Seity RJ, Mödder U, Freund HL (1999) Diffusion- and perfusion-weighted MRI: the DWI/PWI mismatch region in acute stroke. *Stroke* 30: 1591–1597

89   Reese T, Porszasz R, Baumann D, Bochelen D, Boumezbeur F, McAllister KH, Sauter A, Bjelke B, Rudin B (2000) Cytoprotection does not preserve brain functionality in rats during acute post-stroke phase despite evidence of non-infarction provided by MRI. *NMR Biomed* 13: 361–370

90   Rausch M, Hiestand P, Foster CA, Baumann D, Cannet C, Rudin M (2004) Predictability of FTY720 efficacy in experimental autoimmune encephalomyelitis by *in vivo* macrophage tracking: clinical implications for ultrasmall superparamagnetic iron oxide-enhanced magnetic resonance imaging. *J Magn Reson Imag* 20: 16–24

91   Hoehn M, Küstermann E, Blunk J, Wiedermann D, Trapp T, Wecker S, Föcking M, Heinz A, Hescheler J, Fleischmann BK et al (2002) Monitoring of implanted stem cell migration *in vivo*: A highly resolved *in vivo* magnetic resonance imaging investigation of experimental stroke in rat. *Proc Natl Acad Sci USA* 99: 16267–16272

92   Kim DE, Schellingerhout D, Ishii K, Shah K, Weissleder R (2004) Imaging of stem cell recruitment to ischemic infarcts in a murine model. *Stroke* 35: 952–957

93   Benveniste H, Einstein G, Kim KR, Hulette C, Johnson GA (1999) Detection of neuritic plaques in Alzheimer's disease by magnetic resonance microscopy. *Proc Natl Acad Sci USA* 96: 14079–14084

94   Rudin M, Mueggler T, Allegrini P.R, Baumann D, Rausch M. (2003b) Characterization of CNS disorders and evaluation of therapy using structural and functional MRI. *Anal Bioanal Chem* 377: 973–981

95   Zhang J, Yarowsky P, Gordon MN, Di Carlo G, Munireddy S, van Zijl PC, Mori S. (2004) Detection of amyloid plaques in mouse models of Alzheimer's disease by magnetic resonance imaging. *Magn Reson Med* 51: 452–457

96   Jack CR Jr, Petersen RC, Xu YC, O'Brien PC, Smith GE, Ivnik RJ, Boeve BF, Waring SC, Tangalos EG, Kokmen E (1999) Prediction of AD with MRI-based hippocampal volume in mild cognitive impairment. *Neurology* 52: 1397–1403

97   Wadghiri YZ, Sigurdsson EM, Sadowski M, Elliott JI, Li Y, Scholtzova H, Tang CY, Aguinaldo G, Pappolla M, Duff K et al (2003) Detection of Alzheimer's amyloid in transgenic mice using magnetic resonance microimaging. *Magn Reson Med* 50: 293–302

98   Agdeppa ED, Kepe V, Liu J, Flores-Torres S, Satyamurthy N, Petric A, Cole GM, Small GW, Huang SC, Barrio JR (2001) Binding characteristics of radiofluorinated 6-dialkylamino-2-naphthylethylidene derivatives as positron emission tomography imaging probes for beta-amyloid plaques in Alzheimer's disease. *J Neurosci* 21: RC189

99   Hintersteiner M, Frey P, Kinzy W, Kneuer R, Neumann U, Rudin M, Staufenbiel M, Wiederhold KH, Gremlich HU (2005) In vivo detection of amyloid deposits by near-infrared fluorescence imaging using a novel oxazine derivative as contrast agent. *Nature Biotechnolog* 23: 577–583

100   Parvathy S, Davies P, Haroutunian V, Purohit DP, Davis KL, Mohs RC, Park H, Moran TM, Chan JY, Buxbaum JD (2001) Correlation between $A\beta x$-40-, $A\beta x$-42-, and $A\beta x$-43-containing amyloid plaques and cognitive decline. *Arch Neuro* 58: 2025–2032

101   Sturchler-Pierrat C, Abramowski D, Duke M, Wiederhold KH, Mistl C, Rothacher S, Ledermann B, Burki K, Frey P, Paganetti PA et al (1997) Two amyloid precursor protein transgenic mouse models with Alzheimer disease-like pathology. *Proc Natl Acad Sci USA* 94: 13287–13292

102   Sturchler-Pierrat C, Staufenbiel M (2000) Pathogenic mechanisms of Alzheimer's disease analyzed in the APP23 transgenic mouse model. *Ann NY Acad Sci* 920: 134–139

103   Kelly PH, Bondolfi L, Hunziker D, Schlecht HP, Carver K, Maguire E, Abramowski D, Wiederhold KH, Sturchler-Pierrat C, Jucker M et al (2003) Progressive age-related impairment of cognitive behavior in APP23 transgenic mice. *Neurobiol Aging* 24: 365–378

104   Van Dam D, D'Hooge R, Staufenbiel M, Van Ginneken C, Van Meir F, De Deyn PP (2003) Age-dependent cognitive decline in the APP23 model precedes amyloid deposition. *Eur J Neurosci* 17: 388–396

105   Helpern JA, Lee SP, Falangola MF, Dyakin VV, Bogart A, Ardekani B, Duff K, Branch C, Wisniewski T, de Leon MJ et al (2004) MRI assessment of neuropathology in a transgenic mouse model of Alzheimer's disease. *Magn Reson Med* 51: 794–798

106   Müggler T, Meyer-Luehmann M, Rausch M, Staufenbiel M, Jucker M, Rudin M (2004) Restricted diffusion in the brain of transgenic mice with cerebral amyloidosis. *Eur J Neurosci* 20: 811–817

107   Beckmann N, Schuler A, Mueggler T, Meyer EP, Wiederhold KH, Staufenbiel M, Krucker T (2003) Age-dependent cerebrovascular abnormalities and blood flow disturbances in APP23 mice modeling Alzheimer's disease. *J Neurosci* 23: 8453–8459

108   Müggler T, Sturchler-Pierrat C, Baumann D, Rausch M, Staufenbiel M, Rudin M (2002) Dynamic CBV imaging in amyloid precursor protein transgenic mice. *J Neurosci*ence 22: 7218–7224

109   Müggler T, Baumann D, Rausch M, Staufenbiel M, Rudin M (2003) Age-dependent impairment of somatosensory response in the amyloid precursor protein 23 transgenic mouse model of Alzheimer's disease. *J Neurosci* 23: 8231–8236

110   Burgermeister P, Calhoun ME, Winkler DT, Jucker M (2000) Mechanisms of cerebrovascular amyloid deposition. Lessons from mouse models. *Ann NY Acad Sci* 903: 307–316

111   Winkler DT, Bondolfi L, Herzig MC, Jann L, Calhoun ME, Wiederhold KH, Tolnay M, Staufenbiel M, Jucker M (2001) Spontaneous hemorrhagic stroke in a mouse model of cerebral amyloid angiopathy. *J Neurosci* 21: 1619–1627

112   Graves EE, Ripoll J, Weissleder R, Ntziachristos V (2003) A submillimeter resolution fluorescence molecular imaging system for small animal imaging. *Med Phys* 30: 901–911

113   Dawson J, Miltz W, Mir AK, Wiessner C (2003) Targeting monocyte chemoattractant protein-1 signalling in disease. *Expert Opin Ther Targets* 7: 35–48

114   Lehrmann E, Christensen T, Zimmer J, Diemer NH, Finsen B (1997)Microglial and macrophage reactions mark progressive changes and define the penumbra in the rat neocortex and striatum after transient middle cerebral artery occlusion. *J Comp Neurol* 386: 461–476

115   Feuerstein G, Wang X, Barone F (1998) The role of cytokines in the neuropathology of stroke and neurotrauma. *Neuroimmunomodulation* 5:143–149

116   Hemmer B, Archelos JJ, Hartung HP (2002) New concepts in the immunopathogenesis of multiple sclerosis. *Nat Rev Neurosci* 3: 291–301

117   Barkhof F, van Walderveen M (1999) Characterization of tissue damage in multiple sclerosis by nuclear magnetic resonance. *Philos Trans R Soc Lond B Biol Sci* 354: 1675–1686

118   Boneschi FM, Rovaris M, Comi G, Filippi M (2004) The use of magnetic resonance imaging in multiple sclerosis: lessons learned from clinical trials. *Mult Scler* 10: 341–347

119   Cercignani M, Bozzali M, Iannucci G, Comi G, Filippi M (2001) Magnetisation transfer ratio and mean diffusivity of normal appearing white and grey matter from patients with multiple sclerosis. *J Neurol Neurosurg Psychiatry* 70: 311–317

120   Gold R, Hartung HP, Toyka KV (2000) Animal models for autoimmune demyelinating disorders of the nervous system. *Mol Med Today* 6: 88–91

121   Hawkins CP, Munro PM, MacKenzie F, Kesselring J, Tofts PS, du Boulay EP, Landon DN, McDonald WI (1990) Duration and selectivity of blood-brain barrier breakdown in chronic relapsing experimental allergic encephalomyelitis studied by gadolinium- DTPA and protein markers. *Brain* 113 (Pt 2): 365–378

122   Tofts PS, Kermode AG (1991) Measurement of the blood-brain barrier permeability and leakage space using dynamic MR imaging. 1. Fundamental concepts. *Magn Reson Med* 17: 357–367

123   Veldhuis WB, Floris S, van der Meide PH, Vos IM, de Vries HE, Dijkstra CD, Bar PR, Nicolay K (2003) Interferon-beta prevents cytokine-induced neutrophil infiltration and attenuates blood-brain barrier disruption. *J Cereb Blood Flow Metab* 23: 1060–1069

124   Henkelman RM, Stanisz GJ, Graham SJ (2001) Magnetization transfer in MRI: a review. *NMR Biomed* 14: 57–64

125   Graham SJ, Henkelman RM (1997) Understanding pulsed magnetization transfer. *J Magn Reson Imag*ing 7: 903–912

126   't Hart BA, Vogels J, Bauer J, Brok HP, Blezer E (2004) Non-invasive measurement of brain damage in a primate model of multiple sclerosis. *Trends Mol Med* 2004 10: 85–91

127   Rausch M, Hiestand P, Baumann D, Cannet C, Rudin M (2003) MRI-based monitoring of inflammation and tissue damage in acute and chronic relapsing EAE. *Magn Reson Med* 50: 309–314

128   Dousset V, Delalande C, Ballarino L, Quesson B, Seilhan D, Coussemacq M, Thiaudiere

E, Brochet B, Canioni P, Caille JM (1999) *In vivo* macrophage activity imaging in the central nervous system detected by magnetic resonance. *Magn Reson Med* 41: 329–333

129   Dousset V, Doche B, Petry KG, Brochet B, Delalande C, Caille JM (2002) Correlation between clinical status and macrophage activity imaging in the central nervous system of rats. *Acad Radiol* 9 Suppl 1: S156–S159

130   Dousset V, Gomez C, Petry KG, Delalande C, Caille JM (1999) Dose and scanning delay using USPIO for central nervous system macrophage imaging. *MAGMA* 8: 185–189

131   Barber PA, Foniok T, Kirk D, Buchan AM, Laurent S, Boutry S, Muller RN, Hoyte L, Tomanek B, Tuor UI (2004) MR molecular imaging of early endothelial activation in focal ischemia. *Ann Neurol* 56: 116–120

132   Sipkins DA, Gijbels K, Tropper FD, Bednarski M, Li KC, Steinman L (2000) ICAM-1 expression in autoimmune encephalitis visualized using magnetic resonance imaging. *J Neuroimmunol* 104: 1–9

133   Damadian R. (1971) Tumor detection by nuclear magnetic resonance. *Science* 171: 1151–1153

134   Siegel R, Tolesvai L, Rudin M (1988) Partial inhibition of the growth of transplanted Dunning rat prostate tumors with the longacting somatostatin analogue sandostatin (SMS 201–995) *Cancer Res.* 48: 4651–4655

135   Furr BJ (1996) The development of Casodex (bicalutamide): preclinical studies. Eur Urol 29 (Suppl 2): 83–95

136   Rudin M, Briner U, Doepfner W (1988) Quantitative magnetic resonance imaging of estradiol-induced pituitary hyperplasia in rats. *Magn Reson Med* 7: 285–291

137   Qin Y, Van Cauteren M, Osteaux M, Schally, AV, Willems G (1992) Inhibitory effect of somatostatin analogue RC-160 on the growth of hepatic metastases of colon cancer in rats: a study with magnetic resonance imaging. *Cancer Res* 51: 6025–6030

138   Sherley JL, Kelly TJ (1988) Regulation of human thymidine kinase during the cell cycle. *J Biol Chem* 263: 8350–8358

139   van Eijkeren ME, Thierens H, Seuntjens J, Goethals P, Lemahieu I, Strijckmans K (1996) Kinetics of [methyl-11C]thymidine in patients with squamous cell carcinoma of the head an neck. *Acta Oncol* 35: 737–741

140   Van der Borght T, Labar D, Pauwels S, Lambotte L (1991) Production of [2-11C]thymidine for quantification of cellular proliferation with PET. *Appl Radiat Isot* 42: 103–104

141   Mankoff DA, Shields AF, Link JM, Graham MM, Muzi M, Peterson LM, Eary JF, Krohn KA (1999) Kinetic analysis of 2-[11C]thymidine PET imaging studies: validation studies. *J Nucl Med* 40: 614–624

142   Shields AF, Grierson JR, Kozawa SM, Zheng M (1996) Development of labeled thymidine analogs for imaging tumor proliferation. *Nucl Med Biol* 23: 17–22

143   Carnochan P, Brooks R (1999) Radiolabelled 5'-iodo'2'deoxyuridine: a promising alternative to [18F]-2-fluoro-deoxy-D-glucose for PET studies of early response to anticancer treatment. *Nucl Med Biol* 26: 667–672

144   Sato K, Kameyama M, Ishiwata K, Katakura R, Yoshimoto T (1992) Metabolic changes of glioma following chemotherapy: An experimental study using four PET tracers. J Neuro-Oncol 14: 81–89

145   Miyagawa T, Oku T, Uehara H, Desay R, Beattie B, Tjuvajew j. Blasberg R (1998) 'Facilitated' amino acid transport is upregulated in brain tumors. *J Cerebr Blood Flow Metab* 18: 500–509

146   Busch H, Davis JR, Honig GR, Anderson DC, Nair PV, Nyhan WL (1995) The uptake of a

variety of amino acids into nuclear proteins of tumors and other tissues. *Cancer Res* 19: 1030–1039

147   Coenen HH, Kling P, Stocklin G (1989) Cerebral metabolism of L-[2-18F]fluorotyrosine. *J Nucl Med* 30: 1867–1372

148   Negendank WG (1992) Studie of human tumors by MRS: a review. *NMR Biomed* 5: 303–324

149   Hara T, Kosaka N, Kishi H (1998) PET imaging of prostate cancer using carbon-11-choline. *J Nucl Med* 39: 990–995

150   Price DT, Coleman RE, Liao RP, Robertson CN, Polscik TJ, DeGrado TR (2002) Comparison of [18F]fluorocholine and [18F]fluorodeoxyglucose for positron emission tomography of androgen dependent and androgen independent prostate cancer. *J Urology* 168: 273–280

151   Warburg O, Wind F, Negalein E (1927) The metabolism of tumours in the body. *J Physiol* 8: 519–530

152   Semenza GL (1999) Regulation of mammalian O2 homeostatsis by hypoxia-inducible factor 1. *Ann Rev Cell Dev Biol* 15: 551–578

153   Dang CV, Semenza GL (1999) Oncogenic alterations in metabolism. *Trend Biochem Sci* 24: 68–72

154   Wahl RL, Zasadny K, Helvie M, Hutchins GD, Weber B, Cody R (1993) Metabolic monitoring of breast cancer chemohormonotherapy using positron emission tomography: initial evaluation. *J Clin Oncol* 11: 2101–2111

155   Schelling M, Avril N, Nahrig J, Kuhn W, Römer W, Sattler D, Werner M, Dose J, Jänicke F, Graeff H, Schwaiger M (2000) Positron emission tomography using fluorodeoxyglucose for monitoring primary chemotherapy in breast cancer. *J Clin Oncol* 18: 1689–1695

156   Stroobants S, Goeminne J, Seegers M, Dimitrijevic S, Dupont P, Nuyts J, Martens M, van der Borne B, Cole P, Sciot R et al (2003) 18f Positron emission tomography for the early prediction of response in advanced soft tissue sarcoma treated with imatinib mesylate (Gleevec ®). *Eur J Cancer* 39: 2012–2020

157   Kaiser WA (1883) MR mammography. *Radiologie* 33: 292–299

158   Tofts PS and Kermode AG (1991) Measurement of the blood-brain barrier permeability and leakage space using dynamic MR Imaging: 1. Fundamental concepts. *Magn Reson Med* 17: 357–367

159   Rudin M, Beckmann N, Sauter A (1997) Analysis of tracer transit in rat brain after carotid artery and femoral vein administration using linear system theory. *Magn Reson Imag* 15: 551–558

160   Drevs J, Müller-Driver R, Wittig C, Fuxius S, Esser N, Hugenschmidt H, Konerding MA, Allegrini PR, Wood J, Hennig J et al (2002) PTK787/ZK 222584, a specific vascular endothelial growth factor receptor tyrosine kinases inhibitor, affects the anatomy of the tumor vascular bed and the functional vascular properties as detected by dynamic enhanced magnetic resonance imaging. *Cancer Res* 62: 4015–4022

161   Brown LF, Berse B, Jackman RW, Tognazzi K, Manseau EJ, Senger DR, Dvorak HF (1993) Expression of vascular permeability factor (vascular endothelial growth factor) and its receptors in adenocarcinomas of the gastrointestinal tract. *Cancer Res* 53: 4727–4735

162   Carmeliet P, Ferreira V, Breier G, Pollefeyt S, Kieckens L, Gertsenstein M, Fahrig M, Vandenhoeck A, Harpal K, Eberhardt C et al (1996) Abnormal blood vessel development and lethality in embryos lacking a single VEGF allele. *Nature* 380: 435–439

163   Brasch R, Pham C, Shames D, Roberts T, van Dijke K, van Bruggen N, Mann J, Ostrow-

itzki S, Melnyk O (1997) Assessment of tumor angiogenesis using macromolecular MRE imaging contrast media. *J Magn Reson Imag* 7: 68–74

164 Rudin M, McSheehy PMJ, Allegrini PR, Kindler-Baumann D, Bequet M, Brecht K, Brueggen J, Ferretti S, Schaeffer F, Schnell C, Wood J (2005) PTK787 / ZK222584, a tyrosine kinase inhibitor of vascular endothelial growth factor receptor, reduces uptake of the contrast agent GdDOTA by murine orthotopic B16/BL6 melanoma tumours and inhibits their growth *in vivo*. *NMR Biomed* 18: 308–321

165 Morgan B, Thomas AL, Drevs J, Hennig J, Buchert M, Jivan A, Horsfield MA, Mross K, Ball HA, Lee L et al (2003) Dynamic contrast-enhanced magnetic resonance imaging as a biomarker for the pharmacological response of PTK787/ZK 222584, an inhibitor of the vascular endothelial growth factor receptor tyrosine kinases, in patients with advanced colorectal cancer and liver metastases: results from two phase I studies. *J Clin Oncol* 21:3955–3964

166 Martin SJ, Reutelingsperger CP, McGahon AJ, Rader JA, van Schie RC, LaFace DM, Green DR (1995) Early redistribution of plasma membrane phosphatidylserine is a general feature of apoptosis regardless of the initiating stimulus: inhibition by overexpression of Bcl-2 and Abl. *J Exp Med* 182: 1545–1556

167 Fadok VA, de Cathelineau A, Daleke DL, Henson PM, Bratton DL (2001) Loss of phospholipid asymmetry and surface exposure of phosphatidylserine is required for phagocytosis of apoptotic cells by macrophages and fibroblasts. *J Biol Chem*, 276: 1071–1077

168 Koopman G, Reutelingsperger CPM, Kuijten GAM, Keehnen RMJ, Pals ST, van Oers MHJ (1994) Annexin V for flow cytometric detection of phosphatidylserine expression on B cells undergoing apoptosis. *Blood* 84: 1415–1420

169 Blankenberg FG, Katsikis PD, Tait JF, Davis RE, Naumovski L, Ohtsuki K, Kopiwoda S, Abrams MJ, Darkes M, Robbins RC et al (1998) *In vivo* detection and imaging of phosphatidylserin expression during programmed cell death. *Proc Natl Acad Sci USA* 95: 6349–6354

170 Zhao M, Beauregard DA, Loizou L, Davletov B, Brindle KM (2001) Non-invasive detection of apoptosis using magnetic resonance imaging and a targeted contrast agent. *Nat Med* 7: 1241–1244

171 Dumont EA, Reutelingsperger CP, Smits JF, Daemen MJ, Doevendans PA, Wellens HJ, Hofstra L (2001) Real-time imaging of apoptotic cell-membrane changes at the single-cell level in the beating murine heart. *Nat Med* 7: 1352–1355

172 Petrovsky A ,Schellenberger E, Josephson L, Weissleder R, Bogdanov A (2003) Near-infrared gluorescent imaging of tumor apoptosis. *Cancer Res* 63: 1936–1942

173 Schellenberger EA, Bogdanov A Jr, Petrovsky A, Ntziachristos N, Weissleder R, Josephson L (2003) Optical imaging of apoptosis as a biomarker of tumor response to chemotherapy. *Neoplasia* 5: 187–192

174 Hammill AK, Uhr JW, Scheuermann RH (1999) Annexin V staining due to loss of membrane asymmetry can be reversible and precede commitment to apoptotic cell death. *Exp Cell Res* 251: 16–21

175 Laxman B, Hall DE, Bhojani MS, Hamstra DA, Chevenert TL, Ross BD, Rehemtulla A (2002) Noninvasive real-time imaging of apoptosis. *Proc Natl Acad Sci USA* 99: 16551–16555

176 Williams SNO, Anthony ML, Brindle KM (1998) Induction of apoptosis in two mammalian cell lines results in increased levels of fructose-1,6-bisphosphate and CDP-choline as determined by 31P MRS. *Magn Reson Med* 40: 411–420

177 Hakumäki JM, Brindle KM (2003) Techniques: Visualizing apoptosis using nuclear magnetic resonance. *Trends Pharm Sci* 24: 146–149

178 Chevenert TL, McKeever PE, Ross BD (1997) Monitoring early response of experimental brain tumors to therapy using diffusion magnetic resonance imaging. *Clin Cancer Res* 3: 1467–1466

179 Chevenert TL, Stegman LD, Taylor JMG, Robertson PL, Greenberg HS, Rehemtulla A, Ross BD (2000) Diffusion magnetic resonance imaging: an early surrogate marker of therapeutic efficacy in brain tumors. *J Natl Cancer Inst* 92: 2029–2036

180 Tung CH, Mahmood U, Bredow S, Weissleder R (2000) In vivo imaging of proteolytic enzyme activity using a novel molecular reporter. *Cancer Res* 60: 4953–4958

181 Mahmood U, Tung CH, Bogdanov A, Weissleder R (1999) Near-infrared optical imaging of protease activity for tumor detection. *Radiology* 213: 866–870

182 Bremer C, Tung CH, Weissleder R (2001) *In vivo* molecular target assessment of matrix metalloproteinase inhibition. *Nat Med* 7: 743–748

183 Bouvet M, Wang J, Nardin SR, Nassirpour N, Yang M, Baranov E, Jiang P, Moossa AR, Hoffman RM (2000) Real-time optical imaging of primary tumor growth and multiple metastatic events in a pancreatic cancer orthotopic model. *Cancer Res* 62: 1534–1540

184 Rehemtulla A, Stegman LD, Cardozo SJ, Gupta S, Hall DE, Contag CH, Ross BD (2000) Rapid and quantitative assessment of cancer treatment response using *in vivo* bioluminescence imaging. *Neoplasia* 2: 491–495

185 Gambhir SS, Hershman HR, Cherry SR, Barrio JR, Satyamurthy N, Toyokuni T, Phelps ME, Larson SM, Balatoni J, Finn R et al (2000) Imaging transgene expression with radionuclide imaging technologies. *Neoplasia* 2: 118–138

186 Barck KH, Lee WP, Diehl LJ, Ross J, Gribling P, Zhang Y, Nguyen K, van Bruggen N, Hurst S, Carano RA (2004), Quantification of cortical bone loss and repair for therapeutic evaluation in collagen-induced arthritis, by micro-computed tomography and automated image analysis. *Arthritis Rheum* 50: 3377–3386

187 Morenko BJ, Bove SE, Chen L, Guzman RE, Juneau P, Bocan TM, Peter GK, Arora R, Kilgore KS (2004) In vivo micro computed tomography of subchondral bone in the rat after intra-articular administration of monosodium iodoacetate. *Contemp Top Lab Anim Sci* 43: 39–43

188 Ford NL, Thornton MM, Holdsworth DW (2003) Fundamental image quality limits for microcomputed tomography in small animals. *Med Phys* 30: 2869–2877

189 Beckmann N, Bruttel K, Mir AK, Rudin M (1995) Noninvasive 3D MR microscopy as a tool in pharmacological research: application to a model of rheumatoid arthritis. *Magn Reson Imag*ing 13: 1013–1317

190 Dawson J, Gustard S, Beckmann N (1999) High-resolution three-dimensional magnetic resonance imaging for the investigation of knee joint damage during the time course of antigen-induced arthritis in rabbits. *Arthritis Rheum* 42: 119–128

191 Jacobson PB, Morgan SJ, Wilcox DM, Nguyen P, Ratajczak CA, Carlson RP, Harris RR, Nuss M (1999) A new spin on an old model: *in vivo* evaluation of disease progression by magnetic resonance imaging with respect to standard inflammatory parameters and histopathology in the adjuvant arthritic rat. *Arthritis Rheum* 42: 2060–2073

192 Faure P, Doan BT, Beloeil JC (2003) *In-vivo* high resolution three-dimensional MRI studies of rat joints at 7 T. *NMR Biomed* 16: 484–493

193 Harris RR, Black L, Surapaneni S, Kolasa T, Majest S, Namovic MT, Grayson G, Komater V, Wilcox D, King L, Marsh K, Jarvis MF, Nuss M, Nellans H, Pruesser L, Reinhart GA,

Cox B, Jacobson P, Stewart A, Coghlan M, Carter G, Bell RL (2004) ABT-963 [2-(3,4-difluoro-phenyl)-4-(3-hydroxy-3-methyl-butoxy)-5-(4-methanesulfonyl-phenyl)-2H-pyridazin-3-one], a highly potent and selective disubstituted pyridazinone cyclooxgenase-2 inhibitor. *J Pharmacol Exp Ther* 311: 904-12

194   Badger AM, Griswold DE, Kapadia R, Blake S, Swift BA, Hoffman SJ, Stroup GB, Webb E, Rieman DJ, Gowen M et al (2000) Disease-modifying activity of SB 242235, a selective inhibitor of p38 mitogen-activated protein kinase, in rat adjuvant-induced arthritis. *Arthritis Rheum* 43: 175–183

195   Badger AM, Blake S, Kapadia R, Sarkar S, Levin J, Swift BA, Hoffman SJ, Stroup GB, Miller WH, Gowen M, Lark MW (2001) Disease-modifying activity of SB 273005, an orally active, nonpeptide alphavbeta3 (vitronectin receptor) antagonist, in rat adjuvant-induced arthritis. *Arthritis Rheum* 44: 128–137

196   Beckmann N, Bruttel K, Schuurman H, Mir AK (1998) Effects of Sandimmune neoral on collagen-induced arthritis in DA rats: characterization by high resolution three-dimensional magnetic resonance imaging and by histology. *J Magn Reson* 131: 8–16

197   Calvo E, Palacios I, Delgado E, Ruiz-Cabello J, Hernandez P, Sanchez-Pernaute O, Egido J, Herrero-Beaumont G (2001) High-resolution MRI detects cartilage swelling at the early stages of experimental osteoarthritis. *Osteoarthritis Cartilage* 9: 463–472

198   Tessier JJ, Bowyer J, Brownrigg NJ, Peers IS, Westwood FR, Waterton JC, Maciewicz RA (2003) Characterization of the guinea pig model of osteoarthritis by *in vivo* three-dimensional magnetic resonance imaging. *Osteoarthritis Cartilage* 11: 841–853

199   Lohmander LS (1994) Articular cartilage and osteoarthritis. The role of molecular markers to monitor breakdown, repair and disease. *J Anat* 184: 477–492

200   Donahue KM, Burstein D, Manning WJ, Gray ML (1994) Studies of Gd-DTPA relaxivity and proton exchange rates in tissue, *Magn Reson Med* 32: 66–76

201   Laurent D, Wasvary J, O'Byrne E, Rudin M (2003) In vivo qualitative assessments of articular cartilage in the rabbit knee with high-resolution MRI at 3 T. *Magn Reson Med* 50: 541–549

202   Kim DK, Ceckler TL, Hascall VC, Calabro A, Balaban RS (1993) Analysis of water-macromolecule proton magnetization transfer in articular cartilage. *Magn Reson Med* 29: 211–215

203   Vahlensieck M, Dombrowski F, Leutner C, Wagner U, Reiser M (1994)Magnetization transfer contrast (MTC) and MTC-substraction: enhancement of cartilage lesions and intra-cartilaginous degeneration *in vitro*. *Skeletal Radiol* 23: 535–539

204   Gray ML, Burstein D, Lesperance LM, Gehrke L (1995) Magnetization transfer in cartilage and its constituent macromolecules. *Magn Reson Med* 34: 319–325

205   Gaffney K, Cookson J, Blades S, Coumbe A, Blake D (1998) Quantitative assessment of the rheumatoid synovial microvascular bed by gadolinium-DTPA enhanced magnetic resonance imaging. *Ann Rheum Dis* 57: 152–157

206   Cutolo M (1999) Macrophages as effectors of the immunoendocrinologic interactions in autoimmune rheumatic diseases. *Ann NY Acad Sci* 876: 32–41

207   Dardzinski BJ, Schmithorst VJ, Holland SK, Boivin GP, Imagawa T, Watanabe S, Lewis JM, Hirsch R (2001) MR imaging of murine arthritis using ultrasmall superparamagnetic iron oxide particles. *Magn Reson Imaging* 19: 1209–1216

208   Beckmann N, Falk R, Zurbrugg S, Dawson J, Engelhardt P (2003) Macrophage infiltration into the rat knee detected by MRI in a model of antigen-induced arthritis. *Magn Reson Med* 49: 1047–1055

209   Lutz AM, Seemayer C, Corot C, Gay RE, Goepfert K, Michel BA, Marincek B, Gay S, Weishaupt D (2004) Detection of synovial macrophages in an experimental rabbit model of antigen-induced arthritis: ultrasmall superparamagnetic iron oxide-enhanced MR imaging. *Radiology* 233: 149–157

210   Hansch A, Frey O, Sauner D, Hilger I, Haas M, Malich A, Brauer R, Kaiser WA (2004) *In vivo* imaging of experimental arthritis with near-infrared fluorescence. *Arthritis Rheum* 50: 961–967

211   Lai WF, Chang CH, Tang Y, Bronson R, Tung CH (2004) Early diagnosis of osteoarthritis using cathepsin B sensitive near-infrared fluorescent probes. *Osteoarthritis Cartilage* 12: 239–244

212   Wunder A, Tung CH, Muller-Ladner U, Weissleder R, Mahmood U (2004) *In vivo* imaging of protease activity in arthritis: a novel approach for monitoring treatment response. *Arthritis Rheum* 50: 2459–2465

213   Cavanaugh D, Johnson E, Price RE, Kurie J, Travis EL, Cody DD (2004) *In vivo* respiratory-gated micro-CT imaging in small-animal oncology models. *Mol Imaging* 3: 55–62

214   Hu J, Hawort, ST, Molthen RC, Dawson CA (2004) Dynamic small animal lung imaging via a postacquisition respiratory gating technique using micro-cone beam computed tomography. *Acad Radiol* 11: 961–970

215   Langheinrich AC, Leithauser B, Greschus S, Von Gerlach S, Breithecker A, Matthias FR, Rau WS, Bohle RM (2004) Acute rat lung injury: feasibility of assessment with micro-CT. *Radiology* 233: 165–171

216   Bergin CJ, Pauly JM, Macovski A (1991) Lung parenchyma: projection reconstruction MR imaging. *Radiology* 179: 777–781

217   Beckmann N, Tigani B, Mazzoni L, Fozard JR (2003) Magnetic resonance imaging of the lung provides potential for non-invasive preclinical evaluation of drugs. *Trends Pharmacol Sci* 24: 550–554

218   Gewalt SL, Glover GH, Hedlund LW, Cofer GP, MacFall JR, Johnson GA (1993) MR microscopy of the rat lung using projection reconstruction. *Magn Reson Med* 29: 99–106

219   Hedlund LW, Cofer GP, Owen SJ, Allan Johnson G (2000) MR-compatible ventilator for small animals: computer-controlled ventilation for proton and noble gas imaging. *Magn Reson Imaging* 18: 753–759

220   Beckmann N, Tigani,B, Mazzoni,L, Fozard JR (2001) MRI of lung parenchyma in rats and mice using a gradient-echo sequence. *NMR Biomed* 14: 297–306

221   Beckmann N, Tigani B, Ekatodramis D, Borer R, Mazzoni L, Fozard JR (2001) Pulmonary edema induced by allergen challenge in the rat: noninvasive assessment by magnetic resonance imaging. *Magn Reson Med* 45: 88–95

222   Renzi PM, Olivenstein R, Martin JG (1993) Inflammatory cell populations in the airways and parenchyma after antigen challenge in the rat. *Am Rev Resp Dis* 147: 967–974

223   Hannon JP, Tigani B, Williams I, Mazzoni L, Fozard JR (2001) Mechanism of airway hyperresponsiveness to adenoside induced by allergen challenge in actively sensitized Brown Norway rats. *Br J Pharmacol* 132: 1509–1523

224   Tigani B, Schaeublin E, Sugar R, Jackson AD, Fozard JR, Beckmann N (2002) Pulmonary inflammation monitored non-invasively by MRI in freely breathing rats. *Biochem Biophys Res Commun* 292: 216–221

225   Tigani B, Cannet C, Zurbrugg S, Schaeublin E, Mazzoni L, Fozard JR, Beckmann N (2003) Resolution of the oedema associated with allergic pulmonary inflammation in rats. *Br J Pharmacol* 140: 239–246

226 Tigani B, Di Padova F, Zurbrugg S, Schaeublin E, Revesz L, Fozard JR, Beckmann N (2003) Effects of a mitogen-activated protein kinase inhibitor on allergic airways inflammation in the rat studied by magnetic resonance imaging. *Eur J Pharmacol* 482: 319–324

227 Watson, RW, Redmond HP, Bouchier-Hayes D (1994) Role of endotoxin in mononuclear phagocyte-mediated inflammatory responses. *J Leukoc Biol* 56: 95–103

228 Yang RB, Mark MR, Gray A, Huang H, Xie MH, Zhang M, Goddard A, Wood WI, Gurney AL, Godowski PJ (1998) Toll-like receptor-2 mediates lipopolysaccharide-induced cellular signalling. *Nature* 395: 284–288

229 Albelda SM, Smith CW, Ward PA. (1994) Adhesion molecules and inflammatory injury. *FASEB J* 8: 504–512

230 Tesfaigzi Y, Fischer MJ, Martin AJ, Seagrave J (2000) Bcl-2 in LPS- and allergen-induced hyperplastic mucous cells in airway epithelia of Brown Norway rats. *Am J Physiol Lung Cell Mol Physiol* 279: L1210–L1217

231 Harkema JR, Hotchkiss JA (2000) In vivo effects of endotoxin on intraepithelial muco-substances in rat pulmonary airways. Quantitative histochemistry. *Am J Pathol* 141: 307–317

232 Beckmann N, Tigani B, Sugar R, Jackson AD, Jones G, Mazzoni L, Fozard JR (2002) Non-invasive detection of endotoxin induced mucus hypersecretion in rat lung by magnetic resonance imaging. *Am J Physiol Lung Cell Mol Physiol* 283: L22

233 Martin JG, Duguet A, Eidelman DH (2000) The contribution of airway smooth muscle to airway narrowing and airway hyperresponsiveness in disease. *Eur Respir J* 16: 349–354

234 Halayko AJ, Amrani Y (2003) Mechanisms of inflammation-mediated airway smooth muscle plasticity and airways remodeling in asthma. *Respir Physiol Neurobiol* 137: 209–222

235 Beckmann N, Cannet C, Zurbruegg S, Rudin M, Tigani B (2004) Proton MRI of lung parenchyma reflects allergen-induced airway remodeling and endotoxin-aroused hyporesponsiveness: a step towards ventilation studies in spontaneously breathing rats. *Magn Reson Med* 52: 258–268

236 Edelman RR, Hatabu H, Tadamura E, Li W, Prasad PV (1996) Noninvasive assessment of regional ventilation in the human lung using oxygen-enhanced magnetic resonance imaging. *Nature Med* 2: 1236–1239

237 Stock KW, Chen Q, Morrin M, Hatabu H, Edelman RR (1999) Oxygen-enhanced magnetic resonance ventilation imaging of the human lung at 0.2 T and 1.5 T. *J Magn Reson Imaging* 9: 838–841

238 Pauwels RA, Kips JC, Peleman RA, van der Straeten ME (1990) The effect of endotoxin inhalation on airway responsiveness and cellular influx in rats. *Am Rev Respir Dis* 141: 540–545

239 Kips JC, Lefebvre RA, Peleman RA, Joos GF, Pauwels RA (1995) The effect of a nitric oxide synthase inhibitor on the modulation of airway responsiveness in rats. *Am J Respir Crit Care Med* 151: 1165–1169

240 Kobzik L, Bredt DS, Lowenstein CJ, Drazen J, Gaston B, Sugarbaker D, Stamler JS (1993) Nitric oxide synthase in human and rat lung: immunocytochemical and histochemical localization. *Am J Respir Cell Mol Biol* 9: 371–377

241 Moller HE, Chen XJ, Saam B, Hagspiel KD, Johnson GA, Altes TA, de Lange EE, Kauczor HU (2002) MRI of the lungs using hyperpolarized noble gases. *Magn Reson Med* 47: 1029–1051

242 Stupar V, Berthezene Y, Canet E, Tournier H, Dupuich D, Cremillieux Y (2003) Helium3

polarization using spin exchange technique: application to simultaneous pulmonary ventilation/perfusion imaging in small animals. *Invest Radiol* 38: 334–340

243   Viallon M, Cofer GP, Suddarth SA, Moller HE, Chen XJ, Chawla MS, Hedlund LW, Cremillieux Y, Johnson GA (1999) Functional MR microscopy of the lung with hyperpolarized 3He, *Magn Reson Med* 41: 787–792

244   Viallon M, Berthezene Y, Callot V, Bourgeois M, Humblot H, Briguet A, Cremillieux Y (2000) Dynamic imaging of hyperpolarized (3)He distribution in rat lungs using interleaved-spiral scans. *NMR Biomed* 13: 207–213

245   Chen BT, Brau ACS, Johnson GA (2003) Measurement of regional lung function in rats using hyperpolarized 3Helium dynamic MRI. *Magn Reson Med* 49: 78–88

246   Chen BT, Johnson GA (2004) Dynamic lung morphology of methacholine-induced heterogeneous bronchoconstriction, *Magn Reson Med* 52: 1080–1086

247   Dupuich D, Berthezene Y, Clouet PL, Stupar V, Canet E, Cremillieux Y (2003) Dynamic 3He imaging for quantification of regional lung ventilation parameters. *Magn Reson Med* 50: 777–783

248   Barnes PJ (2002) New treatments for COPD. *Nat Rev Drug Discov* 1: 437–446

249   Busch RH, Lauhala KE, Loscutoff SM, McDonald KE (1984) Experimental pulmonary emphysema induced in the rat by intratracheally administered elastase: morphogenesis. *Environ Res* 33: 497–513

250   Chen XJ, Hedlund LW, Moller HE, Chawla MS, Maronpot RR, Johnson GA (2000) Detection of emphysema in rat lungs by using magnetic resonance measurements of 3He diffusion. *Proc Natl Acad Sci USA* 97: 11478–11481

251   Peces-Barba G, Ruiz-Cabello J, Cremillieux Y, Rodriguez I, Dupuich D, Callot V, Ortega M, Rubio Arbo ML, Cortijo M, Gonzalez-Mangado N (2003) Helium-3 MRI diffusion coefficient: correlation to morphometry in a model of mild emphysema. *Eur Respir J* 22: 14–19

252   Berthezene Y, Vexler V, Price DC, Wisner-Dupon J, Moseley ME, Aicher KP, Brasch RC (1992) Magnetic resonance imaging detection of an experimental pulmonary perfusion deficit using a macromolecular contrast agent. Polylysine-gadolinium-DTPA40. *Invest Radiol* 27: 346–351

253   Richard JC, Factor P, Ferkol T, Ponde DE, Zhou Z, Schuster DP (2003) Repetitive imaging of reporter gene expression in the lung. *Mol Imag* 2: 342–349

254   O'Dell WG, McCulloch AD (2000) Imaging three-dimensional cardiac function. *Annu Rev Biomed Eng* 2: 431–456

255   Nahrendorf M, Hiller KH, Hu K, Ertl G, Haase A, Bauer WR (2003) Cardiac magnetic resonance imaging in small animal models of human heart failure. *Med Image Anal* 7: 369–375

256   Rudin M, Pedersen B, Umemura K, Zierhut W (1991) Determination of rat heart morphology and function *in vivo* in two models of cardiac hypertrophy by means of magnetic resonance imaging. *Basic Res Cardiol* 86: 165–174

257   Ryf S, Spiegel MA, Gerber M, Boesiger P (2002) Myocardial tagging with 3D-CSPAMM. *J Magn Reson Imaging* 16: 320–325

258   Masood S, Yang GZ, Pennell DJ, Firmin DN (2000) Investigating intrinsic myocardial mechanics: the role of MR tagging, velocity phase mapping, and diffusion imaging. *J Magn Reson Imaging* 12: 873–883

259   Jay TM, Lucignani G, Crane AM, Jehle J, Sokoloff L (1988) Measurement of local cere-

bral blood flow with [14C]iodoantipyrine in the mouse. *J Cereb Blood Flow Metab* 8: 121–129

260   Cook NS, Zerwes HG, Pally C, Rudin M, Hof RP (1993) Spirapril and cilazapril inhibit neointimal lesion development but cause no detectable inhibition of lumen narrowing after carotid artery balloon catheter injury in the rat. *Blood Press* 2: 322–331

261   Pruessmann KP (2004) Parallel imaging at high field strength: synergies and joint potential. *Top Magn Reson Imaging* 15: 237–244

262   Bock NA, Konyer NB, Henkelman RM (2004) Multiple-mouse MRI. *Magn Reson Med* 49: 158–167

263   Heiss WD, Graf R, Grond M, Rudolf J (1998) Pathophysiology of the ischemic penumbra--revision of a concept. *Cell Mol Neurobiol* 18: 621–638

264   Nicholson JK, Connelly J, Lindon JC, Holmes E (2002) Metabonomics: a platform for studying drug toxicity and gene function. *Nat Rev Drug Discov* 1: 153–161

Progress in Drug Research, Vol. 62
(Markus Rudin, Ed.)
©2005 Birkhäuser Verlag, Basel (Switzerland)

Risk identification and management: MRI as a research tool in toxicology studies of new chemical entities

By Mark W. Tengowski[1]
and John J. Kotyk[2]

Pfizer Global Research and Development, Pfizer, Inc.
[1]2800 Plymouth Road 16-1A/6
Ann Arbor, MI 48105, USA
<mark.w.tengowski@pfizer.com>
[2]700 Chesterfield, Parkway West
Saint Louis, MO 63017, USA

Glossary of abbreviations

BOLD, blood oxygen level dependent imaging; CT, computed tomography; Gd-DTPA, gadolinium diethylene-triamine-pentaacetic acid; MR, magnetic resonance; NCEs, new chemical entities; OCT, optical coherence tomography; PET, positron emission tomography; RF, radio frequency; US, ultrasound.

1 Introduction

Today's biotechnology and pharmaceutical industries have created an ever-expanding funnel of new discovery targets and new chemical entities (NCEs). This tremendous increase in new, potentially valuable therapeutic agents is beginning to overwhelm the capacity of most drug research and development efforts. Such demands are forcing project teams to establish faster, improved methods that enable key decisions to be made at an earlier stage of compound development.

Bioimaging technologies offer one solution to address these expanding needs in drug discovery and development. The impact these technologies can make on the drug portfolio in the pharmaceutical business can be appreciated in two ways: (1) expediting decision making processes; and, (2) reducing resource waste associated with compound attrition. Bioimaging technologies can assist project teams in making decisions regarding NCE selection, dose levels, efficacy, proof of concept, and confidence in mechanism and safety. Bioimaging methods also are beginning to show promise as biomarkers of disease in that they can be applied to animal models of human diseases. In a perfect world, drugs being considered for development would be free of toxicities. In reality, however, toxicity issues and the risks associated with them are real and must be understood and managed, if possible, before embarking on expensive clinical trials and further development. In this capacity, bioimaging methods have the potential to answer animal toxicity, pharmacodynamics, and pharmacokinetics questions that may help identify poor efficacy or toxicity, thus allowing the advancement of safe compounds with a more rapid production of high-quality therapeutics and a reduction in overall developmental costs of an NCE.

In early NCE development, bioimaging can be applied in a variety of animal models of disease to investigate novel compound structures and subsequent confidence in target and development rationale. Bioimaging also can provide efficacy endpoints and biomarkers to evaluate lead NCEs. By exploring, measuring, and characterizing the continuum between safety and efficacy, these efforts can reduce candidate attrition to bridge early NCE optimization studies with non-clinical toxicology studies enabling better Go/NoGo decisions to be made prior to moving NCEs into clinical trials. Bioimaging techniques used in preclinical studies also have the potential to translate well into human situations. Numerous examples of these ideas and their applications are provided in the contributing chapters of this book. This chapter focuses upon the business and science behind risk identification and management using bioimaging, in particular magnetic resonance imaging (MRI), in the preclinical drug development process.

2   Magnetic resonance imaging

MRI offers several advantages over other bioimaging techniques employed in today's biomedical research, e.g., positron emission tomography (PET), computed tomography (CT), ultrasound (US), and optical coherence tomography (OCT). Using MRI, the proton-detected magnetic resonance (MR) signal relies on an absorption/emission rather than a transmission phenomenon, meaning the properties of the MR signal are intrinsic to the tissue being examined, rather than to a foreign, possibly labeled substance introduced into the subject. Thus, since the intensity and contrast-to-noise characteristics of the MR signal are based on properties related to the tissue (e.g., fat, bound or free water), any process that leads to an alteration in the physical or chemical microenvironment of the hydrogen within the tissue has the potential to provide a tool to assess NCE-induced pathophysiological effects/interactions.

MRI technologies utilize non-ionizing radio frequency (RF) signals, and therefore do not cause tissue destruction, and face exposure limitations incurred by PET and CT technologies, e.g., X-rays, radionuclides. As a non-destructive technique, MRI lends itself well to making serial measurements in the same subject over extended periods of time. The spatial resolution of an MR image is a function of the strength of the external magnetic fields (main and gradient) applied during the experiment and the arrangement, geometry, and sensitivity of the RF detection coil relative to the tissue under investigation. Since RF signals lose little energy while passing through tissues, there is essentially no loss in resolution as a function of tissue depth. In addition, the MR signal is relatively free of focus or parallax problems commonly associated with transmission techniques, e.g., OCT, PET [1]. Unfortunately MRI is an inherently insensitive technique compared to other bioimaging methods, a disadvantage that is partially overcome by its low risk nature and the ability to scan or signal average for longer periods of time with deeper tissue penetration.

Like other non-invasive bioimaging techniques, *in vivo* MR techniques can be applied in several different ways. MRI can be used to acquire molecular, biochemical, physiological, and anatomical information in experimental animals and humans. These methods can generate two-dimensional (2D) or three-dimensional (3D) image data on soft tissues that complement information obtained using other modalities, such as CT and PET. MRI studies of various soft tissues, such as liver, brain, kidneys, heart, and reproductive organs are routinely performed in the clinic. Such information has been used to detect tumor metastasis [2–4], measure volumes of individual brain structures [5–8], evaluate muscle volume as an assessment of disuse atrophy [9, 10], cardiomyopathy [11], or congenital defect [12]. With the advent of ultra-fast ECG-gated imaging and specialized protocols, high-resolution MRI of the heart and coronary arteries is becoming a common clinical tool [13, 14]. Reconstruction of 3D MRI data can provide accurate non-invasive assessment of lumen diameters and/or volume [15, 16] and can allow us to detect changes in atherosclerotic plaque location and composition [17]. Similarly, 3D MRI of bone joints can provide accurate assessments of articular cartilage volume and matrix integrity, synovial fluid, bone edema, and ligamentous structures [18].

Functional and physiological information also can be obtained using MRI. Functional MRI (commonly called fMRI) utilizes the difference in the magnetic properties of oxygenated and deoxygenated blood to measure changes in blood flow in the brain [19, 20]. This type of imaging (also known as BOLD or blood oxygen level dependent imaging) can provide information on oxygen utilization, i.e., identify neuronally active regions of the brain. As specific areas in the brain are stimulated, blood flow and oxygenated hemoglobin increases to these areas can be monitored as small changes in the MR signal. While the complete mechanisms behind the BOLD effect need to be better understood, there appears to be a real physiological basis relating blood flow and oxygenation changes. fMRI methods have proven valuable in assessing therapeutic efficacy in stroke [21], have proven useful in measuring abnormalities in activation patterns in Schizophrenia [22], and provide insight into tumor microvasculature, both in terms of blood oxygenation and perfusion [23, 24]. Diffusion/perfusion-weighted imaging also allows one to assess blood flow and cellular diffusion characteristics that have been shown to be very sensitive prognostic indicators of the severity of stroke [25]. As novel imaging protocols and pulse sequences are developed, functional and physiological imaging of the brain, and other tissue, has the potential to become more routine in NCE drug safety studies.

Numerous contrast agents are available and have demonstrated a wide range of applications in MRI studies. For example, Gd-enhanced MRI is used to detect active multiple sclerosis lesions and monitor clinical response in patients [26]. The combination of lesion volume and anatomic location in these studies provides valuable clinical information that can be used to correlate symptoms with clinical outcome. Alternatively, the use of MR contrast agents allow one to obtain accurate measures of vascular physiology and changes in tissue morphology from tumors and inflammation [27, 28]. Gd-DTPA has been used in humans to perform MR angiography [29, 30], measure changes in blood flow, blood volume, or capillary/vascular permeability in tumors. Localized biochemical changes in the articular cartilage also can be measured using a well-established, clinically accepted dGEMRIC protocols that employ Gd-DTPA to provide an indirect measure of glycosaminoglycan concentration in the cartilage. As with other non-invasive modalities, MRI protocols with contrast agents allow repeated measurements to be made in the same patient or animal during longitudinal studies. The most commonly used low molecular weight MR contrast agent is gadopentate dimeglumine (Gd-DTPA, Magnevist®, Schering AG). However, other high molecular weight, selective or molecularly-targeted agents, and iron oxide species are becoming increasingly important in drug development efforts [31–35].

One of the greatest potential roles MRI may play in drug discovery and development is its ability to produce novel measures (imaging biomarkers) that help expedite decision-making processes. Since MRI can provide detailed, non-invasive localized information with good resolution about the progression (and regression) of tissue disease [36], it offers unique capabilities as a biomarker to probe a toxic effect a NCE may have in a therapeutic study. Experimental examples of such a marker could include: disease progression studies in Alzheimer's disease using diffusion tensor imaging approaches [37], progression studies in joint inflammation/disorders, such as osteoarthritis (discussed above), and alterations in mass occupying lesions such as tumors. Potentially of greater importance is the capacity of MRI, in conjunction with molecularly targeted contrast agents, to yield information on the cellular and molecular functional integrity and pathophysiology of tissue. These mechanism-based biomarkers could lay the groundwork for proof-of-concept and proof-of-mechanism studies. Other functional measures might include: regional blood flow indicating the degree of vascularization of tumors, muscle strain in the heart wall, and regional changes in cerebral blood flow following pharmacological treatment. While many of these applications have not yet been fully validated or accepted as biomarkers, clinical endpoints, or surrogate markers by the FDA, they cannot be overlooked for their potentially useful role in driving the internal decisions to evaluate NCEs.

3   Bioimaging in safety sciences

A major factor contributing to the attrition of NCEs in the pharmaceutical industry's development pipeline is a result of positive toxicology findings that cannot be managed with current assays or tools. In many cases, a lack of mechanistic understanding behind toxic effects, or the absence of a reliable clinical biomarker, necessitates the elimination of an attractive compound from further study. Thus, an important goal for pharmaceutical companies is to improve their ability to assess toxicological effects, identify/manage the risks of moving forward with an NCE, and reduce loss or attrition of compounds from the drug discovery pipeline.

Within the range of toxicities typically observed for NCEs, the liver, brain, kidney, and heart are organs frequently affected. The liver, a major target for toxicity effects, can display manifestations such as fatty liver, glycogen deposition, hepatocyte necrosis, and cholestasis. Toxic effects in the nervous system tend to target the neuron, axon, myelinating cell, or the neurotransmitter system. Although attrition due to kidney toxicity or damage is fairly uncommon, i.e., in chronic, late-stage development, considerable resources already have been expended by the time renal findings are detected. Toxic findings in the heart can be very serious and, in many cases, occur too late to be of use as a clinical marker due to delayed release of serum markers of cardiac damage and the limited capacity for the heart to repair itself.

To improve development of efficacious and safe NCEs, faster, more accurate investigational methods need to be established to assess preclinical pharmacological activity and safety. A myriad of MRI methods offer attractive ways in which to achieve this goal, especially in early phases of development. MRI techniques can accommodate a variety of animal models and offer the opportunity to carry forward essentially the same validated methodology into early human studies. Imaging is routinely used for diagnostics in the clinic, and acceptance by the general public is very high. When surveyed, internists identified MRI and CT scanning as their top choice for a technology that has transformed the way physicians practice medicine [38]. Unfortunately, the adoption and acceptance of imaging methods by clinicians to manage toxicology risks has been slow, even though the ability to investigate and understand drug effects remains critical to drug development scientists.

When applied appropriately, imaging has the potential to provide feedback early in the drug discovery pipeline, allowing quicker, more effective decisions for compound selection. Improved confidence in efficacy, mechanism, and safety could lead to elimination of NCEs early in the discovery process as opposed to later in the process. Along these lines, the following sections highlight examples where MRI technology has played an important role in drug development, particularly how these methods have helped overcome problems and manage risks associated with liver, brain, kidney, and heart toxicology during the development of NCEs. In cases where examples of MRI-derived toxicity are not available, suggestions and some speculation are provided as an indicator of how one might consider moving forward to develop an imaging marker of toxicity.

3.1   Safety imaging in the liver

Because of its anatomic location and function, the liver is a major concern when investigating toxic injury during testing of NCEs. By residing between the gut and the body, the liver 'filters' or detoxifies the venous blood coming from the stomach and intestine (via the portal vein) before entering the circulation. From a safety perspective, the liver also is the key organ responsible for metabolizing or biotransforming NCEs, ultimately leading to clearance of the NCE, or possibly, to the generation of an actual toxic chemical species that results in secondary safety concerns. By understanding how the liver handles NCEs, how they percolate through liver sinusoids, and how they might directly or indirectly induce pathologies, a better level of risk identification and management can be obtained during the study of NCEs.

MRI provides a useful tool to help manage risks associated with liver disease. MRI has been used to identify/stage hepatic tumors [39], diagnose cirrhosis [40], and measure liver iron toxicity (and the correlation between cardiac and liver iron levels [41]). This approach provides a particularly valuable tool in safety studies when routine serum chemistry measures, e.g., enzyme levels, are not detected, or where surrogate markers for toxicity cannot be defined. For example, hepatic steatosis [42], a commonly occurring preclinical finding in drug safety studies, does not always correlate with elevations in hepatic serum enzymes. Similarly, histological change in livers of preclinical species might correlate well with increased serum transaminase levels; however, this correlation is often not observed for all animals at the dose level being investigated. The identification of fatty liver in laboratory animal species also can be a common finding produced by strain, diet, stress, or NCE during drug safety studies. The development of non-invasive methods to detect the prodromal onset, progression, and recovery from such a finding could provide a valuable aid in early determination of compound toxicity [43].

Using MRI, it is possible to evaluate normal versus fatty liver tissue by exploiting the chemical shift differences between fat and water protons. One method to accomplish this [44] acquires two images with a delay between the RF pulse and gradient echoes, such that the phase shift between the water and the fat MR signals is either in-phase or out-of-phase, respectively. The difference image obtained by manipulating these two components can be used to generate separate images for both water and fat. Another protocol, the three-point Dixon method [45–47] can also be used to produce fat or water edited MR images. Finding ways to utilize MRI in liver safety studies provides a potentially new biomarker for understanding early toxicity, which may support a clinical program via appropriate risk management. Although not discussed in this article, magnetic resonance spectroscopy (MRS) constitutes a complementary attractive tool with which to probe liver metabolism and related toxicity.

Further validation must be addressed before quantitative *in vivo* data discerning absolute fat/water ratios (as opposed to relative ratios) can be used to monitor liver toxicity. Both a distribution of signal relaxation times for fatty tissue and inter-patient variability can lead to discrepancies between the measured and the true fat content. Respiratory motion and organ movement also have confounding effects, potentially shifting voxels outside of the imaging plane during a single ventilatory cycle. For large voxels studies used in human studies (~0.5 mm in-plane and ~1.0 mm slice thickness resolution), these detrimental affects are smaller than they are in animal studies where smaller voxel dimensions are needed (~100 μm in-plane resolution and ~500 μm thick slices). Acquisition of appropriate preclinical MRI data with resolution sufficient to minimize these effects is often difficult to achieve. However, it should be noted even these sampling errors are significantly improved over those associated using alternative percutaneous biopsy procedures. Ultimately, the degree to which *in vivo* preclinical fatty liver findings can be translated to clinical efforts and used to manage risks in safety studies depends upon the biological similarities between humans and the animal species under investigation, and whether or not preclinical imaging paradigms truly mimic clinical procedures.

3.2   Safety imaging in the brain

Typical disease states of the brain include stroke, cancer, or neurodegeneration. These states, as well as the structural and functional changes that result from the disease processes, represent important clinical indications and pathologies associated with brain tissue that can accompany administration of NCEs. A major target for drug discovery efforts in a wide variety of neurological and psychiatric disorders are γ-aminobutyric acid (GABA) receptors that are expressed in many neurons and brain tissues. The specific sites and mechanisms for these and other targets are beyond the scope of this chapter and are discussed elsewhere [48–52].

Vigabatrin (Sabril®) is probably the best-known CNS compound that possesses a drug safety liability and has been successfully advanced into the clinic. Vigabatrin has not been approved for use in the USA, but is marketed as an anticonvulsive in many countries around the world. It functions as an irreversible inhibitor of GABA transaminase, and was designed to enhance CNS function by increasing brain cerebral spinal fluid concentrations of GABA. Vigabatrin is orally absorbed with a plasma half-life approximating

6 hours with the kidney being the major route of elimination (65% of the administered dose is found unchanged in the urine at 24 h). Chronic administration of vigabatrin (g-vinyl GABA) in rats and in dogs [53–55] produces reversible microvacuolation (intramyelinic edema) in discrete brain regions. Histological changes are most notable in the columns of the fornix and regions of the hypothalamus, thalamus, optic tract, and hippocampus. Intramyelin edema is a histological change that is included in a diverse group of white matter pathologies termed leukodystrophies. Advanced lesions progress to axonal necrosis. Inflammatory changes are rarely observed in leukodystrophies [56]. In many cases, leukodystrophies occur in juveniles [57], yet genetic derangements do appear in adults [58].

MRI has been shown to be a sensitive technique for detecting pathologies of white matter. For instance, Barkhof and Scheltens [59] have demonstrated useful MRI tools for detecting the onset and recovery from drug-induced structural changes. In a study using rats treated with vigabatrin (250 mg/kg/day) [60], cerebellar white matter lesions were detected and quantitated via T_2-weighted relaxation time constant MRI measurements. Changes in both morphology and relaxation time constants in these lesions correlated with histopathology. Preece et al. [61] has extended this investigation using diffusion-weighted measurements (DWI) methods to show that DWI may be a sensitive alternative for detecting and monitoring lesions in cerebellar and cortical white matter. In a canine study, Weiss et al. [62] showed dogs treated chronically with vigabatrin (300 mg/kg/day) for 15 weeks, displayed an increased T_2- and decreased T_1-weighted signals for the treatment group relative to the control group, with the most prominent changes from baseline observed for the columns of the fornix and to a lesser degree in the surrounding hypothalamus and thalamus. Subsequent analysis of *ex vivo* brain tissues showed these data correlated highly with the presence of histopathology and electrophysiological assessment.

When applied in longitudinal CNS studies, MRI is a valuable tool for probing and, hopefully, understanding the reversibility of a histopathologic tissue finding – a key component to risk management. Peyster et al. [63] investigated the reversal of vigabatrin-induced microvacuolation which has been well established in rats and dogs. In this study, beagle dogs were given an oral dose of vigabatrin (300 mg/kg/day) to reproduce the microvacuolation and were subsequently monitored *in vivo* during return to baseline over a 16-week period. This study compared the changes in T_2 signal intensities with histopathology. Notable pathology findings were observed after 4–5 weeks of treatment, which correlated nicely with increases observed in T_2 signal intensities. These observations were even more prominent after 7 weeks and increased further at 12 weeks. The reversal animal groups in this study displayed decreases in both MRI T_2 intensity and microvacuolation at 12 weeks, and a near complete reversal of T_2 changes to normal. In addition, a complete recovery of histopathology findings was detected at 16 weeks. Hence, these preclinical efforts suggest that MRI provides a sensitive, non-invasive probe or biomarker of reversible intramyelin edema.

Since intramyelin edema is potentially a very serious clinical risk, extension of the preclinical MRI findings to monitor *in vivo* toxic effects in humans provides a critical component important for seeking drug approval. Regardless of the extent and basis for the toxicity observed in animals, the ability to manage the clinical risk justified moving forward with development of vigabatrin. Without this capability the clinical study may not have been undertaken, or the decision to stop development may have been made, either of which would have been costly to the drug company. Interestingly, throughout development and post-marketing phases of vigabatrin, intramyelin edema has not been observed in the human brain [64], and no definitive cases of vigabatrin-induced changes in human brains have been reported [65]. The story behind the development of vigabatrin is one example where a false-positive toxicology decision was averted, permitting clinicians and patients to benefit from advancement, and eventual approval of a safe and effective therapy.

3.3 Safety imaging in the kidney

Before fully understanding how to apply MRI technologies to the kidney, one must recognize the kidney, unlike the liver, is not a solid organ, but rather a collection of many individual nephrons packed into a structure grossly called the kidney. The kidney maintains homeostasis by filtering the blood and conserving important molecules through active and passive mechanisms creating urine. Like the liver, it can act as a filter for the NCE and its metabolites. In addition to preserving the fluid and electrolyte balance of the body, the cells of the nephron are the site of production for two hormones, renin and erythropoietin. Renin is an enzyme that is part of a greater hemomodulatory/vasoconstrictor system that converts angiotensinogen to angiotensin I. Erythropoietin is a critical signal in the synthesis and release of red blood cells from the bone marrow. In these capacities, the kidney serves as an endocrine organ; therefore morphologic changes or disease in this organ may manifest themselves in distant locations. For MRI to be used in drug safety studies of the kidney, the initial investigations might best focus on either morphologic (i.e., necrosis) or functional (i.e., renal hypertension that causes a reduction in blood flow thereby reducing glomerular filtration rate) effects. Thus, a good understanding of urine production and MRI contrast agent distribution and clearance can provide insight for morphologic and functional end points.

One of the most common observations associated with NCE-induced nephrotoxicity is acute renal failure. Normally the tight junctions of the cells along the nephron prevent systemic uptake of nitrogenous wastes. However, during compromised renal function, these junctions loosen (i.e., decreases in glomerular filtration rate) during which time excess urea can accumulate in the blood resulting in and increase blood urea nitrogen (BUN), a common serum chemistry marker used to estimate renal funtion. Depending on duration, these effects can lead to acute or chronic renal failure. Downstream of the glomerulus, pathological events can produce a cast or obstruction within the tubule which also can reduce renal blood flow and glomerular filtration rate. Lastly, toxic agents themselves could either directly or indirectly damage tubular cells, again reducing the efficiency of the tight cellular junctions thereby permitting toxic agents to interact with a new compartment of extracellular water. Understanding these effects on renal function in the context of histopathology, available serum chemistries, and urinalysis assays, forms a foundation for developing MRI biomarkers as predictive endpoints of toxicity for NCEs.

Since perfusion is key to renal function, the ability to measure this process using MRI offers an attractive approach for evaluating morphology, tissue integrity, and homeostatic function. Numerous MRI methods exist for measuring renal perfusion, which include: the use of dynamic contrast-enhanced approaches using MRI contrast agents, the application of arterial-spin labeling protocols, and the implementation of either diffusion or phase-mapping pulse sequences. The advantages and disadvantages for each of these methods vary, along with the degrees of technical/physical complexity related to implementing them. Ultimately, the results obtained with each of these

269

approaches provide the ability to probe pathological and functional changes in the kidney. For discussion, examples using the MRI contrast agent approach are described below.

Vallee et al. [66] demonstrated a simple model of renal blood flow can be used to generate realistic quantitative clinical data on renal perfusion. These methods used a standard T1-weighted fast gradient echo MRI sequence to collect data following an intravenous bolus injection of Gd-DTPA. In a variety of human patients (well-functioning native kidneys, transplanted kidneys, significant renal artery stenosis, and renal failure), dynamic contrast enhanced images of the kidney show that the wash-in phase of the contrast agent approximated the absolute renal blood flow when corrected against values from the aorta signal. Differences in cortical blood flow were measured for normal functioning kidneys (2.54 ± 1.16 ml/min per gram), for kidneys in the presence of pre-renal stenosis (1.09 ± 0.75 ml/min per gram), and for kidneys experiencing renal failure (0.51 ± 0.34 ml/min per gram). Using pre-renal stenosis and post-renal obstruction and reperfusion animal surgical models, Pedersen et al. [67] utilized this first-pass contrast agent uptake approach to estimate the integrated renal blood flow of the kidney in the rat (note: an appendix is included in Pedersen's paper describing the mathematics used to estimate renal blood flow and contrast agent clearance.) Similar to Vallee's efforts, this MRI method is amenable to rapid image acquisition and straightforward image analysis procedures and yields accurate measures of renal damage as a function in blood flow and glomerular filtration. If decreased renal blood flow is a possible sequelae observed during testing, then investigations into MRI methods for a renal blood flow safety biomarker is an attractive approach, especially given that these MRI methods have demonstrated translatability from humans to animal models.

Cisplatin, a chemotherapy routinely used to treat testicular, bladder, lung, esophagus, stomach, and ovarian cancers offers another example illustrating how MRI has been used to probe renal toxicity for new drugs. Unfortunately, Cisplatin demonstrates nephrotoxicity limiting its usefulness in the clinic, except a last resort. The exact mechanism behind Cisplatin nephrotoxicity is unknown, but may involve metabolic biotransformation or may be related to molecular structure. *In vitro* studies into the mechanism suggest that Cisplatin inhibits DNA synthesis and possibly transport functions. Thus, Cisplatin may also interfere with the normal proliferative response following injury. Kobayashi et al. [68] generated data using a mouse model and a gadolinium dendrimer MRI contrast agent, to suggest that MRI was able to identify which mice had detectible nephrotoxicity following treatment with Cisplatin. In addition, differences and changes in the MRI contrast for bands in the inner and outer regions of the cortex or medulla appeared to correlate with histopathology. Since each of these regions displays unique cell types and functions, is it not surprising that image contrast differences were detected in the MRI [69] study.

The non-invasive *in vivo* capability of MRI to monitor changes in renal perfusion allows the safety scientist to monitor the functional or morphological onset, progression and regression of toxic insults. By exploiting the changes in tissue contrast that accompany these effects and correlating this information with classical histopathological results, biomarkers of safety (functional or anatomic) can be developed to help manage and evaluate toxic responsiveness in the same animal, possibly over extended periods of time. MRI provides localized or regionally specific information, which can be more easily compared to histological results. In this capacity, MRI methods offer distinct advantages over traditional methods that measure global functional response of renal perfusion using agents like para-aminohippurate and inulin.

Combination of imaging results with a relatively new discipline called metabonomics provides a very attractive way to further investigate NCE effects in the liver. Metabonomics yields a comprehensive profile of (endogenous) metabolites of urine, or any other body fluid using spectroscopic techniques such as NMR or mass spectrometry. Comparing the respective fingerprints of drug-treated and control animals using statistical tools such as principal component or discriminate analysis identifies metabolic aberrations. Advance spectroscopic investigation may allow the identification of deregulated metabolites, and thus, contribute to the elucidation of the underlying mechanism leading to toxicological effects and/or provide a pretrial marker for imminent damage. Using classical toxicological tools, extensive toxicology studies of the metabolites would be required to identify the inciting structure responsible for producing the morphologic change detected in an imaging study, resulting in an alteration of renal function. It is because of its holistic, multivariate information content that the application of metabonomics techniques to the drug development process will increase in use.

3.4   Safety imaging in the heart

The heart is an organ of critical importance in drug safety studies of NCEs. As the pump for the cardiovascular system, it has limited capacity for repair following damage, therefore, special consideration must be given to cardio-vascular pathologies. Some functionally-based pathologies of the heart exist and are manageable in early clinical trials, such as alterations in electrical activity via electrocardiogram collection. Yet structural histopathology such as cardiomyocyte inflammation, degeneration, and necrosis lack prodromal markers of safety and are difficult to monitor. Conventional serum bio-markers for myocardial damage such as troponin T and troponin I exist in kit form [70]. Their usefulness in safety studies of the heart, however, may be lim-ited as these biomarkers are only liberated from cardiomyocytes following cell necrosis. From a safety perspective, indicators of cardiomyocyte necrosis will likely be too late in the toxic process to evaluate an NCE.

Doxorubicin is one example of a drug that demonstrates a myocardial safety liability. Doxorubicin is used clinically to treat a wide spectrum of tumors. Unfortunately, toxic effects thought to be induced by oxygen free radical formation and oxidative stress in the cardiomyocyte, limit the Dox-orubicin dose and cumulative exposure. The Doxorubicin-associated toxic effects alter cardiomyocyte form and function, eventually producing degen-eration, disorganization, and vacuolation of individual cardiac myofibrils. As a result, Doxorubicin provides a number of exemplary, well-documented examples of potential problems to consider when managing cardiotoxicity for studies of NCEs. Various MRI measures have been used to probe toxic effects and can be considered as biomarkers in cardiotoxicity studies. These include changes in: regional myocardium wall thickness, ejection fraction, and myocardial perfusion (via enhancement following MRI contrast admin-istration) [71, 72].

To help build confidence in the predictive value MRI provides in cardio-vascular studies, it would be useful to temporally correlate MRI measures to cardiac troponin levels and histopathology. In some cases, direct experi-mental induction of cardiotoxicity in preclinical studies with subsequent MRI examination can provide important information for developing an imaging biomarker. Ultimately, a detectible or predictive MRI result is desired that cor-relates with the histopathology, i.e., end morphologic changes, and is absent in healthy control samples. Understanding the breadth of cardiac toxicity and the manifestations of MRI in detecting these differences has the potential to reduce the level of false-positive decisions in screening trials.

While preclinical experiments involving known toxicants may seem far removed from building a safety biomarker to predict toxicity, cataloguing MRI measure(s) against known toxicants can be an important component in developing an imaging safety biomarker strategy. Such an approach can be especially important in the absence of knowing which specific cardiotoxicity effects might occur for a given class of NCEs. For example, constant-rate infusion of isoproterenol, acting as a positive ionotrope, produces a reversible left ventricular hypertrophy in non-clinical species [73, 74]. Using isoproterenol as a negative control for Doxorubicin-like cardiac disease demonstrates what one may want to avoid when attempting to produce an imaging biomarker of safety. By investigating other classes of cardiotoxins (i.e., anesthetics, hERG channel potentiators) or agents that alter organ perfusion (i.e., peripheral vasoconstrictors; α_2 agonists like medetomidine) or vasodilatory agents (NO potentiators like nitroglycerin) as a mechanism for surrogate onset, we can establish a clearer understanding and specificity for MRI biomarkers of toxicity. Being able to identify cytotoxic drugs without a cardiac liability will be particularly important in cancer therapeutics. Ultimately, the advent of an imaging biomarker to help screen for cardiotoxicity will contribute to understanding a compound's efficacy, as well as its safety profile.

4   Conclusions

In conclusion, application of MRI to toxicity studies of NCEs provides an attractive opportunity for the pharmaceutical industry. These methods can yield information early in the discovery pipeline to help increase confidence measures (mechanism, rationale, safety), and allow quicker, more effective Go/NoGo decisions to be reached during selection of a new drug. Such impact early in the discovery cycle lead to lower attrition rates later in the development process and can offer powerful risk management and predictive biomarker capabilities. These ideas become particularly important business drivers for the pharmaceutical industry, especially when the technologies can be translated from preclinical work to clinical practice.

Risk management tools also enable NCEs to advance into early clinical trials, when they might otherwise be stopped in non-clinical development as a result of an unmanageable safety finding. The ability to monitor real-time drug safety in the same subject during longitudinal exposure could preclude the need for cross-sectional serial take-off groups and dramatically reduce clinical costs. In this manner, subjects serve as their own control, hopefully reducing inter-subject variability, promoting accurate assessment of toxicity and/or its regression, and providing an early indication into the dose metrics for longer, costlier chronic studies.

Overall, the combination of the ideas described in this article can lead to more rapid, cheap production of new high-quality therapeutics. Although no clear regulatory guidance and few practical examples demonstrating these principles exist, the time and cost savings that pharmaceutical companies can realize by developing and adapting these technologies will ultimately bene-fit the patient and translate to reducing global healthcare management costs.

Acknowledgements

We would like to acknowledge the input and support from our colleagues and collaborators: John Burkhardt, Curt Matherne, Teresa McShane, Wayne Carter, Al Johnson, Larry Hedlund, Xiaowei Zhang, and Elizabeth Arner.

References

1   Spoor F, Jeffery N, Zonneveld F (2000) Using diagnostic radiology in human evolution-ary studies. *J Anat* 197: 61–76
2   Halvorsen RA, Jr., Yee J, McCormick VD (1996) Diagnosis and staging of gastric cancer. *Semin Oncol* 23: 325–335
3   Woodard PK, Dehdashti F, Putman CE (1998) Radiologic diagnosis of extrathoracic metastases to the lung. *Oncology (Huntington)* 12: 431–438
4   Nagashima T, Suzuki M, Yagata H, Hashimoto H, Shishikura T, Imanaka N, Ueda T, Miyazaki M (2002) Dynamic-enhanced MRI predicts metastatic potential of invasive ductal breast cancer. *Breast Cancer* 9: 226–230
5   Kim SG, Ogawa S (2002) Insights into new techniques for high resolution functional MR. *Curr Opin Neurobiol* 12: 607–615
6   Miller DH, Barkhof F, Frank JA, Parker GJ, Thompson AJ (2002) Measurement of atrophy in multiple sclerosis: pathological basis, methodological aspects and clinical relevance. *Brain* 125: 1676–1695
7   Caviness VS, Jr., Lange NT, Makris N, Herbert MR, Kennedy DN (1999) MRI-based brain volumetrics: emergence of a developmental brain science. *Brain Dev* 21: 289–295
8   Lawrie SM, Abukmeil SS (1998) Brain abnormality in schizophrenia. A systematic and

quantitative review of volumetric magnetic resonance imaging studies. *Br J Psychiatry* 172: 110–120

9   Belozerova I, Shenkman B, Mazin M, Leblanc A (2001) Effects of long-duration bed rest on structural compartments of m. soleus in man. *J Gravit Physiol* 8: P71–P72

10   Cockman MD, Jones MB, Prenger MC, Sheldon RJ (2001) Magnetic resonance imaging of denervation-induced muscle atrophy: effects of clenbuterol in the rat. *Muscle Nerve* 24: 1647–1658

11   di Cesare E (2003) MRI assessment of right ventricular dysplasia. *Eur Radiol* 13: 1387–1393

12   Sato M, Yagasaki T, Kora T, Awaya S (1998) Comparison of muscle volume between congenital and acquired superior oblique palsies by magnetic resonance imaging. *Jpn J Ophthalmol* 42: 466–470

13   Nikolaou K, Poon M, Sirol M, Becker CR, Fayad ZA (2003) Complementary results of computed tomography and magnetic resonance imaging of the heart and coronary arteries: a review and future outlook. *Cardiol Clin* 21: 639–655

14   Saeed M (2001) New concepts in characterization of ischemically injured myocardium by MRI. *Exp Biol Med* 226: 367–376

15   Hanni M, Lekka-Banos I, Nilsson S, Haggroth L, Smedby O (1999) Quantitation of atherosclerosis by magnetic resonance imaging and 3-D morphology operators. *Magn Reson Imaging* 17: 585–591

16   Ruehm SG, Corot C, Vogt P, Kolb S, Debatin JF (2001) Magnetic resonance imaging of atherosclerotic plaque with ultrasmall superparamagnetic particles of iron oxide in hyperlipidemic rabbits. *Circulation* 103: 415–422

17   Hockings PD, Roberts T, Galloway GJ, Reid DG, Harris DA, Vidgeon-Hart M, Groot PH, Suckling KE, Benson GM (2002) Repeated three-dimensional magnetic resonance imaging of atherosclerosis development in innominate arteries of low-density lipoprotein receptor-knockout mice. *Circulation* 106: 1716–1721

18   Peterfy CG (1996) MR imaging. *Baillieres Clinical Rheumatology* 10: 635–678

19   Logothetis NK (2002) The neural basis of the blood-oxygen-level-dependent functional magnetic resonance imaging signal. *Phil Trans R Soc Lond* 357: 1003–1037

20   Detre JA, Wang J (2002) Technical aspects and utility of fMRI using BOLD and ASL. *Clin Neurophysiol* 113: 621–634

21   Mullins PG, Reid DG, Hockings PD, Hadingham SJ, Campbell CA, Chalk JB, Doddrell DM (2001) Ischaemic preconditioning in the rat brain: a longitudinal magnetic resonance imaging (MRI) study. *NMR in Biomedicine* 14: 204–209

22   Volz HP, Gaser C, Hager F, Rzanny R, Mentzel HJ, Kreitschmann-Andermahr I, Kaiser WA, Sauer H (1997) Brain activation during cognitive stimulation with the Wisconsin Card Sorting Test--a functional MRI study on healthy volunteers and schizophrenics. *Psychiatry Res* 75: 145–157

23   Sinha S, Sinha U (2002) Functional magnetic resonance of human breast tumors: diffusion and perfusion imaging. *Ann NY Acad Sci* 980: 95–115

24   Huber P, Peschke P, Brix G, Hahn EW, Lorenz A, Tiefenbacher U, Wannenmacher M, Debus J (1999) Synergistic interaction of ultrasonic shock waves and hyperthermia in the Dunning prostate tumor R3327-AT1. *Int J Cancer* 82: 84–91

25   Huisman TA (2003) Diffusion-weighted imaging: basic concepts and application in cerebral stroke and head trauma. *Eur Radiol* 13: 2283–2297

26   Miller DH, Filippi M, Fazekas F, Frederiksen JL, Matthews PM, Montalban X, Polman CH (2004) Role of magnetic resonance imaging within diagnostic criteria for multiple sclerosis. *Ann Neurol* 56: 273–278

27   Weinmann HJ, Ebert W, Misselwitz B, Schmitt-Willich H (2003) Tissue-specific MR contrast agents. *Eur J Radiol* 46: 33–44

28   Pearlman JD, Laham RJ, Post M, Leiner T, Simons M (2002) Medical imaging techniques in the evaluation of strategies for therapeutic angiogenesis. *Curr Pharm Des* 8: 1467–1496

29   Kluge A, Dill T, Ekinci O, Hansel J, Hamm C, Pitschner HF, Bachmann G (2004) Decreased pulmonary perfusion in pulmonary vein stenosis after radiofrequency ablation: assessment with dynamic magnetic resonance perfusion imaging. *Chest* 126: 428–437

30   Baer FM, Theissen P, Schneider CA, Kettering K, Voth E, Sechtem U, Schicha H (1999) MRI assessment of myocardial viability: comparison with other imaging techniques. *Rays* 24: 96–108

31   Botnar RM, Perez AS, Witte S, Wiethoff AJ, Laredo J, Hamilton J, Quist W, Parsons EC, Jr, Vaidya A, Kolodziej A et al. (2004) In vivo molecular imaging of acute and subacute thrombosis using a fibrin-binding magnetic resonance imaging contrast agent. *Circulation* 109: 2023–2029

32   Barber PA, Foniok T, Kirk D, Buchan AM, Laurent S, Boutry S, Muller RN, Hoyte L, Tomanek B, Tuor UI (2004) MR molecular imaging of early endothelial activation in focal ischemia. *Ann Neurol* 56: 116–120

33   Artemov D (2003) Molecular magnetic resonance imaging with targeted contrast agents. *J Cell Biochem* 90: 518–524

34   Shapiro EM, Skrtic S, Sharer K, Hill JM, Dunbar CE, Koretsky AP (2004) MRI detection of single particles for cellular imaging. *Proc Natl Acad Sci USA* 101: 10901–10906

35   Moffat BA, Reddy GR, McConville P, Hall DE, Chenevert TL, Kopelman RR, Philbert M, Weissleder R, Rehemtulla A, Ross BD (2003) A novel polyacrylamide magnetic nanoparticle contrast agent for molecular imaging using MRI. *Mol Imaging* 2: 324–332

36   Hockings PD, Roberts T, Campbell SP, Reid DG, Greenhill RW, Polley SR, Nelson P, Bertram TA, Kramer K (2002) Longitudinal magnetic resonance imaging quantitation of rat liver regeneration after partial hepatectomy. *Toxicol Pathol* 30: 606–610

37   Lee BC, Mintun M, Buckner RL, Morris JC (2003) Imaging of Alzheimer's disease. *J Neuroimaging* 13: 199–214

38   Fuchs VR, Sox HC Jr (2001) Physicians' views of the relative importance of thirty medical innovations. *Health Affairs* 20: 30–42

39   Awaya H, Ito K, Honjo K, Fujita T, Matsumoto T, Matsunaga N (1998) Differential diagnosis of hepatic tumors with delayed enhancement at gadolinium-enhanced MRI: a pictorial essay. *Clin Imaging* 22: 180–187

40   Murakami T, Mochizuki K, Nakamura H (2001) Imaging evaluation of the cirrhotic liver. *Semin Liver Dis* 21: 213–224

41   Beutler E, Hoffbrand AV, Cook JD (2003) Iron deficiency and overload. *Hematology*: 40–61

42   Mortele KJ, Ros PR (2001) Imaging of diffuse liver disease. *Semin Liver Dis* 21: 195–212

43   Hockings PD, Changani KK, Saeed N, Reid DG, Birmingham J, O'Brien P, Osborne J, Toseland CN, Buckingham RE (2003) Rapid reversal of hepatic steatosis, and reduction of muscle triglyceride, by rosiglitazone: MRI/S studies in Zucker fatty rats. *Metabolism* 5: 234–243

44   Zhang X, Tengowski M, Fasulo L, Botts S, Suddarth SA, Johnson GA (2004) Measurement

of fat/water ratios in rat liver using 3D three-point dixon MRI. *Magn Reson Med* 51: 697–702

45   Dixon WT (1984) Simple proton spectroscopic imaging. *Radiology* 153: 189–194

46   Glover GH (1991) Multipoint Dixon technique for water and fat proton and suscepti-bility imaging. *J Magn Reson Imaging* 1: 521–530

47   Glover GH, Schneider E (1991) Three-point Dixon technique for true water/fat decom-position with B0 inhomogeneity correction. *Magn Reson Med* 18: 371–383

48   Rudolph U, Mohler H (2004) Analysis of GABAA receptor function and dissection of the pharmacology of benzodiazepines and general anesthetics through mouse genetics. *Ann Rev Pharmacol Toxicol* 44: 475–498

49   Vacher CM, Bettler B (2003) GABA(B) receptors as potential therapeutic targets. *Curr Drug Target CNS Neurol Disord* 2: 248–259

50   Johnston GA, Chebib M, Hanrahan JR, Mewett KN (2003) GABA(C) receptors as drug targets. *Curr Drug Target CNS Neurol Disord* 2: 260–268

51   Aragon C, Lopez-Corcuera B (2003) Structure, function and regulation of glycine neu-rotransporters. *Eur J Pharmacol* 479: 249–262

52   Sonnewald U, Qu H, Aschner M (2002) Pharmacology and toxicology of astrocyte-neu-ron glutamate transport and cycling. *J Pharm Exp Ther* 301: 1–6

53   Grant SM, Heel RC (1991) Vigabatrin. A review of its pharmacodynamic and pharma-cokinetic properties, and therapeutic potential in epilepsy and disorders of motor con-trol. *Drugs* 41: 889–926

54   Sabers A, Gram L (1992) Pharmacology of vigabatrin. *Pharmacol Toxicol* 70: 237–243

55   Schechter PJ (1989) Clinical pharmacology of vigabatrin. *Brit J Clin Pharmacol* 27: 19S–22S

56   Summers BA, Cummings JF, de Lahunta A (1995) Hereditary, familial, and idiopathic degenerative diseases. In: N Coon (ed): *Veterinary Neuropathology*, Mosby-Year Book, Inc., St. Louis, 281–350

57   Malm G, Ringden O, Winiarski J, Grondahl E, Uyebrant P, Eriksson U, Hakansson H, Skjeldal O, Mansson JE (1996) Clinical outcome in four children with metachromatic leukodystrophy treated by bone marrow transplantation. *Bone Marrow Transplant* 17: 1003–1008

58   Matsuyama W, Kuriyama M, Nakagawa M, Kanazawa H, Takenaga S, Ijichi S, Osame M (1996) Choroideremia with leukoencephalopathy and arylsulfatase A pseudodeficiency. *J Neurol Sci* 138: 161–164

59   Barkhof F, Scheltens P (2002) Imaging of white matter lesions. *Cerebrovasc Dis* 13: 21–30

60   Jackson GD, Williams SR, Weller RO, van Bruggen N, Preece NE, Williams SC, Butler WH, Duncan JS (1994) Vigabatrin-induced lesions in the rat brain demonstrated by quanti-tative magnetic resonance imaging. *Epilepsy Res* 18: 57–66

61   Preece NE, Houseman J, King MD, Weller RO, Williams SR (2004) Development of viga-batrin-induced lesions in the rat brain studied by magnetic resonance imaging, histol-ogy, and immunocytochemistry. *Synapse* 53: 36–43

62   Weiss KL, Schroeder CE, Kastin SJ, Gibson JP, Yarrington JT, Heydorn WE, McBride RG, Sussman NM, Arezzo JC (1994) MRI monitoring of vigabatrin-induced intramyelinic edema in dogs. *Neurology* 44: 1944–1949

63   Peyster RG, Sussman NM, Hershey BL, Heydorn WE, Meyerson LR, Yarrington JT, Gib-son JP (1995) Use of *ex vivo* magnetic resonance imaging to detect onset of vigabatrin-induced intramyelinic edema in canine brain. *Epilepsia* 36: 93–100

64   Agosti R, Yasargil G, Egli M, Wieser HG, Wiestler OD (1990) Neuropathology of a human hippocampus following long-term treatment with vigabatrin: lack of microvacuoles. *Epilepsy Res* 6: 166–170

65   Cohen JA, Fisher RS, Brigell MG, Peyster RG, Sze G (2000) The potential for vigabatrin-induced intramyelinic edema in humans. *Epilepsia* 41: 148–157

66   Vallee JP, Lazeyras F, Khan HG, Terrier F (2000) Absolute renal blood flow quantification by dynamic MRI and Gd-DTPA. *Eur Radiol* 10: 1245–1252

67   Pedersen M, Shi Y, Anderson P, Stodkilde-Jorgensen H, Djurhuus JC, Gordon I, Frokiaer J (2004) Quantitation of differential renal blood flow and renal function using dynamic contrast-enhanced MRI in rats. *Magn Reson Med* 51: 510–517

68   Kobayashi H, Kawamoto S, Jo SK, Sato N, Saga T, Hiraga A, Konishi J, Hu S, Togashi K, Brechbiel MW, Star RA (2002) Renal tubular damage detected by dynamic micro-MRI with a dendrimer-based magnetic resonance contrast agent. *Kidney Int* 61: 1980–1985

69   Hedlund LW, Maronpot RR, Johnson GA, Cofer GP, Mills GI, Wheeler CT (1991) Magnetic resonance microscopy of toxic renal injury induced by bromoethylamine in rats. *Fundam Appl Toxicol* 16: 787–797

70   Collinson PO, Boa FG, Gaze DC (2001) Measurement of cardiac troponins. *Ann Clin Biochem* 38: 423–449

71   Wassmuth R, Lentzsch S, Erdbruegger U, Schulz-Menger J, Doerken B, Dietz R, Friedrich MG (2001) Subclinical cardiotoxic effects of anthracyclines as assessed by magnetic resonance imaging-a pilot study. *Am Heart J* 141: 1007–1013

72   Ochiai K, Ishibashi Y, Shimada T, Murakami Y, Inoue S, Sano K (1999) Subendocardial enhancement in gadolinium-diethylene-triamine-pentaacetic acid-enhanced magnetic resonance imaging in aortic stenosis. *Am J Cardiol* 83: 1443–1446

73   Kitagawa Y, Yamashita D, Ito H, Takaki M (2004) Reversible effects of isoproterenol-induced hypertrophy on in situ left ventricular function in rat hearts. *Am J Physiol Heart Circ Physiol* 287: H277–H285

74   Slawson SE, Roman BB, Williams DS, Koretsky AP (1998) Cardiac MRI of the normal and hypertrophied mouse heart. *Magn Reson Med* 39: 980–987

Progress in Drug Research, Vol. 62
(Markus Rudin, Ed.)
©2005 Birkhäuser Verlag, Basel (Switzerland)

Pharmacokinetic studies with PET

By Mats Bergström[1,2] and Bengt Långström[1,3]

[1]Uppsala Imanet, GE Health Care
Box 967
SE-751 09 Uppsala, Sweden
<Mats.Bergstrom@Uppsala.Imanet.se>
[2]Department of Pharmaceutical Biosciences
Uppsala University
Uppsala, Sweden
[3]Department of Organic Chemistry
Uppsala University
Uppsala, Sweden

Glossary of abbreviations
BBB, blood-brain-barrier; CSF, cerebrospinal fluid; PD, pharmacodynamics; PET, positron-emission tomography; PK, pharmacokinetics; SUV, standardized uptake value.

1   Introduction

Assessment of pharmacokinetics (PK) is a cornerstone in the understanding of drug behavior and a necessary ingredient in drug development. With present available methods, PK is, in most cases, equivalent with plasma kinetics of drugs. However, the concentration which is inducing the therapeutic effect is in most cases tissue concentration of drug and its time course in the organ of interest, which may differ from plasma kinetics. The multiple factors governing the exchange of drug between plasma and tissue, will inevitably lead to a situation in which the maximum tissue concentration is obtained later than the maximum plasma concentration and usually with a different magnitude. Additionally, the egress from tissue is delayed as compared to elimination of drug from plasma. The drug in tissue will in turn interact with the target system with a finite on- and off-rate and this will induce an additional delay in time of maximum target interaction as compared to time of maximum tissue concentration and a retarded time course for fading off of the target interaction.

Hence there is a complicated relation between administration and effect, including its rate of onset, magnitude and duration. However, for the promotion of a new drug, decisions on its formulation, administration route, dosage and dosing interval needs to be made. Traditionally plasma PK has been the most important parameter, which can be determined experimentally in humans as a means to fill the knowledge gap between administration and effect. Biomarkers are of utmost interest as potentially filling this gap with information. In this sense, PET can give important contributions since it can give both PK information and a set of biomarker values, including direct effects on the target system and secondary cellular effects (Fig. 1). It is our belief that PK/PD modeling should always be included in drug development, as it is already today, since this allows predictions during the course of development, which may guide the up-coming experiments. This includes, e.g., planning of phase I and phase II studies with respect to dose selection, group sizes, times, etc. At a later stage this modeling would aid in

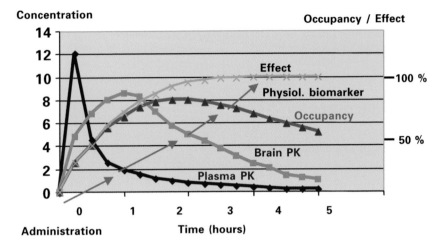

Figure 1.
A purpose of pharmacology is to explain the relation between administration and effect of the drug, with respect to rate of onset, magnitude and rate of off-set. This complex relation needs a range of assessments from plasma and organ PK, interaction with target system to physiological biomarkers for a full understanding and for modeling to extrapolate to different conditions of drug administration and different cohorts of patients.

assessment of impacts of changing formulations and of population heterogeneity.

PET may have a very important role to play in supplying essential information for setting up and for refinements of PK/pharmacodynamics (PD) models. Hence, PET with a labeled drug can measure directly the drug concentration in tissue and define the exchange parameters in a tissue PK-to-plasma PK model, and thereby build up the first part of the PK/PD model. Built upon this, the first extension to include interaction with the target system can be added, and here PET can contribute with occupancy or enzyme inhibition information. The final part, the relation between interaction with the primary molecular target and therapeutic effect is often more complicated, depending on the character of the drug effect. Also here, PET could contribute with important information, utilizing surrogate marker methods such as cerebral metabolism or tumor DNA synthesis.

The present communication focuses on different ways of utilizing PET for the assessment of PK, and attempts to explain the benefits, the technical performance and use of the results [1–9].

2   Alternative or complementary methods

PET is in many instances an excellent method, which can give important information during drug development, but is generally not the only method, which should be considered. Especially during the preclinical phase a range of other methods are used. Still we believe that it is an advantage to include preclinical PET studies, because it simplifies the integration between preclinical and clinical trials [10–13].

In humans, however, there are in general limited possibilities to obtain organ kinetics of drugs by alternative methods to PET.

2.1   Extrapolation from animals

The most common means to assess organ kinetics in humans is to extrapolate information gained in animals. In its simplest form, autoradiographic or organ sampling studies in rodents are used for this purpose. In more advanced settings, drug administrations to higher species are followed by sacrifice, extraction and analysis of compound in selected organs. To refine the extrapolation from animals, human plasma PK data together with modeling is utilized.

A limitation of these methods is that species-specific processes can confound these extrapolations. Of special concern here is the transport over the blood-brain-barrier (BBB), which can include specific carrier and efflux systems, the protein sequence of which can vary among species and render the BBB properties species specific. The dominant species differences typically relate to variable metabolism, absorption and elimination.

2.2   PK modeling

A kinetic analysis of human PK data can indicate the existence of different compartments, and in some cases these mathematically deduced compartments can be associated with certain organs. By including a set of assumptions regarding the plasma-to-tissue exchange, the organ kinetics might be simulated based on plasma PK.

2.3   Microdialysis

Microdialysis is an excellent method to analyze drug concentration and kinetics in the tissue interstitium, primarily utilized in brain in animals. Very sparse examples are available on its use in humans, since ethical aspects, especially for brain, preclude its wider application [14]. However, microdialysis has been suggested to be used routinely in the supervision of acute trauma patients, and this also opens up the prospect of assessing brain kinetics of neuroactive drugs in acute care patients [15–18].

It may be appropriate to utilize microdialysis in the evaluation of drug distribution in cancer and other diseases with microdialysis probes inserted into the pathological tissue [16–18].

Methodological difficulties in microdialysis include problems of absolute calibration of concentration, and the fact that only the concentration in the interstitium is measured. However, this does indeed make microdialysis an important complement to PET, whereas PET only measures the total tissue concentration, see below in Limitations.

2.4   Cerebrospinal fluid sampling

The only way to have access to drug-containing components representative for brain in humans, under reasonable ethics conditions, is to tap the cerebrospinal fluid (CSF) via lumbar puncture. Using this method, drug concentration in CSF can be measured after administration to allow estimates of whether a drug enters the brain. The technique is, however, affected by a number of methodological issues which are not easily taken care of. The concept assumes that spinal CSF drug concentration is representative for brain interstitial concentration. This might not necessarily be true because of the flow pattern of CSF from choroid plexus via a pulsating ventricular system with uncertain mixing with brain tissues and possible absorption and dilution during the path to the spinal fluid compartment.

Furthermore, lipophilic substances are expected to have a quite different concentration within the water like CSF as compared to a glycoprotein-rich interstitial space in the brain, and further different from the lipid-rich cell membrane and cell contents.

2.5 Biopsy or surgery

In rare cases, surgery or biopsy samples have been utilized for the assessment of drug concentration in cancer. This method would only be sparsely available and only allow one time point after drug administration.

3 PET with mixed labeled and unlabeled drug

A labeled entity containing an appropriate positron-emitting radionuclide is usually produced with very high specific radioactivity, typically of the order of 10–200 GBq/μmole [19]. This means that of the order of 1 per 7000 molecules is radioactive, the remaining are unlabeled native drug compound. However, in PET only the radioactive nuclides which undergo decay are measured, and these are taken as representatives for the unlabeled molecules. With time after administration, the unlabeled molecules undergo metabolism and elimination in the body. The labeled ones are included in exactly the same processes, but additionally undergo radioactive decay. This latter factor is predictably related to the half-life of the radionuclide and is readily corrected for. Hence, after the decay correction, the ratio between radioactive and non-radioactive molecules is constant and the concentration of non-radioactive molecules is directly given from the radioactivity measurement divided by this ratio, determined before administration.

A proper PK study should be made under conditions simulating those of a clinical dosing, i.e., with an appropriate administered dose [20–32]. The PET tracer in a patient batch, labeled plus unlabeled, typically constitute about 1–10 μg, which when given alone after administration would lead to typical plasma concentrations of the order of 10–100 pM. With a therapeutic dose of typically 1–100 mg, the plasma concentration of the drug is rather in the range of 0.1–10 μM. It is very common that several of the processes involved in absorption, distribution, metabolization, and excretion (ADME), or specific binding to molecular targets differ considerably at these two extremes of concentrations. Therefore, a proper PET study to elucidate the PK of a drug, should be made under the same conditions as in the therapeutic setting, i.e., the PET tracer should be mixed with the therapeutic dose and the two administered together. Also in this case, the ratio between radioactive and non-radioactive molecules would after decay correction be constant and the drug concentration can be obtained readily by division of the radioactivity measure with this ratio.

3.1 Standardized uptake values

PET measures directly the radioactivity concentration in a tissue expressed in Bq/ml. Since this value is dependent upon the amount of administered radioactivity as well as body weight, it is common in PET to generate a normalized value, standardized uptake value (SUV), enabling comparisons between studies performed with different amount of given radioactivity and in individuals with different weight:

$$SUV = \frac{measured\ radioactivity\ concentration\ (Bq/ml)}{administered\ radioactivity\ (kBq)\ per\ body\ weight\ (kg)} \qquad (1)$$

This entity SUV is very useful in PK studies. With the conservation of the relation between radioactivity and drug, the

$$\frac{measured\ radioactivity\ concentration}{drug\ concentration} = \frac{administered\ radioactivity}{administered\ drug}$$

Substitution of this expression into eq. (1) gives:

$$drug\ concentration\ (\mu g/ml) = SUV \cdot (administered\ drug\ (mg)\ per\ body\ weight\ (kg) \qquad (2)$$

An example: A drug was labeled and the labeled entity mixed with 50 mg native drug and co-administered to a volunteer in a PET study. The individual's body weight was 70 kg. The PET study was performed and showed at 40 min after administration an SUV value in the brain of 1.4. This means that the concentration of drug in brain at this time point was $1.4 \times (50/70) = 1.0\ \mu g/ml$.

3.2 Intravenous administration

Even if most drugs are administered orally, there is a clear advantage in PET to use intravenous (i.v.) administration, the reason behind is related to radiation exposure. Typically a PET study is associated with the administration of about 300–700 MBq. Evenly distributed in the human, this gives a radiation exposure of about 2–4 mSv. This is two to three times the yearly exposure from natural radiation and medical use of radiation to the population and is basically harmless.

When given i.v., it is expected that the radioactivity is rapidly distributed all over the body with the blood stream and the radiation dose to different organs would be relatively similar within about a factor of 10. If, however, the radioactive substance is given orally or as an inhalation, there is a possibility that most of the radioactivity could expose a very small volume of the mucosa, and there could be a local very high radiation dose. To avoid this, oral administration or inhalation studies are typically performed with 5–50 MBq. These doses are usually sufficient for nice imaging of the drug at the deposition sites, but systemic delivery to distant sites, e.g., the brain might be so low that adequate imaging and measurement is not possible.

For this reason PET is especially suitable for studies of i.v. administered drugs, but as indicated below there are also possibilities to recalculate information from an i.v. PET study and apply it to another administration route of the drug.

In a PK PET study with i.v. administration the drug needs to be formulated for i.v. administration. It can often be an advantage to administer the drug plus tracer as a slow infusion, to avoid sampling errors introduced when very sharp kinetic peaks appear, and to better mimic the plasma kinetics of a therapeutic dose. For example, if there is non-linearity of target organ distribution, it is better that the plasma PK has a relevant concentration kinetic pattern. A computerized pump system might be used to simulate the PK from another administration route, still utilizing an i.v. administration.

The PET study typically includes the dynamic imaging over the target and other regions as well as sampling of radioactivity PK in plasma (Fig. 2). The target organ drug concentration and its time course might be derived directly by multiplication of the measured SUV by given dose per kg as indicated above. Alternatively the plasma-to-target organ relation is modeled to extract important parameters such as influx rate and distribution volume, or alternatively the modeling is utilized to simulate the target organ kinetics from other PK profiles (Fig. 3). This is especially important if the formulation is changed during evolution of a project. The PK modeling allows a determi-

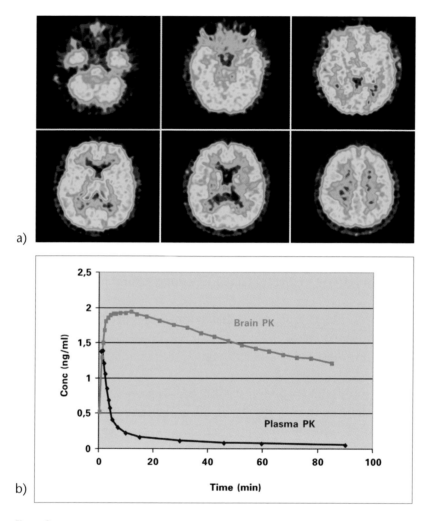

Figure 2.
(a) PET images after administration of an NK1-receptor antagonist, using co-administration of labeled and cold compound. High uptake is observed in brain tissue. (b) Radioactivity in brain and plasma is used for a recalculation to drug concentration, allowing the kinetics to be described in quantitative terms.

nation of the impact on organ kinetics from the change in formulation. The modeling also allows a population kinetic approach for evaluation of how individual variability affects the organ distribution, e.g., if high metabolizers with rapid clearance of a drug still have sufficiently high target organ concentration of the drug.

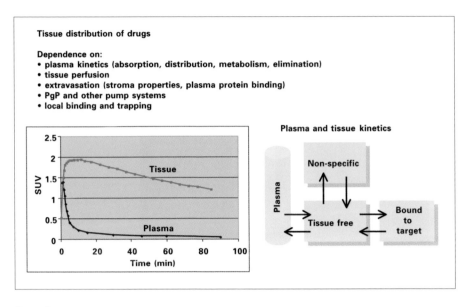

Tissue distribution of drugs

Dependence on:
- plasma kinetics (absorption, distribution, metabolism, elimination)
- tissue perfusion
- extravasation (stroma properties, plasma protein binding)
- PgP and other pump systems
- local binding and trapping

Figure 3.
With respect to tissue kinetics of drugs, it is necessary to consider the different factors contributing to the drug uptake, residence and elimination and also the compartmentalization and cellular, sub-cellular distribution.

3.3 Inhalation

PET is a very attractive alternative for the study of inhaled drugs [26, 33–40]. A major factor is that the drug itself might be labeled and, therefore, the results are fully representative for the drug deposition and disposition, in contrast to scintigraphy with ^{99m}Tc-labeled particles where the results are more representative for the properties of the inhaler.

PET is a fully three-dimensional technique and the very high spatial and temporal resolution and excellent absolute quantification adds to the possibility to perform high-quality assessments of site of deposition and rate and route of disposition (Fig. 4). Even with rather low amounts of administered radioactivity, of the order of 5–20 MBq, good quality images are generated and quantitative values are obtained with better than 10% accuracy and precision. However, with inhaled drugs, one must realize that the inter-individual variability can be rather large, and to have representative results the group sizes should be at least six to ten.

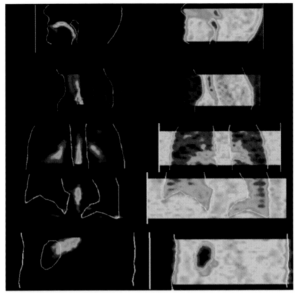

a) **¹¹C-nicotine   Transmission scan**

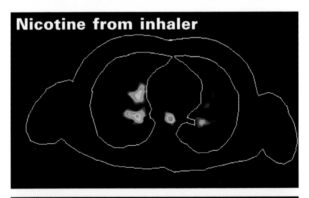

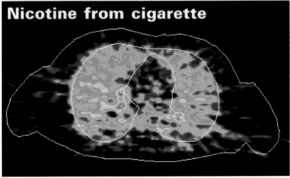

b)

Combined with CT and a mathematical description of the lung anatomy, the relative distributions from trachea to alveoli can be determined after inhalation. This has been utilized to demonstrate superiority of one construction of inhaler as compared to another [26, 36, 37, 39].

The route of absorption and transport to blood could be described for an anti-migraine medication, confirming that a rapid absorption across the nasal mucosa contributed to a rapid systemic availability (Fig. 5). Scans over the full gastrointestinal tract indicated that a portion of the drug was absorbed through this route, but with a significant delay in reaching systemic circulation.

The study of inhaled pharmaceuticals should include an assessment of plasma PK, made both for the unlabeled and the labeled drug. Comparison of these two could reveal if there is a contribution by radiolabeled metabolites. It is often not possible to make a good metabolite analysis for radioactive compounds in inhalation studies since with the low amount of administered radioactivity, the radioactivity concentration in blood is generally very low.

It can sometimes be an advantage to perform an independent measurement of the vascular pool at the deposition sites. Especially lung and nasal mucosa are very blood rich and it might be necessary to separate the contribution of blood-borne radioactivity. This part is readily assessed by multiplying the relative blood volume, as determined in a separate PET study, with the whole blood concentration of radioactivity.

It is in most instances of value to analyze the data with a kinetic model, taking into consideration rate of disposition balanced against the potential distribution of drug from blood into the organ of interest, be it the lung or the mucosa. Such model is best set up based on complementary data from a separate PET study in which the labeled drug is given i.v. and rates and magnitudes of distribution from plasma to organ is evaluated.

Figure 4.
(a) After the administration of ^{11}C-labeled nicotine from an inhaler, PET with sequential movements over different sectors of the body, allow determination of residence of drug at different anatomical positions and different time points. The right image shows corresponding transmission scans for anatomical identification. (b) Transaxial slices over the chest show minimal deposition in the lung after administration of nicotine via the inhaler as compared to administration of nicotine via a cigarette.

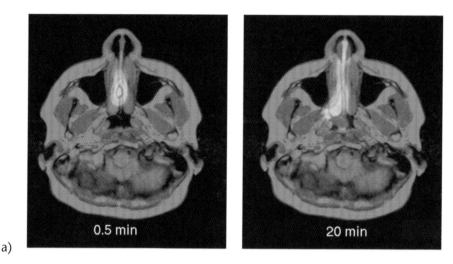

a)

Emission images overlapped on MRI

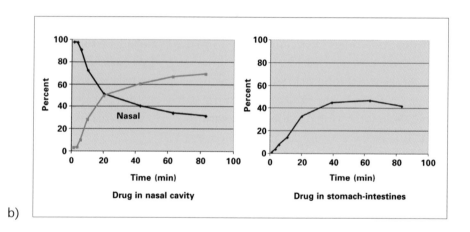

b)

Figure 5.
An ^{11}C-labeled anti-migraine drug administered as a nasal spray shows deposition in the nasal passage, as evidenced when overlapping the PET images on the corresponding MRI images (a). Quantitative values over the nasal passage shows a 100% immediate deposition with 30% absorbed or disposed within the first 10 minutes (b). About 10% has reached the stomach-intestines within the first 10 min, while plasma concentration has reached close to its maximum. The study supports that about 20–30% of the drug reaches the systemic circulation via the nasal mucosa during the first 10 min.

3.4 Oral administration

There are only a few studies documented in which oral administration of labeled drugs have been evaluated [28, 41, 42]. Reasons for this include that the short half-life precludes formulation in tablets, and it is often assumed that the rate of resorption is too slow to allow PET studies, especially when using ^{11}C as radionuclide. Furthermore, the crucial information to be obtained from an oral administration study is usually degree and rate of systemic availability and this information can be gained from a traditional drug administration PK sampling study. There are, however, instances when imaging, with its possibility to evaluate regional residence of drug, can add to the understanding of drug behavior. It can be possible to follow a drug through the intestinal tract, and evaluate dynamically how much is resorbed in different segments of the intestines. It is also possible to evaluate liver uptake and accumulation into and emptying of the gall bladder, and thereby describe hepatic recirculation. The PET- or accelerator mass spectrometry (AMS)-microdosing concepts with super-high sensitivity could be used for the acceleration of drug development and allow oral absorption and bioavailability to be evaluated in drug candidates with limited toxicology backup, and thereby be time saving in the drug development [43, 44]. Finally it can be of pedagogic value to describe drug fate from administration until it reaches the target organ. Such information is best utilized if it is backed up with PK modeling, allowing simulations of impact of changes in formulation, differences in populations, etc.

Indeed, formulation issues are sometimes difficult to handle due to the short time allowed by the decay of radioactivity and this might limit the applicability of PET. Suspensions, liquids and encapsulated suspensions and liquids can be handled, and in such cases a dominant resorption may be at hand within the time span allowed by the radioactive decay, typically 2 h for ^{11}C and 8 h for [18]F.

Studies of orally administered ^{11}C-labeled vinpocetine showed a rapid resorption after about 30-min delay and, via the circulation, an uptake in the brain was measured [23, 24, 42]. In own studies, we verified the systemic kinetics of an ^{18}F-labeled drug, formulated as a suspension in a gelatinized capsule, and its kinetics in organs of interest (Fig. 6). Since in these studies the labeled and unlabeled drug is co-administered, radioactivity measure-

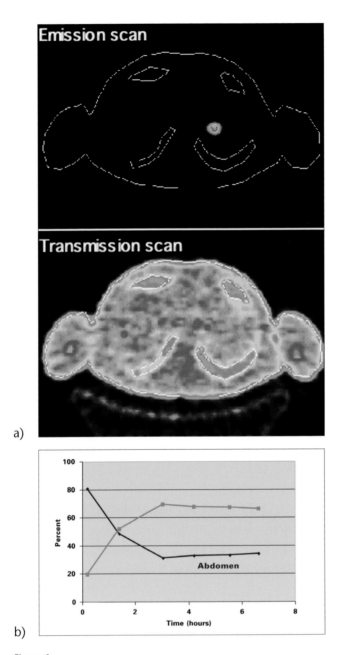

a)

b)

Figure 6.
(a) An ^{18}F-labeled drug, administered as a capsule is localized with PET on its route via the gastrointestinal tract. Transmission scan is used for a crude anatomical localization. (b) Within the first hour about 50% and within 3 h about 70% of the drug is absorbed from the intestines.

ments with PET describing the residual amounts in intestines and distribution to organs, is readily converted to drug amounts and concentrations.

4 PET with i.v. and drug with another administration route

In many cases it is not possible to use the same administration route for PET as in the therapeutic application of a drug. It might not even be desirable, due to the fact that the optimal information in a PET study is achieved with i.v. administration. This does, however, not imply that a PET PK study is meaningless under such conditions, in fact, there is a very useful way to include a PET PK study in drug development and understanding also with orally administered drugs. The PET study with i.v. administration of the labeled drug can record the kinetics of the drug in an organ up to a time set by the half-life of the radionuclide. In the same PET study, the plasma kinetics is recorded, preferably with radiometabolite evaluation to derive a radioactivity PK profile. These data are then combined in an organ PK model to describe the relation between the plasma kinetics and the organ kinetics. This model, together with its parameters can then be applied on the PK profile obtained for the unlabeled drug with its actual administration route to calculate drug concentration and PK in organs [45].

4.1 PK modeling of PET data

The modeling in PET studies has traditionally utilized arterial sampling, from which plasma kinetics together with the measured organ kinetics have been used in a compartment model, describing the changes in concentration and exchange between compartments by differential equations [46–48]. The parameters of the model have been obtained by optimization of fitting of the calculated to the actual tissue curve.

We have suggested a modification to this mode of analysis when applied to a PK study, based on the fact that usually venous blood sampling is utilized in drug PK studies. Since there may be a clear difference in the arterial and venous plasma PK data, especially in the early time points after i.v. administration, the relation between arterial plasma PK and organ PK might not be the same as between venous plasma PK and organ PK. However, arterial plasma PK is best utilized for the simplest description of transfer and exchange of drug with the organ.

To solve this dilemma, we propose the use of venous blood sampling in the PET study, which in fact greatly simplifies the ethical aspects of PET studies. Instead a mathematical "virtual" arterial plasma PK profile is introduced. If, additionally, a convolution modeling instead of compartment modeling is introduced, the concept becomes easily understood and easily applied.

The organ PET data are assumed to be represented by an impulse response from an infinitesimally small capillary plasma exposure, convolving the full capillary plasma time-activity data:

$$B(t) = A(t) \otimes I(t) \tag{3}$$

where $B(t)$ represents organ time-activity data, $A(t)$ capillary plasma time-activity data, $I(t)$ the impulse response from capillary to organ tissue (transfer function) and the symbol $\otimes$ denotes convolution.

A correction must be made for the fact that arterial and capillary time-activity data differ from venous time-activity data. This is made with the assumption that an impulse response can be defined to represent the relation between capillary plasma and venous plasma:

$$V(t) = g(t) \otimes A(t) \tag{4}$$

where $V(t)$ represents venous plasma time-activity data, $g(t)$ the impulse response from capillary to venous plasma at the sampling site. Note that the condition $\int_{-\infty}^{\infty} g(t) \cdot dt = 1$ must hold.

By defining $g^{-1}(t)$ as the inverse of $g(t)$, the expression (3) can be rearranged to:

$$B(t) = \left[g^{-1}(t) \otimes I(t) \right] \otimes V(t) \tag{5}$$

To solve the relation between venous plasma time-activity $V(t)$ and brain time-activity $B(t)$, a program was written in MATLAB, which iteratively fitted data in eq. (5) with $I(t)$ described as an arbitrary tri-exponential function, and $g^{-1}(t)$ described as the inverse of the arterial to venous transfer function, in turn defined by a set of exponential functions.

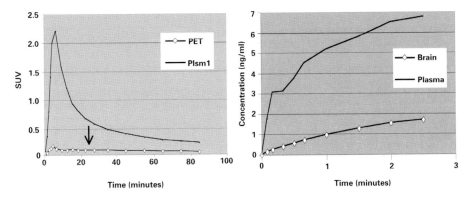

Figure 7.
(a) With the kinetics in plasma and brain determined in an i.v. PET study, an impulse response function is determined such that the brain kinetics corresponds to a convolution of the plasma curve with this function. (b) The convolution of the plasma PK after another administration route with the same impulse response function gives the brain kinetics associated with this administration.

With the assumption that PET data could supply an overall impulse response, describing the relation between organ time-activity data and venous plasma time-activity data, and with the assumption that the relation between organ and plasma is time invariant and linear, organ PK data from another administration route can be obtained as a convolution of its venous plasma PK data with this impulse response (Fig. 7).

$$BD(t) = \left[g^{-1}(t) \otimes I(t) \right] \otimes VD(t) \tag{6}$$

where now $BD(t)$ equals organ kinetics and $VD(t)$ the venous plasma PK of the cold drug, while $[g^{-1}(t) \otimes I(t)]$ is the overall impulse response obtained in the PET study.

The introduction of this "virtual" arterial to venous transform is necessary to obtain a reasonable fit to the organ kinetic data. This becomes clear when observing the arterial and venous PET data together with the organ data. The peak of the venous PK data occurs later that that of the arterial but may also appear later than that of organ PK. It is not possible by a compartment model with a direct exchange between plasma and tissue to describe a situation where the tissue peak comes earlier than the plasma peak, and attempts to fit data would result in a description with clear mismatch at the early time points.

The approach to use PET for a description of a model of relation between organ and plasma is rational and relevant, but some additional precautions are necessary.

The concept relies on the fact that the exchange is dose independent and time invariant. Since exchange with tissue might be dose dependent, e.g., when active molecular pumps are involved in the transfer as in the BBB, a possible influence by the magnitude of plasma concentration must be taken into consideration, either in the modeling or in the performance of the study.

The most appropriate way to perform the study, would be to give the drug by its actual administration route, and at the same time give the PET tracer i.v. with an infusion which is controlled to give a plasma curve equal to the PK data from the drug administration. An alternative simplified scenario is to perform a PET study before administration of the drug, allowing a calculation of the exchange parameters at low drug concentrations, and a new PET study performed at plateau plasma drug concentration. The information from these two studies can be used to evaluate if the tissue exchange is dose independent, and if not, to estimate the exchange with the inclusion of a model for the non-linearity.

When a PET study is performed with the aim to allow a later application of a PK model to drug PK data, it is seldom necessary to obtain data which represent the very rapid phases of exchange. It is therefore more practical to perform the PET study with a prolonged (5–15 min) infusion rather than as a rapid bolus injection of the tracer. With this concept the plasma PK values change more slowly with time and a more sparse blood sampling scheme can be applied without risk of missing peak values and rapidly changing aspects of the plasma curve.

5   PET microdosing

A PET study includes the administration of a small amount of compound, a minor portion of which is labeled with a PET radionuclide. Each of these parts is associated with a certain risk, the drug with possible toxic effects and the radioactivity with a certain radiation hazard. Authorities typically accept a radiation exposure to healthy individuals of the order of 10 mSv, which in a PET trial involves the administration of about 2000 MBq of a ^{11}C-labeled or 600 MBq ^{18}F-labeled compound [49–52]. A high quality PET study with i.v.

administration is performed with about 300–600 MBq for ^{11}C and 150–300 MBq for ^{18}F. The specific radioactivity directly after the synthesis can be as high as 20–200 GBq/µmole, and hence a PET study might be associated with 2–20 nmoles of substance. For small organic molecules this typically means less than 10 µg.

We have introduced the concept of PET microdosing, meaning a trial in humans with PET methodology, where PK information is obtained with the administration of super low amounts of active compound [44, 53, 54]. The PET microdosing would serve either of two objectives:
- To allow early human studies, volunteers or patients, with a new chemical entity with the aim to supply important organ distribution and kinetics information which can aid in the drug selection and development process
- To allow human studies with a tentative or validated PET tracer, serving to elucidate biology, physiology, pathology or drug interaction

Only the first aspect is covered in the present communication.

5.1   Regulatory aspects

Since PET microdosing studies are limited with respect to the population exposed and the doses are very low and given as single administrations, it is reasonable that other criteria are applied with respect to preclinical safety assessments as compared to the development of therapeutic drugs. This has now been accepted by the European regulatory agencies and a limited safety package introduced (http://www.emea.eu.int/pdfs/human/swp/259902en.pdf).

The basic features in the EMEA/CPMP concept include an acute toxicity study in one species with single administration, different dose groups, and evaluation at two time points, 2 days and 2 weeks. The safety margin should be at least 1000 plus allometric scaling as compared to administered dose per kg in the PET study. Furthermore, there should be an evaluation of genotoxicity, in two *in vitro* assays, one of which should be mammalian cells. The genotoxicity assessment is performed according to existing rules (ICH topic 2A and 2B).

In USA, the FDA has opened for a simplified toxicity assessment for imaging agents (http://www.fda.gov/cder/guidance/5742pt2.htm), relatively similar to the European guidelines, with the addition of a study of acute pharmacological effects, and possibly an acute toxicity safety margin of 100 instead of 1000. The preclinical toxicity assessment can be performed with a limited use of animals, in a relatively short time, 3–6 months, and at a limited cost.

We still believe that the regulatory requirements should be modified in some respects, e.g., the genotoxicity studies as specified by ICH (International Conference on Harmonization) require about 4 g of compound, and includes concentrations that are unnecessary high. The requirement to have drug concentrations up to 5 mg/plate means doses which are 25'000'000 times higher than expected in a PET-microdosing study, and if associated with radiolabeled compound would be 10'000 times the lethal radiation dose. There is still an uncertainty in the regulatory document with respect to the desire to perform more than one PET study in the same individual, e.g., to follow sequentially with time the effects of pharmaceuticals. A limit dose concept could save animals, and repeat administrations could make for a more secure toxicity study. Finally, it could be advisable to include a study with the evaluation of potential acute pharmacological effects by the drug.

5.2   Information from a PET-microdosing study

A human PET study performed as a PET-microdosing study would be made with PET imaging over areas of the body of interest. The PET camera typically has a field-of-view of 15 cm, meaning that simultaneously an axial sector of 15 cm is observed. This sector is further subdivided into 63 tomographic slices. It is possible to rapidly switch between different anatomical sectors, and hence also cover other areas and organs. Thus, there is a choice to focus over one part of the body and acquire rapid kinetic data, or to alternate between two or more sectors but cover these with a more sparse kinetics.

In the images, areas of interest are identified and outlined with the cursor, and the tracer kinetics within these areas determined, often expressed as SUV. During the study, typically a number of blood samples would be taken for the determination of tracer concentration and kinetics in whole blood and plasma. A limited number of plasma samples are subjected to metabolite analysis, allowing a calculation of the kinetics of intact (un-metabolized) labeled drug.

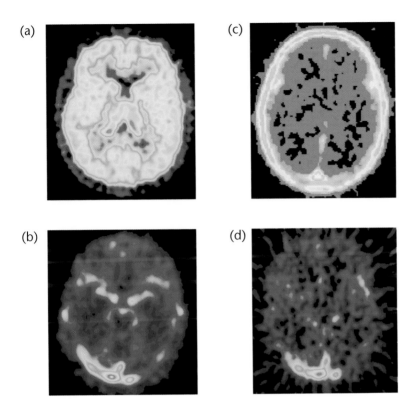

Figure 8.
PET-microdosing studies with three different drugs demonstrate different degrees of passage into the brain. Drug (A) has an excellent uptake in brain, drug (B) a limited but still measurable uptake, whereas drug (C) is only residing in the brain vasculature, as evidenced by comparison with the regional blood volume (D).

The important data coming from a PET-microdosing study include (Fig. 8):
- Plasma kinetics and elimination rate
- Organ distribution
- Concentrations of drug in the organ of interest for therapeutic effect
- Concentration of drug in organs of concern for side effects, physiological or toxic
- Parameters describing exchange between plasma and organ, allowing recalculations for PK from other administration routes or formulations
- In some cases, information that the drug reaches and binds to a defined target can be documented. However, a PET-microdosing study would typically

not allow a determination of which occupancy would result from a certain dose, but a human PET-microdosing study could be used together with PK/PD-modeling and preclinical data to suggest occupancy induced by a certain dose.

PET-microdosing studies could be made with different compounds in the same individual, to allow a more precise comparison, e.g., for selection among lead candidates. PET typically has of the order of 5–10% variability between studies, whereas inter-individual variability can be significantly larger, indicating the superiority of intra-individual comparisons. Such studies must be made sequentially, allowing radioactivity from one study to decay before performing the next study.

5.3   Validation of a labeled new drug

A PET-microdosing study can properly indicate the PK of the compound at tracer doses; however, when the purpose is to use the information to predict the behavior of the drug in clinical use, it will be necessary to attempt to extrapolate the information from micro-dose levels to therapeutic levels. For this reason it is necessary to clarify eventual lack of dose linearity. Studies with this purpose should be made in animals, in a species thought to be representative for the purpose. We prefer to make these studies in monkeys.

The dominant factors which may introduce lack of dose linearity are related to biochemical systems that can be saturated at doses below the therapeutic concentrations:

- Specific binding to receptors and enzymes can occur at nanomolar concentrations
- Specific molecular transporters at nano- to micromolar concentrations
- Metabolizing enzymes in the micromolar range
- "Nonspecific" binding to proteins in the nano- to micro-molar range
- Plasma proteins in the micromolar range
- Physiological effects such as effects on organ blood flow in the nano- to micro-molar range.

Since the PET-microdosing study is performed with typical plasma concentrations of the order of 10–100 pM, specific binding to high-affinity targets can play an important role. The concentration ratio of specifically bound to free drug in tissue is at concentrations significantly lower than the K_D proportional to B_{max} over K_D, and this ratio can be significantly higher than 1. In brain studies with ^{11}C-labeled raclopride ,the striatal dopamine D_2-receptor density is about 10–20 nM, and the K_D of raclopride about 4 nM [55]. We observe a specific to background ratio of about 3–5. Hence, the PET-micro-dosing study would over-estimate the target tissue concentration by a factor of 3–5 as compared to the case of therapeutic application of raclopride when dosed to block 80–90% of the receptors.

In many studies with PET tracers for specific molecular targets, we observe that the plasma curve increases after pharmacological blockade of target [56, 57]. This increase can be a factor of 2. We interpret this as being an effect of blockade of peripheral binding sites. For example, after i.v. administrations the first capillary encounter by the drug is in the lung, and hence a proportionally high binding to targets can occur there. If this binding is blocked pharmacologically, less tracer is cached by the lung and is, therefore, systemically available.

For drugs with specific plasma protein carriers such as steroids, a low binding to liver can be at hand at low concentrations, because plasma protein binding rescues drugs from liver metabolism. At higher drug concentrations this plasma protein binding can be saturated meaning that excess drug is more prone to be taken up by the liver [58].

Non-linear PK is in most cases expressed in plasma PK, and related to dose-dependent effects by systemic elimination and metabolism. This means that the relation of plasma kinetics to eliminating and metabolizing organs, liver and kidney, is changed with changed doses, but not necessarily the relation between other interesting organs and plasma. Therefore, it is in general of interest to model this relation, and these exchange parameters might be unaffected by plasma concentration of drug, even if plasma PK in itself is not. In such cases one would be less concerned by non-linear plasma PK.

An assessment of dose linearity of PK would typically include PET scanning or *ex vivo* measurement of organ tracer kinetics in an animal, coupled with evaluation of plasma PK (Fig. 9). Dose escalation with added tracer and drug would be done with a span from tracer doses to higher than assumed therapeutic doses. The tracer SUV would be the indicator of the tracers concentration in tissue and in studies with added compound, the SUV values would be unchanged if dose linearity exists.

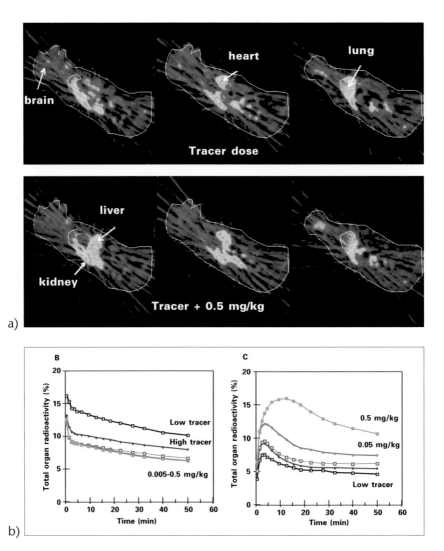

Figure 9.
(a) Sagittal sections in a PET study in monkey utilizing a ^{11}C-labeled drug without and with added cold compound. (b) The relative amount observed in the lung decreases already at low amounts of added compound, suggesting a non-linearity at low concentrations, likely related to blockade of specific binding. (c) The relative amount of drug in the liver is increasing at high amounts of added compound, likely related to redistribution from plasma protein-bound fraction.

Studies in animals or even in humans, in which the specific target binding is blocked by other pharmacological agents which are applicable at therapeutic doses in humans could aid in the interpretation of which factors are involved in the tracers ADME.

Except for dose-linearity evaluation, a crucial point is to evaluate if radioactivity in organs represents intact drug or metabolites thereof. It would be necessary to explore in animal experiments both tissue and plasma radioactivity content with respect to radioactive metabolites. In the human PET-microdosing study it would then be necessary to assay the fraction of intact radioactive compound in plasma at multiple time points. Sometimes it would be necessary to define the exact characters of radioactive metabolites and possibly explore their behavior in separate studies.

6   Mechanistic studies

PET can in some instances be used to elucidate mechanistic aspects of drug distribution. For example, the possible impact of efflux pumps as part of the BBB can be explored utilizing the labeled drug and studies without and with pharmacological blockade of these pump systems, or in a reverse paradigm in which pharmacological challenge with a drug is performed and a PET-tracer for the efflux pump is used to indicate possible effects by the drug on the efflux system [59–61]. In a similar fashion, other types of drug interaction studies can be performed where the potential effect of other pharmaceuticals on a selected drug distribution pattern is explored. These interaction phenomena can sometimes be undesired and induce enhanced side effects, but can also be desired, e.g., by reducing drug concentration in an organ where side effects occur, or increase the drug concentration in the target organ.

Double studies with one PET session performed with the drug labeled in one position and one session with the drug labeled in another position, can be used to explore the impact of metabolism [62–64]. Similar experiments can be made with two enantiomers as part of the exploration of the advantage of using enantiomeric pure compounds [65].

7   Labeling perspectives

The labeling of biologically active molecules used in PET, employing ^{11}C and other short-lived positron-emitting radionuclides has been limited by the short half-life and the access to labeled building blocks [19]. The development of [^{11}C]methyliodide or methyl triflate as a tool to prepare various labeled molecules has been a key factor especially for development of labeled drug molecules or tools for occupancy or inhibition studies. Although a successful method leading to a range of PET tracers for exploration of biology, the selection of the molecules have partly been governed by this limitation in labeling. When the aim is to label a drug candidate, the choices in this respect is relatively limited, since there is a prerequisite that the molecule contains an adequate methyl group. Recently significant alternatives outside methylation, carboxylation or cyanidation reactions have been developed, which is opening up a new scenario [19, 66]. A significant step in the development of labeling with ^{11}C is in our opinion the availability of methods utilizing ^{11}C-CO as a synthon [67–70]. Figure 10 presents schematically a summary of the new dimension of accessible labeled precursors and synthetic methods. This new potential allows a significant number of lead drugs to be labeled with ^{11}C, and furthermore it will improve our possibility to develop appropriate receptor ligands and enzyme substrates. An additional advantage of CO-labeling methods is that they may allow for a significantly higher specific radioactivity as compared to most other reactions.

Labeling with ^{18}F is also attractive for compounds containing suitable fluorine and can sometimes be made with high specific activity using nucleophilic synthetic pathways. Exchange methods can sometimes allow the insertion of ^{18}F into a molecule, but typically at a rather low specific activity. This might, however, not necessarily be of concern in studies with labeled drug except for the PET-microdosing concept.

The increased potentials for labeling drug candidates with ^{11}C open the way for a new possible paradigm in drug development, in which a PET strategy is initiated and run in parallel with the development of the therapeutics. After the first screening, candidates can be selected with additional criteria related to their potentials to be labeled for PET applications. It is especially attractive if a general labeling method can be applied with unaffected pharmacophore and allowance for molecular modifications to increase different pharmacological properties such as lipophilicity and metabolism. Later in the process, some candidates can be promoted to drug candidates, optimizing the requirements for such use, whereas analogues with better PET-related properties can be developed as tracers for the target system.

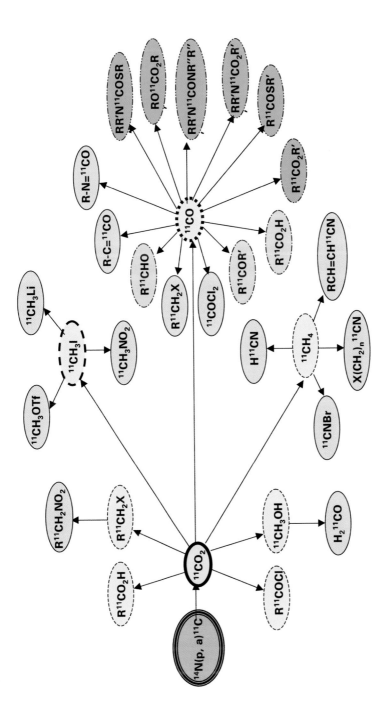

Figure 10.
The versatility of labeling of many chemical structures with ^{11}C has significantly increased with the use of ^{11}CO as synthon.

When labeling of a drug candidate is desired, it is very important also to consider the labeling position. Some labeling positions could more than others lead to labeled metabolites which can confound the interpretation [71].

Since the labeled entity is aimed for use in humans, the product ready for administration must be qualified according to good medical practice (GMP). A working concept for purification, sterilization and validation of the end product has been established, taking into consideration the differences in requirements for PET tracers and conventional drugs.

8   General limitations

PET is an attractive technique since it allows a drug to be labeled with a positron-emitting radionuclide and thereafter in a PET study in humans be investigated with respect to body distribution, including absolute determinations of drug concentration in organs or sub-regions in organs. There are, however, of course also a number of limitations to the method, some of which will be discussed below.

8.1   Resolution, accuracy and precision

PET allows the measurement of tracer concentration within regions, the minimal extent of which is set by the spatial resolution of the PET camera. Typically present PET instruments have a resolution of about 5 mm. This does allow small anatomical details to be imaged and identified, but if the structure has a diameter smaller than about twice the resolution, i.e. about 10 mm, the signal measured will be impaired and not properly reflect the true radioactivity concentration. Even structures as small as 1 mm might be observed, but would typically require that the tracer concentration within the structure is more than 100 times that of the surrounding tissues, and the absolute measure would be severely under-estimated. With structures larger than 10 mm an adequate measure can be obtained, but this requires that the region of interest outlined in the image is reduced radially from the true object edge by about one resolution element, i.e., 5 mm, otherwise the degradation of signal close to the edge would impair the measurement.

PET has an inherent very high accuracy, due to the precise measurements of radioactivity, coupled to the possibility to perform accurate corrections for the major disturbing factors which otherwise would affect the measurement. The dominant correction is for photon attenuation, meaning that only a fraction of photons can emerge out of the body unscattered. This fraction is dependent upon size, shape and composition of the object, and can be of the order of 1/6 for the brain and 1/50 for abdomen sections. A transmission scan would determine these factors and enable an adequate correction. A second disturbing factor is scattered radiation, interpreted as correct signal. This factor can typically be 20–40% and is corrected for by mathematical processing of the raw data. Including all corrections, PET measurements are typically correct with an error within less than 5–10%.

PET images are typically very noisy, due to a limited number of photons detected. Even if the total number of counts is of the order of 10 million, the number of photons per detector combination is rather low. Random fluctuations in the number of photons detected introduce noise in the images, which can be of the order of 10–50%, measured as variations between individual pixels in a uniform area. When averaging over an area, the precision of the average is improved, but in a complicated way related to the pixel-to-pixel variations and number of pixels in the average because of correlation of the noise in the images.

8.2   Cellular and sub-cellular distribution

Although PET can accurately measure the drug concentration in tissue, it is not trivial to relate this concentration to effects on target systems. One reason for this is that the drug might have a very non-uniform cellular and sub-cellular distribution. For example, lipophilic drugs are expected to have a much higher concentration in the lipid-rich cell membranes than in the more water-like extracellular fluid. The reverse may be the case for hydrophilic substances. The drug concentration affecting the target will therefore be dependent upon the exact subcellular position of the target. Similarly, the intracellular concentration can be much lower or much higher than the concentration in the extracellular fluid, e.g., governed by selective in- or out-flux pumps. Also different cell types intermingled can show different intracellular concentrations dependent upon each cell types expression of uptake or efflux systems. Finally, weak bases with high lipophilicity at normal tissue pH conditions but protonizing to polar compounds at low pH can show a very significant accumulation in acidic organelles such as lysosomes and mitochondria. These factors may contribute to a difference in concentration-effect relations when comparing *in vitro* and *in vivo* assays.

8.3   Radioactive metabolites

A major concern in PET is related to the fact that the *in vivo* measurements only represent amount of radioactivity in tissue, with no possibility to discern if the radionuclide is residing in the native drug compound or metabolites thereof. In plasma, however, similar possibilities exist as in regular PK analysis to separate chemical entities, e.g., by HPLC, and determine separately what fraction of total radioactivity is constituted by native labeled compound and by radioactive metabolites.

It is in general advisable to perform validation studies in animals which can be sacrificed, and there evaluate fractions of radioactivity related to intact tracer in the tissue of interest to have a feeling for the potential magnitude of this problem. If needed, additional PET studies can be performed with a radiolabeled metabolite to understand its tissue distribution and kinetics. With respect to CNS active drugs, it is often so that metabolites are more polar than a native lipophilic compound and these might not pass the BBB. However, there are also metabolizing enzymes both within the brain parenchyma and as part of the BBB system, and in such cases metabolites would be formed from the native compound within the brain, and if they are polar they might not leave the brain readily. Kinetic modeling may sometimes be used for a mathematical estimate of the metabolites' organ kinetics and allow a subtraction of their contribution.

8.4   Short follow-up times

The two major radionuclides used in PET and drug development are ^{11}C and ^{18}F with half-lives of 20 and 110 min, respectively. Although radioactivity rapidly decays, it is still usually possible to obtain adequate images and quantitative values up to about 4–5 half-lives, i.e. up to about 90 min for [11]C- and up to 8 h for ^{18}F-labeled material. Ninety minutes might seem to be a rather short time to follow the kinetics of a drug and indeed does not allow all questions raised to be answered in a PK study. However, compared to a total lack of information regarding the organ distribution, still this time-limited information could contribute to a better understanding of the drugs behavior. Under some conditions, the organ kinetics can be extrapolated to times much longer than set by the half-lives. As indicated above, this extrapolation can be aided by utilizing a PK model describing the relation between organ and plasma. If, for example, an equilibrium is achieved in the organ-to-plasma concentration ratio, the extrapolation to longer times would rely on the application of the organ-to-plasma ratio on the plasma PK.

For drugs with questionable BBB penetration, the degree of penetration in a short time interval can give added information, but of course a very slow brain entry might not be possible to discern.

8.5   Radiation dose and specific radioactivity

The amount of radioactivity needed for a high quality PET investigation with i.v. administration of labeled drug, is of the order of 300–500 MBq with ^{11}C and 100–200 MBq with ^{18}F. This radioactivity is associated with about 2 mSv of given radiation dose [49–52], which is fully acceptable also for studies in healthy volunteers, and in turn of the same order as that given by natural radiation from ground and space during about 1 year. It may be desirable to use a higher amount of radioactivity in studies with long duration, especially if metabolite analysis is performed at late time points since these give rather low count rates. Cumulative radioactivity in a study protocol may go up to 2000 MBq for ^{11}C and 600 MBq for ^{18}F, meaning that each individual can be subjected to four to six PET studies. This is a great advantage since it allows intra-individual comparisons between different labeled drugs or the same labeled drug before and after pharmacological challenges.

The specific radioactivity in PET is typically of the order of 20–200 GBq/μmole which means that the administered amount of compound is typically of the order of 1–10 μg. This amount is usually so low that no pharmacological effect is expected. Additionally, it is so low that usually no quantitative binding to the target systems is expected; only a minimal fraction of the target proteins will bind the tracer. For example, in a PET study with ^{11}C-labeled raclopride of the order of a few percent of the dopamine D_2-receptors bind the tracer molecules. In this case the tracer affinity is about 3 nM *in vitro*, 9 nM *in vivo* [55] and the tracer concentration in plasma less than 1 nM. However, there might be cases in which tracer doses are also associated with such high amounts of cold compound that a significant portion of the target system is binding tracer molecules, and this might affect the quantitative values of target binding. This can happen, e.g., with tracers having very high affinity for the target, high picomolar K_D values [72]. To avoid this, the highest possible specific radioactivity is desired so that with reasonable administered radioactivity, the associated cold mass is minimized. This limitation is relatively seldom at hand in human *in vivo* studies but tend to be an important limitation in animal and *in vitro* experiments with PET tracers.

8.6 Limited field of view

A modern PET camera typically has a field of view of about 15 cm. This means that a segment of the body with 15-cm thickness is covered at each time point. This area is reconstructed to a three-dimensional volume in which the radioactivity distribution is given in typically 63 tomographic slices with a 2.5-mm separation. The volume is divided into voxels, volume elements for data storage and visualization with typical dimensions of $4 \times 4 \times 2.5$ mm^3. Slices of this volume can be obtained at any direction for visualization of two-dimensional images.

Multiple acquisitions over the field-of-view can be made according to a desired schedule with the shortest acquisitions being typically 5 s. Practically, such short acquisitions with ^{11}C- and ^{18}F-labeled compounds are too noisy for the images to be meaningful, instead schedules contain acquisitions from parts of minutes to several minutes, altogether constituting sufficient long cover of kinetics. A reasonable compromise, to have good kinetic coverage but not too much data storage, is to make about 15–20 acquisitions within 90 min, with more frequent measurements at the early times when kinetics is changing more rapidly.

It is often desirable to cover more than 15 cm of the body, and it is possible within some seconds to move the patient on the couch and start a new acquisition at another body segment. This, of course, means a measure of radioactivity distribution at another time point than the first measure.

Hence, instead of monitoring kinetics continuously over one body part, sequential movements in-between measurements allow paradigms with more sparse assessments of kinetics, but allowing multiple organs to be evaluated. If desired to cover the full body, excluding the legs, such sequential movements would typically require 20–30 min, where after this coverage can be repeated again.

References

1   Aboagye EO, Price PM, Jones T (2001) *In vivo* pharmacokinetics and pharmacodynamics in drug development using positron-emission tomography. *Drug Discov Today* 6: 293–302

2   Fischman AJ, Alpert NM, Babich JW, Rubin RH (1997) The role of positron emission tomography in pharmacokinetic analysis. *Drug Metab Rev* 29: 923–956

3   Fischman AJ, Alpert NM, Rubin RH (2002) Pharmacokinetic imaging: a noninvasive method for determining drug distribution and action. *Clin Pharmacokinet* 41: 581–602

4   Gupta N, Price PM, Aboagye EO (2002) PET for *in vivo* pharmacokinetic and pharmacodynamic measurements. *Eur J Cancer* 38: 2094–2107

5   Hutchinson OC, Collingridge DR, Barthel H, Price PM, Aboagye EO (2003) Pharmacokinetics of radiolabeled anticancer drugs for positron emission tomography. *Curr Pharm Des* 9: 917–929

6   Klimas MT (2002) Positron emission tomography and drug discovery: contributions to the understanding of pharmacokinetics, mechanism of action and disease state characterization. *Mol Imaging Biol* 4: 311–337

7   Propper DJ, de Bono J, Saleem A, Ellard S, Flanagan E, Paul J, Ganesan TS, Talbot DC, Aboagye EO, Price P et al (2003) Use of positron emission tomography in pharmacokinetic studies to investigate therapeutic advantage in a phase I study of 120-hour intravenous infusion XR5000. *J Clin Oncol* 21: 203–210

8   Roselt P, Meikle S, Kassiou M (2004) The role of positron emission tomography in the discovery and development of new drugs; as studied in laboratory animals. *Eur J Drug Metab Pharmacokinet* 29: 1–6

9   Rubin RH, Fischman AJ (1997) Positron emission tomography in drug development. *Q J Nucl Med* 41: 171–175

10   Bergstrom M, Awad R, Estrada S, Malman J, Lu L, Lendvai G, Bergstrom-Pettermann E, Langstrom B (2003) Autoradiography with positron emitting isotopes in positron emission tomography tracer discovery. *Mol Imaging Biol* 5: 390–396

11   Bergstrom M, Bonasera TA, Lu L, Bergstrom E, Backlin C, Juhlin C, Langstrom B (1998) *In vitro* and *in vivo* primate evaluation of carbon-11-etomidate and carbon-11-metomidate as potential tracers for PET imaging of the adrenal cortex and its tumors. *J Nucl Med* 39: 982–989

12   Bergstrom M, Westerberg G, Langstrom B (1997) 11C-harmine as a tracer for monoamine oxidase A (MAO-A): *in vitro* and *in vivo* studies. *Nucl Med Biol* 24: 287–293

13   Bergstrom M, Westerberg G, Kihlberg T, Langstrom B (1997) Synthesis of some 11C-

labeled MAO-A inhibitors and their *in vivo* uptake kinetics in rhesus monkey brain. *Nucl Med Biol* 24: p. 381–388

14   Stahl M, Bouw R, Jackson A, Pay V (2002) Human microdialysis. *Curr Pharm Biotechnol* 3: 165–178

15   Ederoth P, Tunblad K, Bouw R, Lundberg CJ, Ungerstedt U, Nordstrom CH, Hammarlund-Udenaes M (2004) Blood-brain barrier transport of morphine in patients with severe brain trauma. *Br J Clin Pharmacol* 57: 427–435

16   Bielecka-Grzela S, Klimowicz A (2003) Application of cutaneous microdialysis to evaluate metronidazole and its main metabolite concentrations in the skin after a single oral dose. *J Clin Pharm Ther* 28: 465–469

17   Joukhadar C, Stass H, Muller-Zellenberg U, Lackner E, Kovar F, Minar E, Muller M (2003) Penetration of moxifloxacin into healthy and inflamed subcutaneous adipose tissues in humans. *Antimicrob Agents Chemother* 47: 3099–3103

18   Joukhadar C, Klein N, Dittrich P, Zeitlinger M, Geppert A, Skhirtladze K, Frossard M, Heinz G, Muller M (2003) Target site penetration of fosfomycin in critically ill patients. *J Antimicrob Chemother* 51: 1247–1252

19   Langstrom B, Kihlberg T, Bergstrom M, Antoni G, Bjorkman M, Forngren BH, Forngren T, Hartvig P, Markides K, Yngve U, Ogren M (1999) Compounds labeled with short-lived beta(+)-emitting radionuclides and some applications in life sciences. The importance of time as a parameter. *Acta Chem Scand* 53: 651–669

20   Beshara S, Lundqvist H, Sundin J, Lubberink M, Tolmachev V, Valind S, Antoni G, Langstrom B, Danielson BG (1999) Pharmacokinetics and red cell utilization of iron(III) hydroxide-sucrose complex in anaemic patients: a study using positron emission tomography. *Br J Haematol* 104: 296–302

21   Fischman AJ, Livni E, Babich JW, Alpert NM, Bonab A, Chodosh S, McGovern F, Kamitsuka P, Liu YY, Cleeland R et al (1996) Pharmacokinetics of [18F]fleroxacin in patients with acute exacerbations of chronic bronchitis and complicated urinary tract infection studied by positron emission tomography. *Antimicrob Agents Chemother* 40: 659–664

22   Fischman AJ, Babich JW, Bonab AA, Alpert NM, Vincent J, Callahan RJ, Correia JA, Rubin RH (1998) Pharmacokinetics of [18F]trovafloxacin in healthy human subjects studied with positron emission tomography. *Antimicrob Agents Chemother* 42: 2048–2054

23   Gulyas B, Halldin C, Karlsson P, Chou YH, Swahn CG, Bonock P, Paroczai M, Farde L (1999) Brain uptake and plasma metabolism of [11C]vinpocetine: a preliminary PET study in a cynomolgus monkey. *J Neuroimaging* 9: 217–222

24   Gulyas B, Halldin C, Sandell J, Karlsson P, Sovago J, Karpati E, Kiss B, Vas A, Cselenyi Z, Farde L (2002) PET studies on the brain uptake and regional distribution of [11C]vinpocetine in human subjects. *Acta Neurol Scand* 106: 325–332

25   Islinger F, Bouw R, Stahl M, Lackner E, Zeleny P, Brunner M, Muller M, Eichler HG, Joukhadar C (2004) Concentrations of gemifloxacin at the target site in healthy volunteers after a single oral dose. *Antimicrob Agents Chemother* 48: 4246–4249

26   Lee Z, Berridge MS, Finlay WH, Heald DL (2000) Mapping PET-measured triamcinolone acetonide (TAA) aerosol distribution into deposition by airway generation. *Int J Pharm* 199: 7–16

27   Matarrese M, Salimbeni A, Turolla EA, Turozzi D, Moresco RM, Poma D, Magni F, Todde S, Rossetti C, Sciarrone MT et al (2004) 11C-Radiosynthesis and preliminary human evaluation of the disposition of the ACE inhibitor [11C]zofenoprilat. *Bioorg Med Chem* 12: 603–611

28 Noda A, Takamatsu H, Murakami Y, Yajima K, Tatsumi M, Ichise R, Nishimura S (2003) Measurement of brain concentration of FK960 for development of a novel antidementia drug: a PET study in conscious rhesus monkeys. *J Nucl Med* 44: 105–108

29 Osman S, Rowlinson-Busza G, Luthra SK, Aboagye EO, Brown GD, Brady F, Myers R, Gamage SA, Denny WA, Baguley BC, Price PM (2001) Comparative biodistribution and metabolism of carbon-11-labeled N-[2-(dimethylamino)ethyl]acridine-4-carboxamide and DNA-intercalating analogues. *Cancer Res* 61: 2935–2944

30 Rubin RH, Livni E, Babich J, Alpert NM, Liu YY, Tham E, Prosser B, Cleeland R, Callahan RJ, Correia JA et al (1993) Pharmacokinetics of fleroxacin as studied by positron emission tomography and [18F]fleroxacin. *Am J Med* 94: 31S–37S

31 Saleem A, Harte RJ, Matthews JC, Osman S, Brady F, Luthra SK, Brown GD, Bleehen N, Connors T, Jones T et al (2001) Pharmacokinetic evaluation of N-[2-(dimethylamino) ethyl]acridine-4-carboxamide in patients by positron emission tomography. *J Clin Oncol* 19: 1421–1429

32 Sanderson L, Taylor GW, Aboagye EO, Alao JP, Latigo JR, Coombes RC, Vigushin DM (2004) Plasma pharmacokinetics and metabolism of the histone deacetylase inhibitor trichostatin a after intraperitoneal administration to mice. *Drug Metab Dispos* 32: 1132–1138

33 Bergstrom M, Nordberg A, Lunell E, Antoni G, Langstrom B (1995) Regional deposition of inhaled 11C-nicotine vapor in the human airway as visualized by positron emission tomography. *Clin Pharmacol Ther* 57: 309–317

34 Bergstrom M, Cass LM, Valind S, Westerberg G, Lundberg EL, Gray S, Bye A, Langstrom B (1999) Deposition and disposition of [11C]zanamivir following administration as an intranasal spray. Evaluation with positron emission tomography. *Clin Pharmacokinet* 36, Suppl 1: 33–39

35 Berridge MS, Heald DL, Muswick GJ, Leisure GP, Voelker KW, Miraldi F (1998) Biodistribution and kinetics of nasal carbon-11-triamcinolone acetonide. *J Nucl Med* 39: 1972–1977

36 Berridge MS, Lee Z, Heald DL (2000) Regional distribution and kinetics of inhaled pharmaceuticals. *Curr Pharm Des* 6: 1631–1651

37 Berridge MS, Lee Z, Heald DL (2000) Pulmonary distribution and kinetics of inhaled [11C]triamcinolone acetonide. *J Nucl Med* 41: 1603–1611

38 Dolovich MB (2001) Measuring total and regional lung deposition using inhaled radiotracers. *J Aerosol Med* 14, Suppl 1: S35–S44

39 Lee Z, Berridge MS (2002) PET imaging-based evaluation of aerosol drugs and their delivery devices: nasal and pulmonary studies. *IEEE Trans Med Imaging* 21: 1324–1331

40 Pike VW, Aigbirhio FI, Freemantle CA, Page BC, Rhodes CG, Waters SL, Jones T, Olsson P, Ventresca GP, Tanner RJ et al (1995) Disposition of inhaled 1,1,1,2-tetrafluoroethane (HFA134A) in healthy subjects and in patients with chronic airflow limitation. Measurement by 18F-labeling and whole-body gamma-counting. *Drug Metab Dispos* 23: 832–839

41 Nilsson D, Lennernas H, Fasth KJ, Sundin A, Tedroff J, Aquilonius SM, Hartvig P, Langstrom B (1999) Absorption of L-DOPA from the proximal small intestine studied in the rhesus monkey by positron emission tomography. *Eur J Pharm Sci* 7: 185–189

42 Gulyas B, Halldin C, Sovago J, Sandell J, Cselenyi Z, Vas A, Kiss B, Karpati E, Farde L (2002) Drug distribution in man: a positron emission tomography study after oral administra-

tion of the labeled neuroprotective drug vinpocetine. *Eur J Nucl Med Mol Imaging* 29: 1031–1038

43   Lappin G, Garner RC (2003) Big physics, small doses: the use of AMS and PET in human microdosing of development drugs. *Nat Rev Drug Discov* 2: 233–240

44   Bergstrom M, Grahnen A, Langstrom B (2003) Positron emission tomography microdosing: a new concept with application in tracer and early clinical drug development. *Eur J Clin Pharmacol* 59: 357–366

45   Meikle SR, Matthews JC, Brock CS, Wells P, Harte RJ, Cunningham VJ, Jones T, Price P (1998) Pharmacokinetic assessment of novel anti-cancer drugs using spectral analysis and positron emission tomography: a feasibility study. *Cancer Chemother Pharmacol* 42: 183–193

46   Lammertsma AA, Bench CJ, Hume SP, Osman S, Gunn K, Brooks DJ, Frackowiak RS (1996) Comparison of methods for analysis of clinical [11C]raclopride studies. *J Cereb Blood Flow Metab* 16: 42–52

47   Lammertsma AA, Bench CJ, Price GW, Cremer JE, Luthra SK, Turton D, Wood ND, Frackowiak RS (1991) Measurement of cerebral monoamine oxidase B activity using L-[11C]deprenyl and dynamic positron emission tomography. *J Cereb Blood Flow Metab* 11: 545–556

48   Hume SP, Ashworth S, Opacka-Juffry J, Ahier RG, Lammertsma AA, Pike VW, Cliffe IA, Fletcher A, White AC (1994) Evaluation of [O-methyl-3H]WAY-100635 as an *in vivo* radioligand for 5-HT1A receptors in rat brain. *Eur J Pharmacol* 271: 515–523

49   Seltzer MA, Jahan SA, Sparks R, Stout DB, Satyamurthy N, Dahlbom M, Phelps ME, Barrio JR (2004) Radiation dose estimates in humans for (11)C-acetate whole-body PET. *J Nucl Med* 45: 1233–1236

50   Tang G, Tang X, Wang M, Luo L, Gan M (2004) Radiation dosimetry of O-(3-[18F]fluoropropyl)-L-tyrosine as oncologic PET tracer based on the mice distribution data. *Appl Radiat Isot* 60: 27–32

51   Pauleit D, Floeth F, Herzog H, Hamacher K, Tellmann L, Muller HW, Coenen HH, Langen KJ (2003) Whole-body distribution and dosimetry of O-(2-[18F]fluoroethyl)-L-tyrosine. *Eur J Nucl Med Mol Imaging* 30: 519–524

52   Marthi K, Hansen SB, Jakobsen S, Bender D, Smith SB, Smith DF (2003) Biodistribution and radiation dosimetry of [N-methyl-11C]mirtazapine, an antidepressant affecting adrenoceptors. *Appl Radiat Isot* 59: 175–179

53   Aboagye EO, Luthra SK, Brady F, Poole K, Anderson H, Jones T, Boobis A, Burtles SS, Price P (2002) Cancer Research UK procedures in manufacture and toxicology of radiotracers intended for pre-phase I positron emission tomography studies in cancer patients. *Br J Cancer* 86: 1052–1056

54   Combes RD, Berridge T, Connelly J, Eve MD, Garner RC, Toon S, Wilcox P (2003) Early microdose drug studies in human volunteers can minimise animal testing: Proceedings of a workshop organised by Volunteers in Research and Testing. *Eur J Pharm Sci* 19: 1–11

55   Farde L, Hall H, Pauli S, Halldin C (1995) Variability in D2-dopamine receptor density and affinity: a PET study with [11C]raclopride in man. *Synapse* 20: 200–208

56   Bergstrom M, Fasth KJ, Kilpatrick G, Ward P, Cable KM, Wipperman MD, Sutherland DR, Langstrom B (2000) Brain uptake and receptor binding of two [11C]labeled selective high affinity NK1-antagonists, GR203040 and GR205171--PET studies in rhesus monkey. *Neuropharmacology* 39: 664–670

57   Dobbs FR, Banks W, Fleishaker JC, Valentine AD, Kinsey BM, Franceschini MP, Digenis

GA, Tewson TJ (1995) Studies with [11C]alprazolam: an agonist for the benzodiazepine receptor. *Nucl Med Biol* 22: 459–466

58   Lahteenmaki P, Heikinheimo O, Croxatto H, Spitz I, Shoupe D, Birgerson L, Luukkainen T (1987) Pharmacokinetics and metabolism of RU 486. *J Steroid Biochem* 27: 859–863

59   Elsinga PH, Franssen EJ, Hendrikse NH, Fluks L, Weemaes AM, van der Graaf WT, de Vries EG, Visser GM, Vaalburg W (1996) Carbon-11-labeled daunorubicin and verapamil for probing P-glycoprotein in tumors with PET. *J Nucl Med* 37: 1571–1575

60   Elsinga PH, Hendrikse NH, Bart J, Vaalburg W, van Waarde A (2004) PET Studies on P-glycoprotein function in the blood-brain barrier: how it affects uptake and binding of drugs within the CNS. *Curr Pharm Des* 10: 1493–1503

61   Kurdziel KA, Kiesewetter DO, Carson RE, Eckelman WC, Herscovitch P (2003) Biodistribution, radiation dose estimates, and *in vivo* Pgp modulation studies of 18F-paclitaxel in nonhuman primates. *J Nucl Med* 44: 1330–1339

62   Sundin A, Eriksson B, Bergstrom M, Bjurling P, Lindner KJ, Oberg K, Langstrom B (2000) Demonstration of [11C] 5-hydroxy-L-tryptophan uptake and decarboxylation in carcinoid tumors by specific positioning labeling in positron emission tomography. *Nucl Med Biol* 27: 33–41

63   Bergstrom M, Eriksson B, Oberg K, Sundin A, Ahlstrom H, Lindner KJ, Bjurling P, Langstrom B (1996) *In vivo* demonstration of enzyme activity in endocrine pancreatic tumors: decarboxylation of carbon-11-DOPA to carbon-11-dopamine. *J Nucl Med* 37: 32–37

64   Saleem A, Brown GD, Brady F, Aboagye EO, Osman S, Luthra SK, Ranicar AS, Brock CS, Stevens MF, Newlands E et al (2003) Metabolic activation of temozolomide measured *in vivo* using positron emission tomography. *Cancer Res* 63: 2409–2415

65   Luurtsema G, de Lange EC, Lammertsma AA, Franssen EJ (2004) Transport across the blood-brain barrier: stereoselectivity and PET-tracers. *Mol Imaging Biol* 6: 306–318

66   Rahman O, Kihlberg T, Langstrom B (2004) Synthesis of [11C]/(13C)amines via carbonylation followed by reductive amination. *Org Biomol Chem* 2: 1612–1616

67   Itsenko O, Kihlberg T, Langstrom B (2004) Photoinitiated carbonylation with [(11)C]carbon monoxide using amines and alkyl iodides. *J Org Chem* 69: 4356–4360

68   Karimi F, Langstrom B (2003) Synthesis of 11C-amides using [11C]carbon monoxide and in situ activated amines by palladium-mediated carboxaminations. *Org Biomol Chem* 1: 541–546

69   Kihlberg T, Karimi F, Langstrom B (2002) [(11)C] Carbon monoxide in selenium-mediated synthesis of (11)C-carbamoyl compounds. *J Org Chem* 67: 3687–3692

70   Rahman O, Kihlberg T, Langstrom B (2003) Aryl triflates and [11C]/(13C)carbon monoxide in the synthesis of 11C-/13C-amides. *J Org Chem* 68: 3558–3562

71   Farde L, Ginovart N, Ito H, Lundkvist C, Pike VW, McCarron JA, Halldin C (1997) PET-characterization of [carbonyl-11C]WAY-100635 binding to 5-HT1A receptors in the primate brain. *Psychopharmacology (Berl)* 133: 196–202

72   Olsson H, Halldin C, Farde L (2004) Differentiation of extrastriatal dopamine D2 receptor density and affinity in the human brain using PET. *Neuroimage* 22: 794–803

Progress in Drug Research, Vol. 62
(Markus Rudin, Ed.)
©2005 Birkhäuser Verlag, Basel (Switzerland)

Imaging biomarkers predictive of disease/therapy outcome: ischemic stroke and drug development

By Janet C. Miller and
A. Gregory Sorensen

MGH-HST Center for Biomarkers in
Imaging
Department of Radiology
Massachusetts General Hospital
Boston, MA, USA
<sorensen@nmr.mgh.harvard.edu>

Glossary of abbreviations

ADC, apparent diffusion constant; AIF, arterial input function; CTp, CT perfusion; DWI, MRI diffusion weighted imaging; FH, flow heterogeneity; GAM, generalized additive model; GLM, generalized linear model; MMPs, matrix metalloproteases; MRA, magnetic resonance angiography; mRS, modified Rankin Score; MTT, mean transit time of contrast agent; NIHSS, National Institutes of Health Stroke Scale; PDF, probability density function; PET, positron emission tomography; PWI, perfusion weighted imaging; rADC, apparent diffusion constant relative to contralateral brain; rCBF, estimate of relative blood flow derived from rMTT and rCBV; rCBV, estimate of blood flow derived from area under the curve of T2 hypodensity due to contrast agent, relative to contralateral brain; rMTT, mean time of arrival of contrast agent relative to contralateral brain; rTTP, time of arrival of contrast bolus peak relative to contralateral brain; TIMPs, tissue inhibitors of matrix metalloproteases; t-PA, tissue plasminogen activator; USPIO, ultra-small superparamagnetic iron oxide.

1   Introduction

Despite many promising studies in animal models, the results of clinical trials for ischemic stroke have been remarkable for their lack of success. Only 2 of 85 potential drugs, tested in clinical trials conducted between the 1950s and 1999, have been found to be beneficial; tissue plasminogen activator (t-PA), given within the first 3–6 h after the onset of symptoms, and aspirin, which has a very modest beneficial effect [1]. This is a very high proportion of failures compared to clinical trials for other medical conditions.

This high failure rate of clinical trials for stroke therapy can been attributed to several factors, which have been discussed at length elsewhere [2, 3]. First, etiology, site, and extent of injury in ischemic stroke vary widely but the vast majority of clinical trials did not discriminate between underlying pathologies and included patients with stroke lesions that were widely variable in size and location, a mix of patients with thrombolytic and embolic occlusions, and varying severity and type of symptoms. Second, the time after symptom onset when treatment was started varied widely because the rapid evolution of stroke and the need for prompt treatment were not widely appreciated. Consequently, the statistical power of many of the clinical trials was weak because the population under study was too heterogeneous [1]. This is in stark contrast to preclinical trials, in which the ischemic lesions are highly controlled, treatment is typically initiated at a uniform time soon after injury, and the animals studied are young and healthy. In preclinical trials, drugs have been administered either before or within minutes, not hours, after the ischemic insult and the effects have been assessed within a few days, although it is now known that early effects may not be sustained after a period of weeks. In clinical trials, 3 months is now considered to be the optimal time to assess drug effects [2, 3].

At this time, intravenous t-PA is the only therapy approved by the US Food and Drug Administration (FDA) for acute ischemic stroke. This treatment is limited to a 3-h window after initial symptoms because the risk of hemorrhage upon reperfusion increases with time [4]. Unfortunately, only about 15% of stroke patients arrive soon enough for treatment within this time window. Alternatively, catheter directed intra-arterial t-PA can be given within 3–6 hours after stroke onset. However, the risk of treatment-induced hemorrhage means that many do not meet the criteria for treatment, including those whose symptoms are mild and those being treated with anticoagulant therapy. Thus, only about 2% of stroke victims are currently treated with intravenous t-PA within the requisite time window [5].

Since there are about 700 000 cases of stroke each year in the Unites States alone [6], there is clearly a need for the development of safer therapies. Stroke is the cause of death of about 165 000 people annually and is the most frequent cause of severe disability in the United States. Presently, there are 4.8 million stroke survivors of whom 1.16 million are permanently disabled [7]. The direct and indirect costs of this disease in the Unites States in 2004 have been estimated to be $53.6 billion [8].

Approval of a new drug by the FDA normally depends on the demonstration that the drug improves clinical outcome. Unfortunately, measurement of the clinical outcome of stroke is not an exact science. First, the same degree of tissue injury can cause different degrees of disability, depending on the site of injury. Second, the functions that the clinical scales test relate more to the ability to live independently than functional loss. For example, patients with the same National Institutes of Health Stroke Scale (NIHSS) score are likely to have infarction volumes in the left hemisphere that are significantly smaller than those in the right [9] because the NIHSS places a greater emphasis on deficits of the left hemisphere [10]. Third, similar clinical presentations can be due to occlusions at a variety of different sites [11]. Consequently, there is no consensus as to which of the many assessment scales (Rankin, Barthel, NIHSS, Fugl-Meyer, etc.) are most suitable to use in clinical trials of stroke therapy or the number within these scales that corresponds to recovery [2].

Such difficulties have led some investigators to consider imaging end-points as more objective and perhaps of lower variance, and recommenda-tions have been made that imaging data be included in clinical trials of drug efficacy for stroke [11, 12]. Initial imaging data could be used in patient selec-tion to increase population homogeneity, while differences between acute and outcome (3 months) imaging data could be considered as an outcome measure. Although gathering imaging data may add to the per-patient costs of clinical trials, these imaging techniques are being used more commonly for clinical purposes and, with greater population homogeneity, the trials will have more statistical power and require fewer patients.

A considerable body of work has established correlations between imag-ing data and outcome with the goal of establishing imaging as a surrogate marker. If successful, drug development for stroke may benefit from the FDA Modernization Act of 1997, which allows the approval of drugs for "treat-ment of a serious or life-threatening condition … upon a determination that a product has an effect on a clinical endpoint or on a surrogate endpoint that is reasonably likely to predict clinical benefit" [13].

2   Clinical imaging of stroke

Over the past few years, the effectiveness of a variety of imaging techniques in assessing stroke damage has been demonstrated, and the clinical role of CT and MRI in examining patients with symptoms of stroke has expanded well beyond a non-contrast CT scan to rule out hemorrhage or other causes of stroke-like symptoms. A non-contrast CT scan is still typically the first scan to be performed on patients who present with stroke symptoms. How-ever, MRI has a comparable degree of sensitivity and specificity to CT for detection of cerebral hemorrhage within the first 6 h after symptom onset, using sequences that are sensitive to magnetic inhomogeneities caused by the paramagnetic effects of deoxyhemoglobin [14, 15]. MRI is more accu-rate [16, 17] than CT for detecting post-procedural hemorrhage, and is now routinely used to screen patients after treatment with t-PA because extravasated CT contrast agent cannot be distinguished from hemorrhage [16].

CT angiography (CTA) can be used to visualize the site of occlusion by scanning the brain while injected contrast agent is flowing through the arterial system. This scan can be performed in minutes following non-contrast imaging, and high-resolution (pixel size, 0.4 mm in plane resolution or less) CTA images can be rapidly post-processed into 3-D images, which are used to determine whether the symptoms are due to partial or complete occlusion, dissection, trauma damage, arteriovenous malformation, or aneurysm. CTA images can also show calcification and some arterial wall thickening due to atherosclerotic plaque [18, 19].

CT can also be used to obtain information about tissue level, parenchymal brain perfusion after rapid injection of a small additional dose of contrast for dynamic first-pass bolus imaging (CT perfusion, CTp). From the sequential images acquired as contrast passes through the tissue capillary bed, it is possible to calculate quantitative cerebral blood flow (CBF), blood volume (CBV), and the mean transit time (MTT), on a pixel-by-pixel basis (although as with all tracer kinetic techniques, there is some variance between estimated flow and true flow, greater when the assumptions underlying a given technique are not met). However, CTp imaging is limited by the width of the CT detectors. This typically limits perfusion imaging to a 2-cm thick "slab" of brain per contrast bolus. Future generations of CT scanners, available soon, will have at least double that coverage. In addition, CTA source images can provide blood volume weighted imaging of the entire brain, although these images may have artifacts from unenhanced CT components as well [18].

Diffusion-weighted MR imaging (DWI) is a highly sensitive method of detecting changes due to ischemia [20], which are seen as regions of marked hyperdensity (Fig. 1) in the earliest moments after stroke onset. There is no CT equivalent to DWI, and the degree of accuracy is much greater than for stroke detection with non-contrast CT [20–23]. The sensitivity of DWI for detecting abnormalities associated with stroke in the first 6 h after the appearance of symptoms has been reported as 91–100%, with specificities of 95–100% and positive predictive values of 99% [21–24]. Consequently, DWI is recognized as the gold standard for stroke diagnosis [25].

MR angiography (MRA) is an alternate method to image the site of occlusion stroke by scanning the brain while injected contrast agent is flowing through the arterial system, and rapid post-processing techniques are employed to visualize the circle of Willis and major arteries major arteries as 3-D images. However, the spatial resolution of MRA is not as high as CTA [26, 27].

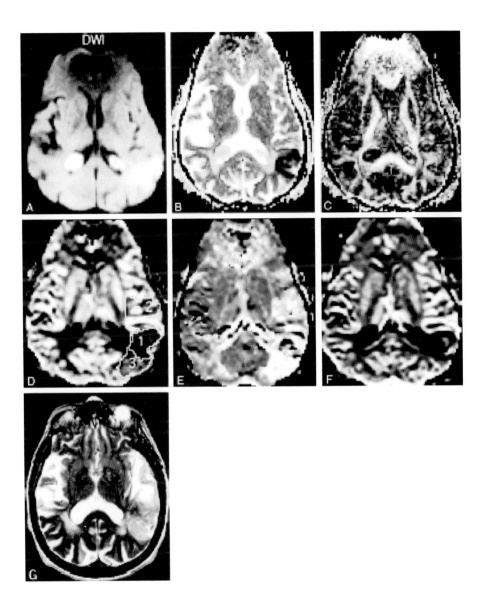

Figure 1.
MRI of 83-year-old woman with aphasia and right-sided weakness, 6 h after stroke onset: A, DWI; B, ADC; C, FA; D, rCBF; E, MTT; F, rCBV. G, follow-up T_2-weighted image, 6 days after stroke onset. In D, region 1 is the "infarct core", the region of hyperintensity in the DW image; region 2 is the "penumbra" that is destined to infarct, the region that is normal in initial DWI but shows perfusion deficit in rCBF and MTT images; region 3 is hypoperfused tissue that remains viable, the region that has perfusion deficit in MTT and rCBF images but is normal on initial DWI and on T_2-weighted follow-up. From [31], with permission.

Table 1.
Non-invasive imaging techniques commonly used for ischemic stroke

	Comments
Non-contrast CT	Low sensitivity for acute stroke
	Will show chronic stroke lesion, intracranial hemorrhage, tumors and other non-stroke lesions
	Easy to obtain
Angiographic CTA and MRA	CTA has higher spatial resolution than MRA
	MRA good for detecting occlusions in the Circle of Willis
MR DWI	Appear as hyperintensity
	Very sensitive for diagnosis of ischemic stroke
	Very high predictive value for infarction
	Observed early after symptom onset, evolves over time through poorly understood physiological changes
	Quantitative apparent diffusion constants (ADC) derived from DWI
CTp imaging	Quantitative dynamic contrast imaging technique for measuring CBF, CBV, MTT, FH
	CT scanning limited to 2 cm "slab" of tissue
	CT contrast agents relatively toxic compared to MRI contrast
MR PWI	Semi-quantitative dynamic contrast imaging technique for measuring rCBF, rCBV, rMTT, FH
	rCBF and rMTT abnormalities with no DWI abnormality is at risk for infarction (ischemic penumbra)
	rCBF and rMTT accuracy dependent on selection of arterial input function (AIF)
	Range of values for rCBF and MTT that progress to infarction have some overlap with range of values that recover
	rCBV not good predictor because of compensatory dilation of blood vessels with poor blood flow
	FH sensitive to the range in size of non-occluded blood vessels and is lower when blood flow is restricted
MR T_2-weighted imaging	No abnormalities observed within the first 6 h after stroke onset
	T_2 abnormality seen after 6 days of stroke onset corresponds to final infarction volume

Unlike CT, MR perfusion-weighted imaging (PWI) can scan nearly the entire brain. PWI can be used to measure several variables (Tab. 1), including relative blood volume (rCBV), blood flow (rCBF), and mean transit time (rMTT) [28]. Thus, PWI can be used to determine the location and volume of the perfusion deficit, the presence of collateral flow, and measure regional variations in the degree of perfusion deficit throughout the stroke lesion. Often, there is a PWI/DWI mismatch [29], in which the PWI lesion is larger than that observed by DWI. Since there is evidence that regions with a PWI deficit but no DWI deficit have the potential to recover (Fig. 1) [30–33], imaging data can provide predictive information that is not possible by clinical examination. The predictive value of DWI/PWI mismatch for progression to infarction without treatment has led to its application in the clinical setting as a factor in decision making about the suitability of thrombolytic therapy [27, 34–36], along with other factors that affect clinical severity and outcome, such as age [37–39] and the location of the ischemic lesion.

Finally, T_2-weighted MRI and CT are used to detect changes that appear at least 6 h after stroke onset that are indicative of permanent infarction (Fig. 1) [20].

As mentioned above, information from imaging, in conjunction with that from clinical examination, is already playing a role in clinical decision making. Consequently, it is not surprising that many authors have recognized the potential of imaging data as a biomarker in clinical trials for stroke therapy [12, 40–43]. With this in mind, several authors have found correlations between lesion volumes measured by MRI and clinical outcome [44–48].

3 Correlations between imaging data and clinical outcome

3.1 Lesion volume

Several studies have demonstrated correlations between the NIHSS and the volume of the initial DWI lesion ($r = 0.67$–0.97, $p \leq 0.0001$–0.01) as well as the NIHSS and the chronic infarction volume measured by T_2-weighted imaging and clinical outcome ($r = 0.77$–0.86, $p \leq 0.0001$–0.05) [44–48].

The initial DWI lesion volume has been equated with the ischemic core because this tissue almost invariably proceeds to infarction [32, 49]. This observation has been confirmed by a retrospective analysis of a randomly selected group of patients. In all cases included in the study, the DWI lesions due to stroke tissue proceeded to infarction, although there was one additional anecdotal case known to the authors in which there was apparent recovery. From this study, Grant et al. [50] estimated that the frequency of full recovery in the absence of chemical thrombolysis was less than 0.4%.

There are other reports of apparent recovery of all or part of the initial DWI lesion with no abnormality visible in follow-up T_2 images. Most of these cases have been associated with recanalization within the first day after stroke onset, usually in response to early thrombolytic therapy [44, 51, 52]. For example, in a recent study of apparent recovery of initial DWI lesions after successful chemical thrombolysis, 11 out of 31 patients who were first imaged within 3 h showed some apparent recovery of tissue, compared to only 3 out of 37 patients, who were first imaged between 3 and 6 h after symptom onset [53]. Therefore, even if apparent full recovery is very rare, the entire region with low DWI values cannot be equated unequivocally with the ischemic core [33, 51–53].

The volume of the final infarct seen in later T_2 images is usually, but not necessarily, significantly greater than the initial DWI lesion [24, 54]. Several studies have demonstrated that the volume of deficit, measured from PWI, in rCBF, rCBV, rMTT, and flow heterogeneity (FH) have good sensitivity and specificity for predicting final infarction volume [24, 55–57]. However, rMTT deficit volume tends to overestimate, whereas rCBV volumes tend to underestimate the final infarct volume [56, 58, 59]. Tissue volumes that have abnormal FH also overestimate final infarction volume but to a lesser extent than MTT [60]. Although these studies show the potential of including imaging in clinical trials, simple volume measurement is of limited use as a surrogate marker because it requires between population studies that require large numbers to achieve clinical significance.

Even though there is a great deal of individual variability in the amount of expansion of the initial DWI lesion, measurement of lesion growth allows within-patient measurements that increase the statistical power of clinical trials. The value of within-patient controls as a measure of stroke outcome was first supported in a study of a neuroprotective agent, citicoline as a treatment for acute stroke therapy. The primary MRI outcome measure in this study was lesion growth from the initial volume of DWI lesions to the volume of infarcted tissue, measured in T_2 images acquired 12 weeks after stroke onset. This study demonstrated that the mean volume increase in the placebo group was fivefold greater than that in the citicoline-treated group, but the variation in the placebo group was very large and the group differences were not statistically significant. However, it should be noted that this trial only included 81 patients and, therefore, the statistical power was low. Nevertheless, there were statistically significant differences between the group treated with citicoline compared to the placebo-treated group in a secondary outcome measure, the decrease in lesion volume from the week 1 DWI lesion volume and the final outcome volume (Tab. 2). This study also demonstrated

Table 2.
MRI data from a clinical trial of citicoline

Variable	Placebo ($n = 40$)	Citicoline ($n = 41$)
Lesion volume (mL)		
Baseline DWI	31.0 ± 5.7	25.7 ± 3.4
Week 1 DWI (larger of b_0 and b_{1000})	57.6 ± 9.3	54.1 ± 8.1
Week 12 T_2-weighted	50.8 ± 9.6	37.0 ± 6.5
Change in lesion volume		
Baseline to week 12 (mL)	18.9 ± 7.0	11.3 ± 4.4
Baseline to week 12 (%)	180.0 ± 107	34.0 ± 18.5
Week 1 to week 12 (mL)	-6.9 ± 2.8	-17.2 ± 2.6*

*$p < 0.01$. Although the differences in lesion volume appear to favor the citicoline-treated group, the variance in lesion size in the placebo group was also large, precluding a statistically significant effect ($p = 0.18$). Adapted from Warach et al. [45].

statistically significant correlations between initial lesion volume and initial NIHSS score, and between the final lesion volume and final NIHSS score, Rankin score, and Barthel index [45].

A similar study on the effect of t-PA therapy on lesion growth and penumbral salvage demonstrated significantly smaller final infarct sizes (T_2-weighted volume at 90 days), recovery of a larger percentage of the MTT volume compared to historical controls, and improved clinical outcome, as measured by a ≥ 7 point improvement the NIHSS score 90 days after stroke onset [30]. In more recent studies in which MRI has been used to study outcomes after t-PA treatment, ethical reasons have prevented the inclusion of placebo- or conservatively treated controls [61, 62]. Although these studies cannot measure the treatment effect per se, imaging can assess the expected effect of treatment, such as thrombolysis leading to recanalization, which MRA studies have shown to occur in patients treated with t-PA when compared with those treated conservatively ($p < 0.001$) [63].

For example, the effect of increased perfusion early after stroke onset, measured by the change in volume of MTT lesions within 1.5–4.5 h after the administration of t-PA, has been shown to correlate with improved clinical outcome [62]. These studies have confirmed that improved clinical outcome is highly correlated with recanalization (Tab. 3) [61, 64]. Nonetheless, residual perfusion deficits, measured by PWI, have been observed in some patients even when MRA images show complete recanalization. Therefore, recanalization of large artery occlusions cannot be equated with complete reperfu-

Table 3.
Comparison of treatment effect versus recanalization on clinical outcome[a]

Treatment effect	TIMI 1–3 n (%)	TIMI 2 + 3 n (%)	Dichotomized mRS = 2 at 90 days	Dichotomized mRS = 1 at 90 days	NIHSS n = 26 mean ± SD	NIHSS n =19 median (range)
No t-PA treatment	17 (33%)	11 (21%)	25 (40%)	17 (27%)		5 (0 – 20)
t-PA treatment	47 (66%)	23 (32%)	46 (61%)	35 (46%)		15 (1 – 40)
p*	< 0.001(63)	0.22(63)	0.017(63)	0.023(63)		<.001(64)
Recanalization effect						
TIMI 2 + 3			67.6%		5.8 ± 6.4	5 (0 – 20)
TIMI 0–1			42.7%		14 ± 2	15 (1 – 40)
p†			0.0016(63)		0.0002(61)	<.001(64)
TIMI 1–3				64%		
TIMI 0				40%	—	
p*				0.001(63)		

*Univariate analysis; †Mann-Whitney U test;
[a]mRS, modified Rankin Scale; TIMI, modified thrombolysis in myocardial infarction criteria (TIMI 0, no recanalization/reperfusion; TIMI 1, minimal recanalization/reperfusion; TIMI 2, incomplete recanalization/reperfusion; TIMI 3, complete recanalization/reperfusion). From [61, 63, 64].

sion as observed with MRA [62]. This apparent contradiction can be explained by the spatial resolution of MRA, which is not sufficient to observe occlusions in small blood vessels.

In addition to recanalization, raising the oxygen partial pressure in brain tissue can improve outcome. For example, raising blood pressure with phenylephrine or saline to a to mean arterial pressure of 130 mg Hg has been shown to decrease the volume of time-to-peak (TTP) lesions and to have some clinical benefit in stroke patients [41]. Secondly, the simple measure of administering normobaric oxygen soon after stroke onset has been shown in a pilot study to have beneficial effects over the first few days, although they did not appear to be sustained over a longer period [65].

Unfortunately, the limitations of using volumetric measurements as a bio-marker could lead to lost opportunities or even misinterpretation. First of all, simple volume measurements do not take advantage of the richness of the data imaging provides on the variations in the degree of deficit within a lesion's boundaries or on the anatomical site of the lesion, which has a major effect on the degree of disability. Secondly, measuring volumes requires judgment, either human or computer-based, to determine the margins of the lesion. This can be particularly problematic for DWI lesions, which can be patchy and ill defined early after the onset of stroke.

3.2   Quantitative imaging biomarkers

One approach to overcome the limitations of a volume-based approach is voxel-by-voxel analysis of quantitative parameters (Tab. 1), which can give a more detailed assessment of the ischemic lesion. Diffusion abnormalities can be quantified from DWI by calculating the apparent diffusion constant (ADC) [66], and there are several quantitative parameters that relate to perfusion [67]. Any quantitative analytical approach needs to assure that the data measurements are accurate and reproducible. In this respect, positron emission tomography (PET) has been held up as the gold standard because tracer kinetics can be applied to the data and attenuation artifacts largely avoided. Attenuation due to CT contrast agents can easily be calibrated, although there may be some image artifacts. However, for MRI, it is important to recognize that variations in protocols and instrument performance make considerable differences in the strength of signals, which makes it harder to compare data obtained on different instruments, especially when programmed to use different imaging protocols.

Variations in the rate of injection of contrast agent will also affect reproducibility. Although power injectors are not normally used for MRI contrast studies, their use to provide a consistent rate of bolus is likely to be beneficial for clinical trials. It is also important to use a consistent method for selecting the arterial input function (AIF), and to correct for the contributions from large blood vessels (partial volume effect); improving the reliability of brain perfusion maps is an area of active research [68, 69].

ADC maps have been shown to have good inter- and intra-observer reproducibility and reliability [70] and to be better in this regard than estimates of DWI lesion volume [71]. Recent methods that suppress the signal from cerebrospinal fluid (CSF) by applying a fluid attenuated inversion recovery (FLAIR) pre-pulse appears to improve the accuracy of ADC measurement (although at the expense of less signal-to-noise per unit time). Using this technique ADC maps and corresponding histograms have been shown to have a narrower range of distribution of ADC values and a somewhat lower mean value than ADC values without the inversion pulse [72]. In addition, scan-rescan reproducibility studies of the distribution of ADC values, measured in healthy individuals, did not show any significant differences even when the subjects were re-positioned [72].

Quantitative studies of perfusion and diffusion have provided considerable insight into the progression of stroke lesions over the first few hours and days. ADC values decrease rapidly over the first few hours, an event that has been associated with cytotoxic edema and cell swelling [73]. During the time frame of decreasing ADC values decrease, the volume encompassing abnormal ADC values increases and is nearly always larger 1 day after the ischemic event compared to that measured within 3 h [44]. Then, starting at about 18.5 h after initial symptoms, ADC values slowly increase, even if recanalization does not occur [37]. However, this apparent normalization does not signify tissue recovery. Rather, it is associated with cell death and membrane lysis, which allows water to move more freely. Therefore, the observation of DWI lesion "recovery" does not, by itself, indicate clinical recovery [73]. ADC normalization is termed "pseudonormalization" if a T_2 lesion is present indicating infarction.

PWI and MRA studies on the duration of perfusion deficit also account for some of the variables that contribute to the natural history of stroke. As many as 20–30% of arterial occlusions resolve spontaneously, without treatment, within the first 6 h; an event that is more likely to occur in cases with embolic rather than local thrombotic occlusions [74, 75]. This compares to recanalization in approximately two-thirds of patients treated with t-PA [30, 63]. Indeed, one study has shown that the correlation between recanalization and clinical outcome had a higher statistical significance than that between t-PA treatment and clinical outcome (Tab. 3) [63].

PWI and CTp data are usually derived from dynamic contrast imaging, in which serial images are acquired as a bolus of contrast agent (which does not pass through the blood-brain barrier) travels through the vasculature of the brain. Non-contrast MRI approaches (typically referred to as arterial spin labeling or ASL) are also in development [76], although none are as widely used as the gadolinium-based MRI approaches. In dynamic contrast imaging, the passage of the bolus results in an attenuation (CT) or enhancement (MRI) curve that is asymmetric because the flow through the microvasculature is slower than that through the arteries (Fig. 2). An AIF must be determined and deconvolution methods used to correct for the earlier arrival time and proportionally greater blood volume and flow in the arteries than in the perfused tissue. In CTp, the attenuation due to contrast is directly related to its concentration (although there may be some attenuation artifacts due to bony structures). However, this is not completely true for PWI because highly concentrated gadolinium contrast agents diminish the T_2 signal, while low concentrations enhance the T_1 signal. Therefore, the PWI enhancement curve has an initial drop and subsequent rise. Although the area under the MRI enhancement curve is proportional to blood volume, it is not an absolute measurement because of the combined T_1 and T_2 effects at the tail end of the enhancement curve. For this and other reasons, MRI estimates of CBV are generally measured relative to that in the normally perfused contralateral brain (rCBV). Nevertheless, measurements of CBV determined by dynamic contrast imaging correlate well with that determined by ^{15}O-CO PET [28], as do measurements of MTT from PWI and PET in patients with chronic carotid occlusive disease [77, 78]. In addition, the reproducibility of PWI for measuring rCBV has been demonstrated in normal volunteers. In these experiments, the mean ratio of blood volume in five hand-drawn regions of interest was 1.08, with a coefficient of variation of 12% and a between scan correlation of 0.84 ($p < 0.0001$) [79].

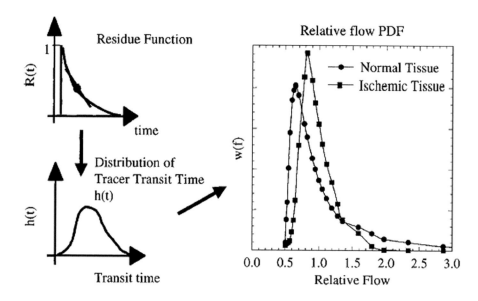

Figure 2.
Calculation of FH. The deconvolution of the tissue concentration–time curve with the AIF yields the R(t) (upper left). The negative slope of the residue function at a given time is the h(t) (lower left). Using the relation CBV + CBF + MTT turns this curve into a distribution of flow (right). In the graph on the right, the x axis displays flow relative to the mean flow and the y axis displays the associated probability – that is, the distribution of relative flow rates, or w(f). The probability density functions of relative flow for normal and ischemic regions in one patient are shown. The functions for the ischemic area indicate a loss of the high-flow component relative to normal tissue. The distribution of flow becomes more narrow, and microscopic flow displays a more uniform velocity pattern, i.e, a more homogeneous distribution of flow. From [60] with permission.

MTT or time-to-peak (TTP) maps can be derived from dynamic contrast MR data corrected with an AIF. Microvascular blood flow relative to the contralateral hemisphere (rCBF) can then be calculated from the relationship: rCBF = rCBV/MTT [80].

In stroke lesions, the arrival time of the contrast agent in the ischemic tissue can be delayed by several seconds, and there is increased dispersion of contrast agent. Therefore, the location of the artery used to measure the AIF influences the estimates of rCBF and MTT, which may appear to be inconsistent with the clinical presentation [81, 82]. For example, if a single AIF is derived from the contralateral hemisphere to an external carotid occlusion, rMTT and rCBF are underestimated because of the delayed arrival from contralateral circulation is not accounted for [83]. On the other hand, an AIF derived from the hemisphere ipsilateral and downstream of a stenosis can produce aberrant under- or overestimations of rCBF and MTT values because contralateral circulation arrives sooner than that predicted by the AIF [84]. Without considering the effect of dispersion, mathematical modeling has demonstrated that if contrast agent arrival into the region of interest is delayed by ≥ 2 s compared to the AIF, rCBF is underestimated by about 35% and, correspondingly, MTT is overestimated by about 60%. Increased dispersion contributes additional under- and overestimation of rCBV and MTT, respectively [85].

Many groups are working to improve the methodology by which CBF is measured with MRI, and in particular to overcome the challenges presented by delay or dispersion of the tracer. Recently, methods have been developed that are insensitive to tracer arrival time using a block circulant matrix [86] or an independent component analysis to determine the local AIF for each voxel [87]. Monte Carlo simulations were used to demonstrate the greater accuracy of the former method for the calculation of rCBF, and to show that these values are insensitive to variability in the selection of AIF. Both methods appear to improve the specificity of PWI for diagnosis, although the data available at this time are limited.

4 Threshold data and predictions of infarction

That there are identifiable thresholds of blood flow that affect outcome was first demonstrated in animal models of stroke. These studies showed that if blood flow drops below a certain threshold, there is insufficient oxygen to produce ATP and maintain homeostasis. As a result, cells rapidly depolarize, lose intracellular potassium, and cell death occurs within minutes. If blood flow is slowed but remains above that threshold, the cells remain metabolically active and can recover if blood flow is restored promptly. However, if blood supply is not restored, the cells die over a period of several days. These studies gave rise to the concept of the "ischemic core" in which cells inevitably die and the "ischemic penumbra", which has the potential to recover [88].

PET has been used to demonstrate that such thresholds exist in human ischemic stroke, using ^{15}O-H_2O imaging using to measure blood flow, $^{15}O_2$ to measure oxygen uptake, and [^{18}F]fluorodeoxyglucose (FDG) to measure metabolic activity. These studies showed that when blood flow drops below a certain rate, the oxygen extraction fraction is very low and there is no metabolic activity. Tissue with these characteristics represents the ischemic core. Where blood flow is below normal but above this threshold, the oxygen extraction fraction is elevated in the acute phase but depressed if the same imaging procedure is repeated more than 3 days after the initiation of symptoms. The conclusion drawn from these studies was that the cells in this region, the ischemic penumbra, were able to compensate to some extent the low rate of cerebral blood flow but, if left underperfused, the cells die and the tissue progresses to infarction [89].

These studies were the first to show that a window of opportunity might exist when restoration of blood flow could salvage tissue that would otherwise progress to infarction [89]. This proved to be correct and there is now evidence that, if blood flow is promptly restored, a substantial portion of the ischemic penumbra will recover [90], and that there is some salvageable tissue for at least 6 h after stroke onset [90, 91].

More recent PET studies have estimated the thresholds of blood flow that, within 95% confidence limits, are predictive of infarction and recovery (4.8 and 14.1 mL/100 g/min, respectively) [92]. However, MRI is a more widely available and practical method for evaluating patients with acute stroke symptoms. Several attempts have been made to define thresholds that would be predictive of infarction and recovery from quantitative imaging measurements of rADC, rCBF and rMTT.

Some studies have found significant differences in ADC values in tissue that progress to infarction compared to that in tissues that recovered [49, 93, 94] For example, Heiss et al. [94] determined an rADC threshold of 0.83, below which infarction could be predicted (95% confidence limits). Overall, they showed that 71% of the infarct volume corresponded to pixels with below threshold values.

Of the hemodynamic parameters, MTT has been shown to be significantly more prolonged ($p < 0.001$) and rCBF lower ($p < 0.05$) in regions that infarcted compared to salvaged tissue [59]. Another biomarker of the state of the microvascular flow, FH, has also been investigated as a predictor of infarction. In any given voxel, rCBF is heterogeneous because the microvessels it encompasses vary in size and have a corresponding range of flow. The distribution in transit times can be incorporated into an algorithm that assigns appropriate flows and rates in parallel vascular paths to describe the heterogeneity

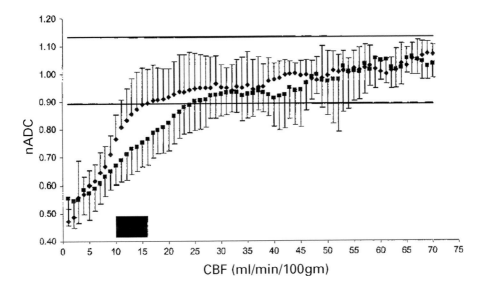

Figure 3.
Relationship between CBF and ADC, normalized to that of the contralateral hemisphere (nADC) in two groups of patients; group A (◆), imaged within 4 h of stroke onset and group B, (■) imaged between 4 and 6.5 h after stroke onset. The vertical lines represent 95% confidence limits and the horizontal line, the nADC value below which CBF decreased sharply. From [97] with permission.

in terms of a probability density function (PDF) [95]. In normal tissue, the PDF is very similar from region to region and from patient to patient. However, in ischemic regions, the PDF peak is narrower and less heterogeneous. Deviations from the normal PDF can be quantified and the regions with abnormal FH can be mapped (Fig. 1). Regions with extremely narrow range of flow rates (very low FH) correlate with regions that progress to infarction [96].

In another approach, PET imaging has been used to estimate thresholds of neural viability that predict infarction and recovery. These studies imaged the distribution of [^{11}C]flumenazenil (FMZ), a ligand that binds to benzodiazapine receptor sub-units of γ-amino butyric acid (GABA). Histograms showing the frequency distribution of CBF values and FMZ binding that predict infarction and recovery show a narrower overlap of values for FMZ binding than for CBF and a steeper positive prediction curve (Figs 2–4) [92], indicating that FMZ binding appears to be well suited to identifying tissue that is likely to progress to infarction. Thus, the 95% limit predictive of cortical

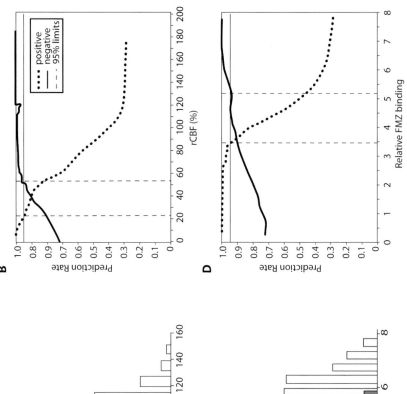

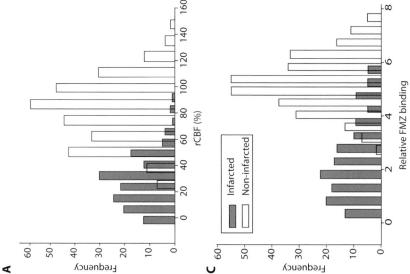

infarction for FMZ binding of ≤ 3.2, relative to normal white matter, corresponded to 84% of the tissue volume that ultimately infarcted.

However, all these methods are limited in value because, no matter how exact, they provide only a snapshot of tissue status at a single point of stroke evolution. For example, Butcher et al. [59] found that there was an inverse correlation ($r = 0.93$, $p < 0.001$) between time of initial MRI scan and MTT delay in salvaged tissue [59]. Furthermore, ADC values have a time-dependent relationship with CBF. For example, the rCBF threshold for significant ADC abnormalities was below 15 mL/100 mL/min in patients within the first 4 h after stroke onset compared to 21.5 mL/100 mL/min when imaged 4 and 6.5 h after stroke onset (Fig. 3) [97]. Therefore, we can conclude that, while these studies provide some insight into stroke evolution, threshold values alone are not sufficiently accurate for use as a surrogate biomarker for drug discovery.

5   The search for more sophisticated biomarkers

None of the correlations described above made full use of the continuum of perfusion and diffusion deficit data. However, it is likely that quantitative measurements that reflect this continuum will be statistically much more powerful than those that rely on volume measurements or cut-off points. In addition, the combination of different MRI parameters may be more powerful than a single parameter. This idea was first proposed by Welch et al. [98] who combined T_2 and DWI to suggest "tissue signatures" that might correlate with various stages of tissue damage. Extending these approaches to include perfusion data was a logical extension of the earliest animal MRI

Figure 4.
rCBF and relative FMZ binding in stroke patients, measured by PET imaging between 1.5 and 11.5 h (mean 6 h) after stroke onset. (A, C) Frequency distribution of CBF (A) and FMZ binding (C) compared to average values in the contralateral hemisphere. Shaded boxes show values that progressed to infarction, as observed in follow-up T_2-weighted MRI, and open columns indicates values in tissue that was not infarcted on follow-up. (B, D) Weighted mean curves across all patients' volume of interest and corresponding 95% probability limits for predicting infarction (positive prediction curve) or non-infarction (negative prediction curve). Relative FMZ binding has less overlap in frequencies in the infarcted and non-infarcted tissue and a steeper positive predictive curve than rCBF.
However, FMZ binds to cortical tissue only and is not able to predict white matter infarction. Redrawn from [92].

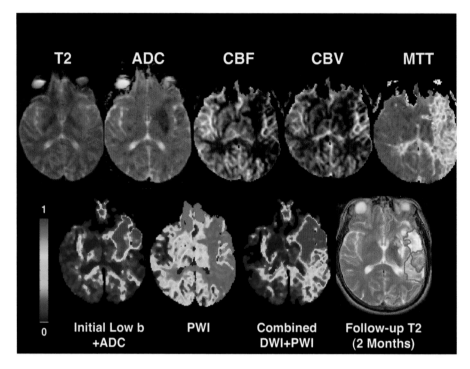

Figure 5.
Images from a patient with acute cerebral ischemia. Top row: Various input images. Bottom row: Risk maps based on T_2 and ADC, PWI, or a combination of DWI and PWI showing a range of risks. Bottom right is the follow-up image with infarct outlined in red. (The green outline shows training regions to teach the model what tissue that did not infarct looked like; further methodology described in [101])

approaches (indeed, the initial DWI work also included PWI). The first example of a correlation study of final infarct size with combined DWI and PWI showed that this method correlated better than that from correlations with one parameter (Fig. 5) [96].

Therefore, more sophisticated means of combining these data have been proposed, with the goal of quantitatively predicting tissue destiny. This approach is, perhaps at first, not necessarily intuitive: if the goal is to predict tissue is salvageable, why focus on predictive models in the absence of therapy? The approach stems from the recognition that the definition of 'salvageable tissue' requires a therapy to perform the salvage, and as there are a potentially infinite number of therapies that might be tried in stroke, the definition of salvageable must always remain tentative and incomplete. In parallel with this, the observation that the DWI/PWI mismatch has variable outcome suggests that some spontaneous tissue recovery can occur. These two facts lead to the concept, then, that a method that quantifies the natural history of tissue destiny can generate error bars around that which is expected to happen in the absence of therapy – and then a given intervention can be compared to see if any tissue was salvaged. By combining DWI, PWI, T_2, and any other predictive variable into a single probability at each voxel, interventions can be tested for efficacy against tissue that typically does not spontaneously recover, tissue that is highly likely to recover, and tissue with highly variable outcome. Such additional variables may be from clinical data, advanced MRI measures of the diffusion tensor [99], perfusion measures such as estimations of variance due to spontaneous low frequency oscillations (< 1 Hz) (which may be due to coordinated capillary vasomotion, and which is absent in ischemic tissue) [100], or CTp data.

5.1 Generalized linear models

Initial attempts to combine multiple datasets used a common and straightforward statistical technique, called generalized linear models (GLMs), to convert DWI and PWI data into voxel-by-voxel maps of the risk of infarction, termed "risk maps" [101]. These GLM approaches have been shown to have high specificity and sensitivity for predicting the threshold values for infarction (Fig. 6) [84, 86, 101].

Therefore, GLMs can be used to test new therapeutic interventions by comparing what the model predicts would happen to each voxel in the absence of therapy with what actually happened, thus using the initial imaging data to allow each patient to act as his or her own control (a so-called change-from-baseline approach). Statistical analysis of change in the positive predictive value of infarction in each voxel indicated by the GLM will demonstrate any treatment effects that change the natural history of the tissue. If the GLM predicts tissue outcome "incorrectly" and more tissue is salvaged than expected, given the combination of diffusion, perfusion, and other imaging changes in that voxel at that time, the positive predictive value will be lowered. These approaches appear quite promising because they suggest much lower variance and, therefore, lower sample sizes for clinical trials than other MRI endpoints such as volumetric approaches.

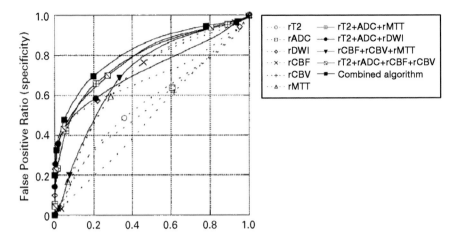

Figure 6.
Performance of (A) thresholding and (B) GLM methods, pooling results across 14 patients. For both methods, the perfusion-based maps (rCBF + rCBV + rMTT) appear more sensitive than the diffusion-based maps (rT$_2$ + rADC + rDWI) at values of high false-positive ratio (FPR). The multivariate algorithms tend to have a higher ROC curve than the univariate algorithms. When perfusion and diffusion data are combined either singly (rT$_2$ + rADC + rMTT) or multiply (rT$_2$ + rADC + rCBF + rCBV, or combined algorithm), an overall increase in sensitivity in areas of high specificity (FPR < 0.2) is seen. Reprinted with permission from [101].

Table 4 provides estimates of sample sizes based on various approaches to testing for a new stroke treatment that might have a 20% effect size in patients, based on our own recent analysis of DWI, PWI, and GLM approaches in a group of 71 patients [102, 103]. Of particular note is that volumetric approaches have substantial variance; this suggests that their value lies more in understanding the biological effects of a new treatment and allowing correlations with animal models than in reducing sample size per se. The voxel-based approach, even with the current initial approach, suggests that much smaller sample sizes can be used.

A number of efforts to advance these approaches have also been suggested [102, 104]; a clear limitation is the assumption of a linear relationship between changes in tissue parameters such as CBV or ADC and risk of infarction. This is likely not the case; CBV may actually increase initially in tissue at risk [105], suggesting that more mathematically sophisticated approaches would be useful. These include generalized additive models (GAMs) [106] and

Table 4.
Potential impact of MRI metrics on size of clinical trials

Sample sizes for various endpoints	Mean $(n = 74)$	SD $(n = 74)$	ES	Total sample size
Inter-patient metrics				
Clinical outcome scores	Typical clinical trials require < 600–5000 patients [129]			
Initial DWI volume (mm^3)	34.3	39.4	0.17	1026
Final infarct volume (mm^3)	54.7	52.7	0.21	734
Intra-patient metrics				
Final T$_2$ – initial DWI (mm^3)	20.5	29.9	0.14	1756
GLM (PPV)	49.6%	29.8%	0.33	281

Note: the NINDs and ECASS trials each had 600–650 patients.
ES, effect size if new therapy shrinks lesion by 20%; GLM, PPV, see text.
Sample size is for a = 0.05, b = 0.8.

other approaches [102]. We have yet to see how MRI derived linear models that take into account variations in the degree of perfusion and diffusion abnormalities, lesion location, and other factors that affect stroke outcome will fare in clinical drug trials for stroke therapy.

6 Future directions for imaging-based approaches

While these linear models show promise, the variance in the link between imaging prediction and actual outcome is not yet ideal, and other fruitful areas of research could be explored. One source of variance that could be incorporated into a predictive model is the location of the infarction. Small lesions in eloquent cortex can have a much larger impact on clinical outcome than large lesions elsewhere in the brain. This leads to low correlations between lesion size and clinical outcome. Indeed, a number of studies of lesion size and clinical outcomes with rigorous guidelines for comparisons show correlations only in the $r^2 = 0.2$–0.4 range. Efforts to link lesion location with size may reduce this variance [102].

Beyond the technical aspects of imaging techniques alone, it is increasingly clear that including clinical parameters, such as age [37] and time from symptom onset [97], will improve predictive value. Other factors, unrelated to the ischemic event have also been shown to contribute to outcome. For example, hyperglycemia is associated with a significantly worse clinical outcome [107, 108]. Genetic factors, such as the -765G → C polymorphism of the cyclooxygenase-2 gene, play a role in both predisposition to stroke and stoke outcome. Individuals who carry this gene variant have been shown to have a significantly lower incidence of stroke and to have lower levels of MMP-9 activity in atherosclerotic plaque. On the other hand, those who carry the apolipoprotein E4 gene are likely to experience a worse stroke outcome, as measured by both expansion of the lesion and poorer clinical outcomes [109, 110]. Therefore, the inclusion of genotypic and phenotypic information will likely become be increasingly important as factors in predictive models.

7   Imaging and targeted drug development

In addition to gathering data on perfusion and diffusion changes due to stroke, several imaging applications have been devised for investigations into stroke physiology and for assessments of the predicted response to targeted drugs. These applications use specialized imaging agents that are designed to visualize a particular physiological characteristic (such as blood vessel permeability) or molecular imaging agents, which are designed to visualize and quantify the distribution and/or activity of a biomolecular target. One example of such an agent, [^{18}F]FMZ, has been mentioned above. In addition, the pharmacokinetics and pharmacodynamics of novel drugs, labeled with a suitable radioisotope, can be investigated with PET or single-photon emission computed tomography (SPECT) [111]. Several such techniques have been developed that are applicable to drug development for stroke therapy.

Drugs development strategies for stroke therapy fall into two main camps, those that restore blood flow and neuroprotective agents that prevent cell death. The latter strategy is based on studies that have shown that cells in the ischemic penumbra are initially metabolically active but are compromised by ionic imbalance, excitotoxicity, and oxidative and nitrosative stress. These perturbations in neurovascular function initiate several cascades of events that result in subcellular injury. Examples of such injurious reactions include increased production of degradative enzymes, such as matrix metalloproteases (MMPs) and t-PA, and the recruitment of leukocytes and platelets, which is initiated by the expression of intercellular adhesion molecules by vascular endothelial cells [112–114].

The degradative activity of MMPs has several adverse effects. First, breakdown of the intracellular matrix is detrimental to cell viability; the cells respond, over hours to days by dying through apoptotic-like cell death mechanisms, expanding the region of infarction. Neurons and oligodendrocytes are especially sensitive to this process [90]. Secondly, MMP-mediated degradation of endovascular intracellular matrix weakens blood vessels. Consequently, high blood levels of MMPs correlate with the increased likelihood of hemorrhagic transformation [115]. Third, MMP activity has been implicated in the rupture of atherosclerotic plaque and, therefore, to initiating stroke and other embolic diseases [116].

Human stroke studies have shown that blood levels of MMP-9 increase during the course of ischemia [114], and that acute MMP-9 levels have a positive correlation with NIHSS outcome [117] and DWI lesion size [113, 115, 117, 118]. Furthermore, there appears to be a link between the concentration of t-PA and up-regulation of the MMP-9, suggesting that t-PA itself up-regulates MMP production [112–114]. This would explain why patients treated with t-PA have higher blood levels of MMP-9 compared to those treated with hypothermia [114]. These lines of evidence have raised hopes that a drug that interferes with MMP activity would be beneficial early in the course of stroke evolution. However, tissue remodeling appears to depend on MMPs to allow the passage of new cells and the development of new blood vessels. Therefore, any successful therapy based on MMP inhibition would have to be aimed at the earliest stages in stroke evolution and be withdrawn to allow for tissue remodeling.

A novel, large diameter MRI contrast agent, monocrystalline iron oxide nanocolloid (MION) has been used to demonstrate the effect of t-PA on hemorrhagic transformation in animal model of stroke. Since MION is normally confined within the vasculature (its intravascular half-life is several hours) but will extravasate from weakened blood vessels, it can be used in steady state susceptibility contrast-enhanced imaging to monitor the degradation of the vascular matrix. This imaging method has been used to demonstrate that t-PA, when given to animals 6 h after onset of ischemia, significantly enhances hemorrhagic transformation in the ischemic area but has no meaningful effect on improving blood flow [119]. Clearly, this imaging method could be useful for monitoring the effect of drugs designed to protect blood vessels from degradation.

Other imaging techniques have been devised to directly visualize *in vivo* activity of MMPs. For example, optical agents have been developed that are minimally fluorescent when they are administered but become highly fluorescent when cleaved by enzyme activity [120–123]. Since these agents fluoresce in the near infrared, which is little absorbed by tissue, they can be detected at depths up to a few centimeters within the body, making it possible to make *in vivo* tomographic images of MMP activity. Optical imaging is an attractive and inexpensive imaging method that is particularly well adapted to preclinical trials in small animals.

Nuclear imaging (PET or SPECT) methods have also been developed to monitor MMP activity, and are better suited to human studies because high energy photons are attenuated by tissue to a much lesser extent than those in the infrared spectrum. Recently, radiolabeled broad spectrum MMP inhibitor has been used to image MMP activity in the arterial walls of apolipoprotein E-deficient mice [124]. In addition, a series of sub-group-specific MMP inhibitors have been developed, which are suitable for molecular imaging of MMP activity with PET or SPECT [125].

Other lines of research into the pathophysiology of stroke have demonstrated that ischemia increases the expression of intercellular adhesion molecules on the vascular endothelium [90]. These adhesion molecules recruit platelets and leukocytes, initiating inflammatory responses and increasing the likelihood of thrombus formation. As a result, re-occlusion following recanalization is a common event in stroke evolution, occurring in an estimated 17% of patients in whom recanalization has been observed [126]. A pivotal event in thrombus formation is the adhesion of fibrinogen to a receptor found on the surface of activated platelets, platelet glycoprotein IIb/IIIa receptor. Antagonists to this receptor have been developed, including abciximab, eptifibatide, and tirofiban, all of which are approved for use in patients with acute coronary syndromes. Trials in animal models have shown that they reduce the infarct volume in ischemic stroke models, and there are some encouraging preliminary results in clinical trials of abciximab and a phase III study is currently underway [127]. Although molecular imaging has not been used to date to monitor the effect of these drugs, a radiolabeled high-affinity glycoprotein IIb/IIIa receptor antagonist has been developed, which has been used in clinical trials of novel diagnostic techniques [128].

These examples of advanced imaging techniques represent a small fraction of the possibilities that could be used for drug development applications. Such applications could be highly valuable for determining whether the drug candidate reaches its target, accumulates in other parts of the body where it could have toxic effects, and has the desired effect on the drug target. Therefore, these imaging techniques could be valuable for the selection of drug candidates that have the highest potential for success and to determine drug dose and schedule.

8 Conclusion

Imaging is currently an important part of the clinical evaluation of stroke patients and for decision making for clinical management. Imaging data are increasingly applied in clinical trials for tasks ranging from identifying appropriate patients for inclusion in the trial to providing endpoints indicative of successful therapy. Innovative imaging data-analytical techniques, especially those for MRI, offer the means to reduce sample size in clinical trials of stroke therapy by providing a change-from-baseline statistical approach. These approaches are particularly valuable in early decision making about the potential efficacy of treatments (go/no-go decision making). Before MRI can be unequivocally established as a surrogate marker in pivotal clinical trials (e.g., as a registration endpoint), it must be demonstrated that the abnormalities seen in images can be shown to directly correspond to the symptoms or the survival of the patient, and that corresponding effects of therapy can be measured reliably both by MRI and clinical examination. Measurement implies quantification of such things as values for the diffusion and perfusion abnormalities as well as lesion volume, while reliability implies that, not only must the abnormalities be consistently present, they must also be numerically similar when assessed by independent readers who may be in different institutions and using different instrumentation. Such multicenter approaches are in various phases for a number of therapies, and soon such tools may become the standard method for stroke trials, which in turn should lead to more efficient evaluations of new therapies for this difficult disease. In addition, future drug trials may benefit from advanced imaging techniques in which molecular processes can be measured and pharmacokinetics and pharmacodynamics can be assessed.

References

1   Kidwell CS, Liebeskind DS, Starkman S, Saver JL (2001) Trends in acute ischemic stroke trials through the 20th century. *Stroke* 32: 1349–1359

2   Gladstone DJ, Black SE, Hakim AM (2002) Toward wisdom from failure: lessons from neuroprotective stroke trials and new therapeutic directions. *Stroke* 33: 2123–2136

3   Hoyte L, Kaur J, Buchan AM (2004) Lost in translation: taking neuroprotection from animal models to clinical trials. *Exp Neurol* 188: 200–204

4   The National Institute of Neurological Disorders and Stroke rt-PA Stroke Study Group (1995) Tissue Plasminogen Activator for Acute Ischemic Stroke. *N Eng J Med* 333: 1581–1587

5   Katzan IL, Hammer MD, Hixson ED, Furlan AJ, Abou-Chebl A, Nadzam DM (2004) Utilization of intravenous tissue plasminogen activator for acute ischemic stroke. *Arch Neurol* 61: 346–350

6   National Center for Health Statistics (2004) *Stroke/cerebrovascular disease.* Center for Disease Control. http://www.cdc.gov/nchs/fastats/stroke.htm (access date June 2005)

7   (2001) Prevalence of Disabilities and Associated Health Conditions Among Adults — United States1999. MMMR 50:120–125

8   National Institutes of Health (2004) *Morbidity & Mortality, Chart book on cardiovascular, lung, and blood diseases.* National Heart, Lung, and Blood Institute, Bethesda, MD. http://www.nhlbi.nih.gov/resources/docs/04a_chtbk.pdf (access date June 2005)

9   Fink JN, Selim MH, Kumar S, Silver B, Linfante I, Caplan LR, Schlaug G (2002) Is the association of National Institutes of Health Stroke Scale scores and acute magnetic resonance imaging stroke volume equal for patients with right- and left-hemisphere ischemic stroke? *Stroke* 33: 954–958

10   Woo D, Broderick JP, Kothari RU, Lu M, Brott T, Lyden PD, Marler JR, Grotta JC, NINDS t-PA Stroke Study Group (1999) Does the National Institutes of Health Stroke Scale favor left hemisphere strokes? *Stroke* 30: 2355–2359

11   Higashida R, Furlan A, Roberts H, Tomsick T, Connors B, Barr J, Dillon W, Warach S, Broderick J, Tilley B, Sacks D; Technology Assessment Committees of the American Society of Interventional and Therapeutic Neuroradiology and the Society of Interventional Radiology (2003) Trial design and reporting standards for intraarterial cerebral thrombolysis for acute ischemic stroke. *J Vasc Interv Radiol* 14: S493–494

12   Warach S (2001) Use of diffusion and perfusion magnetic resonance imaging as a tool in acute stroke clinical trials. *Curr Control Trials Cardiovasc Med* 2: 38–44

13   US Congress (1997) *Food and Drug Administration Modernization Act of 1997.* US Congress, Washington. Public Law 105–115, 105th Congress

14   Fiebach JB, Schellinger PD, Gass A, Kucinski T, Siebler M, Villringer A, Olkers P, Hirsch JG, Heiland S, Wilde P et al, Kompetenznetzwerk Schlaganfall B5 (2004) Stroke magnetic resonance imaging is accurate in hyperacute intracerebral hemorrhage: a multicenter study on the validity of stroke imaging. *Stroke* 35: 502–506

15   Wiesmann M, Mayer TE, Yousry I, Medele R, Hamann GF, Bruckmann H (2002) Detection of hyperacute subarachnoid hemorrhage of the brain by using magnetic resonance imaging. *J Neurosurg* 96: 684–689

16   Greer DM, Koroshetz WJ, Cullen S, Gonzalez RG, Lev MH (2004) Magnetic resonance imaging improves detection of intracerebral hemorrhage over computed tomography after intra-arterial thrombolysis. *Stroke* 35: 491–495

17   Hjort N, Butcher K, Davis SM, Kidwell CS, Koroshetz WJ, Rother J, Schellinger PD, Warach S, Ostergaard L; UCLA Thrombolysis Investigators (2005) Magnetic resonance imaging criteria for thrombolysis in acute cerebral infarct. *Stroke* 36: 388–397

18   Cullen SP, Symons SP, Hunter G, Hamberg L, Koroshetz W, Gonzalez RG, Lev MH (2002) Dynamic contrast-enhanced computed tomography of acute ischemic stroke: CTA and CTP. *Semin Roentgenol* 37: 192–205

19   Ezzeddine MA, Lev MH, McDonald CT, Rordorf G, Oliveira-Filho J, Aksoy FG, Farkas J, Segal AZ, Schwamm LH, Gonzalez RG, Koroshetz WJ (2002) CT angiography with whole brain perfused blood volume imaging: added clinical value in the assessment of acute stroke. *Stroke* 33: 959–966

20   Mullins ME, Schaefer PW, Sorensen AG, Halpern EF, Ay H, He J, Koroshetz WJ, Gonzalez RG (2002) CT and conventional and diffusion-weighted MR imaging in acute stroke: study in 691 patients at presentation to the emergency department. *Radiology* 224: 353–360

21   Lansberg MG, Albers GW, Beaulieu C, Marks MP (2000) Comparison of diffusion-weighted MRI and CT in acute stroke. *Neurology* 54: 1557–1561

22   Gonzalez RG, Schaefer PW, Buonanno FS, Schwamm LH, Budzik RF, Rordorf G, Wang B, Sorensen AG, Koroshetz WJ (1999) Diffusion-weighted MR imaging: diagnostic accuracy in patients imaged within 6 hours of stroke symptom onset. *Radiology* 210: 155–162

23   Fiebach JB, Schellinger PD, Jansen O, Meyer M, Wilde P, Bender J, Schramm P, Juttler E, Oehler J, Hartmann M (2002) CT and diffusion-weighted MR imaging in randomized order: diffusion-weighted imaging results in higher accuracy and lower inter-rater variability in the diagnosis of hyperacute ischemic stroke. *Stroke* 33: 2206–2210

24   Schaefer PW, Hunter GJ, He J, Hamberg LM, Sorensen AG, Schwamm LH, Koroshetz WJ, Gonzalez RG (2002) Predicting cerebral ischemic infarct volume with diffusion and perfusion MR imaging. *AJNR Am J Neuroradiol* 23: 1785–1794

25   Warach S (2003) Stroke neuroimaging. *Stroke* 34: 345–347

26   Schramm P, Schellinger PD, Klotz E, Kallenberg K, Fiebach JB, Kulkens S, Heiland S, Knauth M, Sartor K (2004) Comparison of perfusion computed tomography and computed tomography angiography source images with perfusion-weighted imaging and diffusion-weighted imaging in patients with acute stroke of less than 6 hours' duration. *Stroke* 35: 1652–1658

27   Schellinger PD, Fiebach JB, Hacke W (2003) Imaging-based decision making in thrombolytic therapy for ischemic stroke: present status. *Stroke* 34: 575–583

28   Ostergaard L, Smith DF, Vestergaard-Poulsen P, Hansen SB, Gee AD, Gjedde A, Gyldensted C (1998) Absolute cerebral blood flow and blood volume measured by magnetic resonance imaging bolus tracking: comparison with positron emission tomography values. *J Cereb Blood Flow Metab* 18: 425–432

29   Perkins CJ, Kahya E, Roque CT, Roche PE, Newman GC (2001) Fluid-attenuated inversion recovery and diffusion- and perfusion-weighted MRI abnormalities in 117 consecutive patients with stroke symptoms. *Stroke* 32: 2774–2781

30   Parsons MW, Barber PA, Chalk J, Darby DG, Rose S, Desmond PM, Gerraty RP, Tress BM, Wright PM, Donnan GA, Davis SM (2002) Diffusion- and perfusion-weighted MRI response to thrombolysis in stroke. *Ann Neurol* 51: 28–37

31   Schaefer PW, Ozsunar Y, He J, Hamberg LM, Hunter GJ, Sorensen AG, Koroshetz WJ, Gonzalez RG (2003) Assessing tissue viability with MR diffusion and perfusion imaging. *AJNR Am J Neuroradiol* 24: 436–443

32   Schlaug G, Benfield A, Baird AE, Siewert B, Lovblad KO, Parker RA, Edelman RR, Warach S (1999) The ischemic penumbra: operationally defined by diffusion and perfusion MRI. *Neurology* 53: 1528–1537

33   Kidwell CS, Alger JR, Saver JL (2003) Beyond mismatch: evolving paradigms in imaging the ischemic penumbra with multimodal magnetic resonance imaging. *Stroke* 34: 2729–2735

34   Rordorf G, Koroshetz WJ, Copen WA, Cramer SC, Schaefer PW, Budzik RF Jr, Schwamm LH, Buonanno F, Sorensen AG, Gonzalez G (1998) Regional ischemia and ischemic injury in patients with acute middle cerebral artery stroke as defined by early diffusion-weighted and perfusion-weighted MRI. *Stroke* 29: 939–943

35   Guadagno JV, Calautti C, Baron JC (2003) Progress in imaging stroke: emerging clinical applications. *Br Med Bull* 65: 145–157

36   Latchaw RE, Yonas H, Hunter GJ, Yuh WT, Ueda T, Sorensen AG, Sunshine JL, Biller J, Wechsler L, Higashida R, Hademenos G; Council on Cardiovascular Radiology of the American Heart Association (2003) Guidelines and recommendations for perfusion imaging in cerebral ischemia: A scientific statement for healthcare professionals by the writing group on perfusion imaging, from the Council on Cardiovascular Radiology of the American Heart Association. *Stroke* 34: 1084–1104

37   Copen WA, Schwamm LH, Gonzalez RG, Wu O, Harmath CB, Schaefer PW, Koroshetz WJ, Sorensen AG (2001) Ischemic stroke: effects of etiology and patient age on the time course of the core apparent diffusion coefficient. *Radiology* 221: 27–34

38   Nakayama H, Jorgensen HS, Raaschou HO, Olsen TS (1994) The influence of age on stroke outcome. The Copenhagen Stroke Study. *Stroke* 25: 808–813

39   Jorgensen HS, Reith J, Nakayama H, Kammersgaard LP, Raaschou HO, Olsen TS (1999) What determines good recovery in patients with the most severe strokes? The Copenhagen Stroke Study. *Stroke* 30: 2008–2012

40   Uno M, Harada M, Yoneda K, Matsubara S, Satoh K, Nagahiro S (2002) Can diffusion- and perfusion-weighted magnetic resonance imaging evaluate the efficacy of acute thrombolysis in patients with internal carotid artery or middle cerebral artery occlusion? *Neurosurgery* 50: 28–34; discussion 34–25

41   Hillis AE, Wityk RJ, Beauchamp NJ, Ulatowski JA, Jacobs MA, Barker PB (2004) Perfusion-weighted MRI as a marker of response to treatment in acute and subacute stroke. *Neuroradiology* 46: 31–39

42   Tatlisumak T, Strbian D, Abo Ramadan U, Li F (2004) The role of diffusion- and perfusion-weighted magnetic resonance imaging in drug development for ischemic stroke: from laboratory to clinics. *Curr Vasc Pharmacol* 2: 343–355

43   Barber PA, Parsons MW, Desmond PM, Bennett DA, Donnan GA, Tress BM, Davis SM (2004) The use of PWI and DWI measures in the design of "proof-of-concept" stroke trials. *J Neuroimaging* 14: 123–132

44   Fiehler J, Foth M, Kucinski T, Knab R, von Bezold M, Weiller C, Zeumer H, Rother J (2002) Severe ADC decreases do not predict irreversible tissue damage in humans. *Stroke* 33: 79–86

45   Warach S, Pettigrew LC, Dashe JF, Pullicino P, Lefkowitz DM, Sabounjian L, Harnett K, Schwiderski U, Gammans R (2000) Effect of citicoline on ischemic lesions as measured by diffusion-weighted magnetic resonance imaging. Citicoline 010 Investigators. *Ann Neurol* 48: 713–722

46   van Everdingen KJ, van der Grond J, Kappelle LJ, Ramos LM, Mali WP (1998) Diffusion-weighted magnetic resonance imaging in acute stroke. *Stroke* 29: 1783–1790

47   Lovblad KO, Baird AE, Schlaug G, Benfield A, Siewert B, Voetsch B, Connor A, Burzynski C, Edelman RR, Warach S (1997) Ischemic lesion volumes in acute stroke by diffusion-weighted magnetic resonance imaging correlate with clinical outcome. *Ann Neurol* 42: 164–170

48   Schwamm LH, Koroshetz WJ, Sorensen AG, Wang B, Copen WA, Budzik R, Rordorf G, Buonanno FS, Schaefer PW, Gonzalez RG (1998) Time course of lesion development in patients with acute stroke: serial diffusion- and hemodynamic-weighted magnetic resonance imaging. *Stroke* 29: 2268–2276

49   Oppenheim C, Grandin C, Samson Y, Smith A, Duprez T, Marsault C, Cosnard G (2001) Is there an apparent diffusion coefficient threshold in predicting tissue viability in hyperacute stroke? *Stroke* 32: 2486–2491

50   Grant PE, He J, Halpern EF, Wu O, Schaefer PW, Schwamm LH, Budzik RF, Sorensen AG, Koroshetz WJ, Gonzalez RG (2001) Frequency and clinical context of decreased apparent diffusion coefficient reversal in the human brain. *Radiology* 221: 43–50

51   Kidwell CS, Saver JL, Mattiello J, Starkman S, Vinuela F, Duckwiler G, Gobin YP, Jahan R, Vespa P, Kalafut M, Alger JR (2000) Thrombolytic reversal of acute human cerebral ischemic injury shown by diffusion/perfusion magnetic resonance imaging. *Ann Neurol* 47: 462–469

52   Schaefer PW, Hassankhani A, Putman C, Sorensen AG, Schwamm L, Koroshetz W, Gonzalez RG (2004) Characterization and evolution of diffusion MR imaging abnormalities in stroke patients undergoing intra-arterial thrombolysis. *AJNR Am J Neuroradiol* 25: 951–957

53   Fiehler J, Knudsen K, Kucinski T, Kidwell CS, Alger JR, Thomalla G, Eckert B, Wittkugel O, Weiller C, Zeumer H, Rother J (2004) Predictors of apparent diffusion coefficient normalization in stroke patients. *Stroke* 35: 514–519

54   Beaulieu C, de Crespigny A, Tong DC, Moseley ME, Albers GW, Marks MP (1999) Longitudinal magnetic resonance imaging study of perfusion and diffusion in stroke: evolution of lesion volume and correlation with clinical outcome. *Ann Neurol* 46: 568–578

55   Thijs VN, Adami A, Neumann-Haefelin T, Moseley ME, Marks MP, Albers GW (2001) Relationship between severity of MR perfusion deficit and DWI lesion evolution. *Neurology* 57: 1205–1211

56   Parsons MW, Yang Q, Barber PA, Darby DG, Desmond PM, Gerraty RP, Tress BM, Davis SM (2001) Perfusion magnetic resonance imaging maps in hyperacute stroke: relative cerebral blood flow most accurately identifies tissue destined to infarct. *Stroke* 32: 1581–1587

57   Fiehler J, von Bezold M, Kucinski T, Knab R, Eckert B, Wittkugel O, Zeumer H, Rother J (2002) Cerebral blood flow predicts lesion growth in acute stroke patients. *Stroke* 33: 2421–2425

58   Igarashi H, Hamamoto M, Yamaguchi H, Ookubo S, Nagashima J, Nagayama H, Amemiya S, Katayama Y (2003) Cerebral blood flow index: dynamic perfusion MRI delivers a simple and good predictor for the outcome of acute-stage ischemic lesion. *J Comput Assist Tomogr* 27: 874–881

59   Butcher K, Parsons M, Baird T, Barber A, Donnan G, Desmond P, Tress B, Davis S (2003) Perfusion thresholds in acute stroke thrombolysis. *Stroke* 34: 2159–2164

60   Simonsen CZ, Rohl L, Vestergaard-Poulsen P, Gyldensted C, Andersen G, Ostergaard L

(2002) Final infarct size after acute stroke: prediction with flow heterogeneity. *Radiology* 225: 269–275

61   Nighoghossian N, Hermier M, Adeleine P, Derex L, Dugor JF, Philippeau F, Ylmaz H, Honnorat J, Dardel P, Berthezene Y et al (2003) Baseline magnetic resonance imaging parameters and stroke outcome in patients treated by intravenous tissue plasminogen activator. *Stroke* 34: 458–463

62   Chalela JA, Kang DW, Luby M, Ezzeddine M, Latour LL, Todd JW, Dunn B, Warach S (2004) Early magnetic resonance imaging findings in patients receiving tissue plasminogen activator predict outcome: Insights into the pathophysiology of acute stroke in the thrombolysis era. *Ann Neurol* 55: 105–112

63   Rother J, Schellinger PD, Gass A, Siebler M, Villringer A, Fiebach JB, Fiehler J, Jansen O, Kucinski T, Schoder V et al (2002) Effect of intravenous thrombolysis on MRI parameters and functional outcome in acute stroke <6 hours. *Stroke* 33: 2438–2445

64   Straub S, Junghans U, Jovanovic V, Wittsack HJ, Seitz RJ, Siebler M (2004) Systemic thrombolysis with recombinant tissue plasminogen activator and tirofiban in acute middle cerebral artery occlusion. *Stroke* 35: 705–709

65   Singhal AB, Benner T, Roccatagliata L, Koroshetz WJ, Schaefer PW, Lo EH, Buonanno FS, Gonzalez RG, Sorensen AG (2005) A pilot study of normobaric oxygen therapy in acute ischemic stroke. *Stroke* 36: 797–802

66   Warach S, Gaa J, Siewert B, Wielopolski P, Edelman RR (1995) Acute human stroke studied by whole brain echo planar diffusion-weighted magnetic resonance imaging. *Ann Neurol* 37: 231–241

67   Tofts PS, Brix G, Buckley DL, Evelhoch JL, Henderson E, Knopp MV, Larsson HB, Lee TY, Mayr NA, Parker GJ et al (1999) Estimating kinetic parameters from dynamic contrast-enhanced T(1)-weighted MRI of a diffusible tracer: standardized quantities and symbols. *J Magn Reson Imaging* 10: 223–232

68   Jackson A, Jayson GC, Li KL, Zhu XP, Checkley DR, Tessier JJ, Waterton JC (2003) Reproducibility of quantitative dynamic contrast-enhanced MRI in newly presenting glioma. *Br J Radiol* 76: 153–162

69   Wirestam R, Ryding E, Lindgren A, Geijer B, Holtas S, Stahlberg F (2000) Absolute cerebral blood flow measured by dynamic susceptibility contrast MRI: a direct comparison with Xe-133 SPECT. *Magma* 11: 96–103

70   Rana AK, Wardlaw JM, Armitage PA, Bastin ME (2003) Apparent diffusion coefficient (ADC) measurements may be more reliable and reproducible than lesion volume on diffusion-weighted images from patients with acute ischaemic stroke-implications for study design. *Magn Reson Imaging* 21: 617–624

71   Latour LL, Warach S (2002) Cerebral spinal fluid contamination of the measurement of the apparent diffusion coefficient of water in acute stroke. *Magn Reson Med* 48: 478–486

72   Steens SC, Admiraal-Behloul F, Schaap JA, Hoogenraad FG, Wheeler-Kingshott CA, le Cessie S, Tofts PS, van Buchem MA (2004) Reproducibility of brain ADC histograms. *Eur Radiol* 14: 425–430

73   Sorensen AG (2002) Apparently, diffusion coefficient value and stroke treatment remains mysterious. *AJNR Am J Neuroradiol* 23: 177–178

74   Kassem-Moussa H, Graffagnino C (2002) Nonocclusion and spontaneous recanalization rates in acute ischemic stroke: a review of cerebral angiography studies. *Arch Neurol* 59: 1870–1873

75   Wolpert SM, Bruckmann H, Greenlee R, Wechsler L, Pessin MS, del Zoppo GJ; The rt-PA

Acute Stroke Study Group (1993) Neuroradiologic evaluation of patients with acute stroke treated with recombinant tissue plasminogen activator. *AJNR Am J Neuroradiol* 14: 3–13

76   Chalela JA, Alsop DC, Gonzalez-Atavales JB, Maldjian JA, Kasner SE, Detre JA (2000) Magnetic resonance perfusion imaging in acute ischemic stroke using continuous arterial spin labeling. *Stroke* 31: 680–687

77   Mihara F, Kuwabara Y, Tanaka A, Yoshiura T, Sasaki M, Yoshida T, Masuda K, Matsushima T (2003) Reliability of mean transit time obtained using perfusion-weighted MR imaging; comparison with positron emission tomography. *Magn Reson Imaging* 21: 33–39

78   Kaneko K, Kuwabara Y, Mihara F, Yoshiura T, Nakagawa M, Tanaka A, Sasaki M, Koga H, Hayashi K, Honda H (2004) Validation of the CBF, CBV, and MTT values by perfusion MRI in chronic occlusive cerebrovascular disease: a comparison with 15O-PET. *Acad Radiol* 11: 489–497

79   Henry ME, Kaufman MJ, Lange N, Schmidt ME, Purcell S, Cote J, Perron-Henry DM, Stoddard E, Cohen BM, Renshaw PF (2001) Test-retest reliability of DSC MRI CBV mapping in healthy volunteers. *Neuroreport* 12: 1567–1569

80   Sorensen A, Reimer P (2000) *Cerebral MR perfusion imaging: Principles and current applications*. Thieme, New York

81   Lythgoe DJ, Ostergaard L, William SC, Cluckie A, Buxton-Thomas M, Simmons A, Markus HS (2000) Quantitative perfusion imaging in carotid artery stenosis using dynamic susceptibility contrast-enhanced magnetic resonance imaging. *Magn Reson Imaging* 18: 1–11

82   Thijs VN, Somford DM, Bammer R, Robberecht W, Moseley ME, Albers GW (2004) Influence of arterial input function on hypoperfusion volumes measured with perfusion-weighted imaging. *Stroke* 35: 94–98

83   Yamada K, Wu O, Gonzalez RG, Bakker D, Ostergaard L, Copen WA, Weisskoff RM, Rosen BR, Yagi K, Nishimura T, Sorensen AG (2002) Magnetic resonance perfusion-weighted imaging of acute cerebral infarction: effect of the calculation methods and underlying vasculopathy. *Stroke* 33: 87–94

84   Wu O, Ostergaard L, Koroshetz WJ, Schwamm LH, O'Donnell J, Schaefer PW, Rosen BR, Weisskoff RM, Sorensen AG (2003) Effects of tracer arrival time on flow estimates in MR perfusion-weighted imaging. *Magn Reson Med* 50: 856–864

85   Calamante F, Gadian DG, Connelly A (2000) Delay and dispersion effects in dynamic susceptibility contrast MRI: simulations using singular value decomposition. *Magn Reson Med* 44: 466–473

86   Wu O, Ostergaard L, Weisskoff RM, Benner T, Rosen BR, Sorensen AG (2003) Tracer arrival timing-insensitive technique for estimating flow in MR perfusion-weighted imaging using singular value decomposition with a block-circulant deconvolution matrix. *Magn Reson Med* 50: 164–174

87   Calamante F, Morup M, Hansen LK (2004) Defining a local arterial input function for perfusion MRI using independent component analysis. *Magn Reson Med* 52: 789–797

88   Astrup J, Siesjo B, Symon L (1981) Thresholds in cerebral ischemia: the ischemic penumbra. *Stroke* 12: 723–725

89   Leblanc R (1991) Physiologic studies of cerebral ischemia. Clin Neurosurg 37: 289–311

90   Lo EH, Dalkara T, Moskowitz MA (2003) Mechanisms, challenges and opportunities in stroke. *Nat Rev Neurosci* 4: 399–415

91   Furlan A, Higashida R, Wechsler L, Gent M, Rowley H, Kase C, Pessin M, Ahuja A, Calla-

han F, Clark WM et al (1999) Intra-arterial prourokinase for acute ischemic stroke. The PROACT II study: a randomized controlled trial. Prolyse in Acute Cerebral Thromboembolism. *JAMA* 282: 2003–2011

92   Heiss WD, Kracht LW, Thiel A, Grond M, Pawlik G (2001) Penumbral probability thresholds of cortical flumazenil binding and blood flow predicting tissue outcome in patients with cerebral ischaemia. *Brain* 124: 20–29

93   Bykowski JL, Latour LL, Warach S (2004) More accurate identification of reversible ischemic injury in human stroke by cerebrospinal fluid suppressed diffusion-weighted imaging. *Stroke* 35: 1100–1106

94   Heiss WD, Sobesky J, Smekal U, Kracht LW, Lehnhardt FG, Thiel A, Jacobs AH, Lackner K (2004) Probability of cortical infarction predicted by flumazenil binding and diffusion-weighted imaging signal intensity: a comparative positron emission tomography/magnetic resonance imaging study in early ischemic stroke. *Stroke* 35: 1892–1898

95   King RB, Raymond GM, Bassingthwaighte JB (1996) Modeling blood flow heterogeneity. *Ann Biomed Eng* 24: 352–372

96   Ostergaard L, Sorensen AG, Chesler DA, Weisskoff RM, Koroshetz WJ, Wu O, Gyldensted C, Rosen BR (2000) Combined diffusion-weighted and perfusion-weighted flow heterogeneity magnetic resonance imaging in acute stroke. *Stroke* 31: 1097–1103

97   Lin W, Lee JM, Lee YZ, Vo KD, Pilgram T, Hsu CY (2003) Temporal relationship between apparent diffusion coefficient and absolute measurements of cerebral blood flow in acute stroke patients. *Stroke* 34: 64–70

98   Welch KM, Windham J, Knight RA, Nagesh V, Hugg JW, Jacobs M, Peck D, Booker P, Dereski MO, Levine SR (1995) A model to predict the histopathology of human stroke using diffusion and T2-weighted magnetic resonance imaging. *Stroke* 26: 1983–1989

99   Sorensen AG, Wu O, Copen WA, Davis TL, Gonzalez RG, Koroshetz WJ, Reese TG, Rosen BR, Wedeen VJ, Weisskoff RM (1999) Human acute cerebral ischemia: detection of changes in water diffusion anisotropy by using MR imaging. *Radiology* 212: 785–792

100   Hudetz AG, Biswal BB, Shen H, Lauer KK, Kampine JP (1998) Spontaneous fluctuations in cerebral oxygen supply. An introduction. *Adv Exp Med Biol* 454: 551–559

101   Wu O, Koroshetz WJ, Ostergaard L, Buonanno FS, Copen WA, Gonzalez RG, Rordorf G, Rosen BR, Schwamm LH, Weisskoff RM, Sorensen AG (2001) Predicting tissue outcome in acute human cerebral ischemia using combined diffusion- and perfusion-weighted MR imaging. *Stroke* 32: 933–942

102   Menezes N, Ay H, Lopez M et al (2004) An atlas for prediciting stroke clinical outcome. International Society of Molecular Resonance in Medicine. Twelfth Scientific Meeting: 412

103   Menezes NM, Sorensen AG (2005) *Predicting Stroke Clinical Outcome in the Nondominant Hemisphere Using MRI.* The American Heart Association's 30th International Stroke Conference. New Orleans, LA

104   Menezes NM, Lopez M, Benner T et al (2003) *Geography-based assessment of cerebral infarction improves correlation with clinical outcome.* International Society of Molecular Resonance in Medicine. Toronto, Ontario

105   Derdeyn CP, Videen TO, Yundt KD, Fritsch SM, Carpenter DA, Grubb RL, Powers WJ (2002) Variability of cerebral blood volume and oxygen extraction: stages of cerebral haemodynamic impairment revisited. *Brain* 125: 595–607

106   Wu O, Schwamm L, Koroshetz W et al (2001) *Spatial-temporal cluster analysis of serial diffusion-tensor MRI in human cerebral ischemia.* International Society of Molecular Resonance in Medicine Ninth Scientific Meeting: 316

107   Parsons MW, Barber PA, Desmond PM, Baird TA, Darby DG, Byrnes G, Tress BM, Davis
        SM (2002) Acute hyperglycemia adversely affects stroke outcome: a magnetic resonance
        imaging and spectroscopy study. *Ann Neurol* 52: 20–28
108   Alvarez-Sabin J, Molina CA, Ribo M, Arenillas JF, Montaner J, Huertas R, Santamarina E,
        Rubiera M (2004) Impact of Admission Hyperglycemia on Stroke Outcome After Throm-
        bolysis. Risk Stratification in Relation to Time to Reperfusion. *Stroke* 35: 2493–2498. Epub
        2004 Oct 7
109   Liu Y, Laakso MP, Karonen JO, Vanninen RL, Nuutinen J, Soimakallio S, Aronen HJ (2002)
        Apolipoprotein E polymorphism and acute ischemic stroke: a diffusion- and perfusion-
        weighted magnetic resonance imaging study. *J Cereb Blood Flow Metab* 22: 1336–1342
110   Treger I, Froom P, Ring H, Friedman G (2003) Association between apolipoprotein E4 and
        rehabilitation outcome in hospitalized ischemic stroke patients. *Arch Phys Med Rehabil*
        84: 973–976
111   Fischman AJ, Alpert NM, Rubin RH (2002) Pharmacokinetic imaging: a noninvasive
        method for determining drug distribution and action. *Clin Pharmacokinet* 41: 581–602
112   Lo EH, Broderick JP, Moskowitz MA (2004) tPA and proteolysis in the neurovascular unit.
        Stroke 35: 354–356
113   Montaner J (2003) Cooling matrix metalloproteases to improve thrombolysis in acute
        ischemic stroke. *Stroke* 34: 2171–2172
114   Horstmann S, Kalb P, Koziol J, Gardner H, Wagner S (2003) Profiles of matrix metallo-
        proteinases, their inhibitors, and laminin in stroke patients: influence of different ther-
        apies. *Stroke* 34: 2165–2170
115   Montaner J, Molina CA, Monasterio J, Abilleira S, Arenillas JF, Ribo M, Quintana M,
        Alvarez-Sabin J (2003) Matrix metalloproteinase-9 pretreatment level predicts intracra-
        nial hemorrhagic complications after thrombolysis in human stroke. *Circulation* 107:
        598–603
116   Galis ZS, Khatri JJ (2002) Matrix metalloproteinases in vascular remodeling and athero-
        genesis: the good, the bad, and the ugly. *Circ Res* 90: 251–262
117   Montaner J, Alvarez-Sabin J, Molina C, Angles A, Abilleira S, Arenillas J, Gonzalez MA,
        Monasterio J (2001) Matrix metalloproteinase expression after human cardioembolic
        stroke: temporal profile and relation to neurological impairment. *Stroke* 32: 1759–1766
118   Montaner J, Rovira A, Molina CA, Arenillas JF, Ribo M, Chacon P, Monasterio J, Alvarez-
        Sabin J (2003) Plasmatic level of neuroinflammatory markers predict the extent of dif-
        fusion-weighted image lesions in hyperacute stroke. *J Cereb Blood Flow Metab* 23:
        1403–1407
119   Dijkhuizen RM, Asahi M, Wu O, Rosen BR, Lo EH (2002) Rapid breakdown of microvas-
        cular barriers and subsequent hemorrhagic transformation after delayed recombinant
        tissue plasminogen activator treatment in a rat embolic stroke model. *Stroke* 33:
        2100–2104
120   Bremer C, Tung CH, Weissleder R (2001) *In vivo* molecular target assessment of matrix
        metalloproteinase inhibition. *Nat Med* 7: 743–748
121   Bremer C, Tung CH, Weissleder R (2002) Molecular imaging of MMP expression and ther-
        apeutic MMP inhibition. *Acad Radiol* 9, Suppl 2: S314–315
122   Pham W, Choi Y, Weissleder R, Tung CH (2004) Developing a peptide-based near-
        infrared molecular probe for protease sensing. *Bioconjug Chem* 15: 1403–1407
123   McIntyre JO, Fingleton B, Wells KS, Piston DW, Lynch CC, Gautam S, Matrisian LM
        (2004) Development of a novel fluorogenic proteolytic beacon for *in vivo* detection and

imaging of tumour-associated matrix metalloproteinase-7 activity. *Biochem J* 377: 617–628

124   Schafers M, Riemann B, Kopka K, Breyholz HJ, Wagner S, Schafers KP, Law MP, Schober O, Levkau B (2004) Scintigraphic imaging of matrix metalloproteinase activity in the arterial wall *in vivo*. *Circulation* 109: 2554–2559

125   Breyholz HJ, Schafers M, Wagner S, Holtke C, Faust A, Rabeneck H, Levkau B, Schober O, Kopka K (2005) C-5-disubstituted barbiturates as potential molecular probes for non-invasive matrix metalloproteinase imaging. *J Med Chem* 48: 3400–3409

126   Qureshi AI, Siddiqui AM, Kim SH, Hanel RA, Xavier AR, Kirmani JF, Suri MF, Boulos AS, Hopkins LN (2004) Reocclusion of recanalized arteries during intra-arterial thrombolysis for acute ischemic stroke. *AJNR Am J Neuroradiol* 25: 322–328

127   Lapchak PA, Araujo DM (2003) Therapeutic potential of platelet glycoprotein IIb/IIIa receptor antagonists in the management of ischemic stroke. *Am J Cardiovasc Drugs* 3: 87–94

128   Brouwers FM, Oyen WJ, Boerman OC, Barrett JA, Verheugt FW, Corstens FH, Van der Meer JW (2003) Evaluation of Tc-99m-labeled glycoprotein IIb/IIIa receptor antagonist DMP444 SPECT in patients with infective endocarditis. *Clin Nucl Med* 28: 480–484

129   Higashida RT, Furlan AJ, Roberts H, Tomsick T, Connors B, Barr J, Dillon W, Warach S, Broderick J, Tilley B, Sacks D; Technology Assessment Committee of the American Society of Interventional and Therapeutic Neuroradiology; Technology Assessment Committee of the Society of Interventional Radiology (2003) Trial design and reporting standards for intra-arterial cerebral thrombolysis for acute ischemic stroke. *Stroke* 34: 109–137

Progress in Drug Research, Vol. 62
(Markus Rudin, Ed.)
©2005 Birkhäuser Verlag, Basel (Switzerland)

Clinical drug evaluation using imaging readouts: regulatory perspectives

By David S. Lester

Site Head, WW Clinical Technology
PGRD New Products Development
PGP Pfizer Inc.
685 Third Ave, MS 685/19/8
New York, NY 10017, USA
<david.s.lester@pfizer.com>

Glossary of abbreviations

AD, Alzheimer's disease; cIMT, carotid ultrasound/carotid IMT; CT, computed tomography; CV, cardiovascular; DMAs, disease-modifying agents; DMOADs, disease-modifying osteoarthritis drugs; IMT, intima-medial thickness; IVUS, intravascular ultrasound; JSN, joint space narrowing; MRI, magnetic resonance imaging; MS, multiple sclerosis; OA, osteoarthritis; PET, positron-emission tomography; vMRI, volumetric

1   Introduction

In this chapter, I will refrain from providing a list of the uses of biomedical imaging in drug development, as much of this will be expertly covered by other authors in this volume. Rather, I will focus on specific examples where imaging is recognized as having an impact, and the difficulties that are being and will be experienced in the introduction of innovative technologies into the regulatory arena. I will also discuss present efforts by the regulators, particularly the Food and Drug Administration (FDA), and their activities regarding the use of imaging methodologies into the drug approval process. It should be noted that many of these issues are not unique to biomedical imaging but are common to all innovative approaches that are presently under review for a potential role in the drug development activities associated with regulatory submissions.

Biomedical imaging has changed the way in which medicine is practiced. For example, in 1985, there were between 5 and 10 magnetic resonance imaging (MRI) scans. In 1998, in the US alone, there were over 7 million [1]. The impact of biomedical imaging was celebrated with the US Post Office releasing a stamp recognizing this achievement as one of the 100 most important events of the 20th century. In terms of drug development, there are considerable examples of the use of imaging in drug development in both preclinical and clinical studies, many of which are addressed by other authors in this volume. This chapter focuses on regulatory issues and implications in relation to the development and use of biomedical imaging in clinical drug development. The regulatory environment focuses on phase III clinical studies, drug approval, and in light of increased interest and pressure, phase IV, postmarketing activities. In terms of phase III, some examples of imaging applications presently being utilized are discussed; however, the focus is on the changing environment of drug development, highlighted by new therapeutic strategies targeting disease modification, and the challenges to the various stakeholders in this rapidly developing process. These new trends in drug development are resulting in compounds that are directly targeting specific molecules or pathways that are associated specifically with the disease [2–4]. In order for these disease modification models to succeed, it will be essential to understand and even define or redefine the disease itself. This provides opportunities for application of new clinical endpoints, including clinical molecular imaging approaches.

To exploit these opportunities we must understand the regulatory environment and what will be required by it to gain acceptance of these technologies so that they can have the appropriate impacts.

2   Present regulatory status for specific diseases and therapeutic areas

2.1   Oncology

Early attempts to define tumor responses to therapies began in the 1960s [5]. In the late '70s and early '80s, the World Health Organization (WHO) defined criteria by which such changes could be monitored. However, there were problems in the application of these criteria by various groups as specific interpretations were made [6–9]. In addition, the increased use of CT and MRI and the integration of three-dimensional (3D) data analysis provided additional complexities [6, 7]. Awareness of these issues resulted in many modifications to the original WHO criteria; however, the significant advances in biomedical imaging technologies could not be suitably addressed. In response, in 1994, the European Organization for Research and Treatment of Cancer (EORTC), the National Cancer Institute (NCI) and the National Cancer Institute of Canada, established a task force to develop new guidelines for measuring tumor responses based on intensive analyses of large datasets of patients previously examined [6]. There were 3 years of regular meetings and exchanges of ideas within the task force, followed by a drafted revision that was widely circulated for comments from the biomedical community. This resulted in the second version of the document which was sent out to external reviewers who participated in a consensus meeting in October 1998, to discuss and resolve problems and issues. Representatives from industry, academia and regulatory agencies were present to finalize the third version of the document, which was officially presented to the scientific community in the 1999 American Society for Clinical Oncology. The final version was submitted for official publication in June 1999 to the *Journal of the National Cancer Institute*. Data from collaborative studies of an accumulated 4000 plus patients with tumor response assessment was used to define the measurement criteria. The RECIST criteria are discussed in detail by various authors [6–10]. The criteria were meant to be used for tumor response evaluation as a prospective endpoint in early clinical trials (typically phase II for investigational drugs or regimens). In addition, they could be used as a prospective endpoint in more definitive endpoint trials for patient populations. Under these circumstances, the measured tumor response for the population could be used as a surrogate endpoint to determine clinical benefit. It could also be used in daily clinical practice to evaluate tumor response in relation to continuation of treatment.

The following guidelines were developed: "At baseline, tumor lesions will be classified as measurable (accurate measurement of lesions in one diameter (longest) as > 20 mm with conventional techniques or as > 10 mm with spiral CT), or non-measurable (all other lesions < 20 mm with conventional or < 10 mm with spiral CT). The term "evaluable" is not recommended. Baseline measurements should be between treatment or no more than 4 weeks before treatment. A similar protocol should be used following treatment effects."

Imaging protocols are preferred to clinical examination. X-rays can be used for chest tumors but CT is certainly preferred. CT and MRI are the most recommended methods at present. Ultrasound is generally not recommended. It can be used as an easy routine analysis for superficial tumors as a support to clinical examination. In the documentation [11] there is considerable detail regarding the radiological conditions, the types of responses, and necessary details to standardize the measurements. Four different responses are well documented: complete response, partial response, stable disease and progressive disease [6, 11].

These detailed guidelines provided a standardization of tumor response, which did not necessarily take into account the latest innovations in imaging technology, but which provided a basis for comparison of one RECIST trial to another. RECIST data did not show a good correlation with older WHO criteria [8, 9].

So, after extensive efforts to standardize an approach to tumor response, less than 5 years after this 5-year process was summarized and completed, a new approach has been proposed suggesting a new approach which takes into account the various developments and potentialities of advancing biomedical imaging technologies. These include 3D measurements, imaging contrast agents and multimodal analysis [12]. There were numerous pitfalls with the RECIST criteria that are well recognized by the scientific community.

The use of imaging in oncology highlights a fundamental problem in the application of emerging technologies to the drug development process, that is, the clash between technology development and clinical trial application. Research tends to focus on innovation and development is more refinement and improvement of existing methods. It is difficult to keep a balance. The return on investment to innovative approaches is not easily realized in the business world due to the required duration for development of an appropriate product. In spite of this, pharmaceutical companies continue to be amongst the leading investors in R&D technologies compared to all industries. With the pressures of increasing costs in drug development and increased attrition rates, a major contribution is expected from these innovative and emerging technologies. However, to date, this has only been realized in terms of additional expenses and the return on investment has not been recognized.

2.1.1 Regulatory considerations regarding use of imaging in oncology

The pressure is increasing on regulatory agencies from numerous directions. From the perspective of the general public, whom they are serving regarding health and human services, the emphasis is on increased safety. Advocacy groups continue to encourage more rapid approval of new therapies. From the industry perspective, there is increased pressure to innovate the process. The challenge to the regulatory agencies is to achieve all of these goals simultaneously! The inconsistency is evident in that increased safety generally requires a "risk averse" position, while increasing innovation would infer greater "risk taking".

2.2 Multiple sclerosis

Even though multiple sclerosis (MS) was first described over 130 years ago, the exact diagnosis still remains a challenge. It is the most common neurological disease among young adults. The recent introduction of therapeutic agents has raised the importance for a diagnostic procedure that stands up to the rigors of both clinical practice and interventional clinical trials. Generally, the clinical symptomatology, the typical transient nature of the complaints and the abnormal neurological signs, are sufficient diagnosis [13]. However, they are complicated and the variability in the measures makes it extremely difficult for the development of a therapy. MRI was first used to investigate MS in 1981 [14]. MRI dramatically changed the nature of disease diagnosis and within less than a decade of its first use, it was universally accepted and adopted, and chosen to be the exclusive basis for diagnosis by most clinical neurologists worldwide. MRI was capable of detecting and correlating the number of lesions, their size, and location to the clinical signs and symptoms [13–15]. However, there are reports of poor correlation in terms of diagnosis and distinguishing between MS and disseminated encephalomyelitis. In 2001, McDonald and colleagues provided updated diagnostic criteria that provided a scheme for MS diagnosis, which included clinical signs and symptoms, MRI, and cerebrospinal fluid biochemical markers [16]. The guidelines provide precise technical details regarding the use of MRI in diagnosis.

The sensitivity, reproducibility, metrics and objectivity of MRI are used in conjunction with the more classical endpoints for the monitoring of experimental therapies in the treatment of MS. There is evidence that the enhancement of lesions and the changes of the T_2 load in serial MRI scans may serve as a valid criterion for the relapse rate in patients with relapsing-remitting MS [17]. However, there are limited data as to the correlation between relapse rate and disability accrual. The significant distinction in terms of MRI use for MS must be made between its applications in a clinical trial setting or a clinical diagnosis, in contrast to use in understanding basic mechanisms of the disease [18]. The standards of the measurement are significantly different. Due to the high prevalence of this disease and the pressures to develop therapeutic interventions, MRI has been recognized and utilized extensively in evaluation of therapeutic action as a disease-modifying agent. It has been used in FDA-approved therapies, including subcutaneous interferon-β-1b (IFNβ-1b, Betaseron), IM interferon-β-1a (Avonex), SC interferon-β-1a (Rebif), glatiramer acetate (Copaxone), and mitoxantrone (Novantrone), all of which are known as disease-modifying agents (DMAs) [19]. The label for each of these compounds has included reference to the MRI data, indicating that it has played a major role in the approval process. However, the labels clearly states: "The exact relationship between the MRI patients and the clinical status of the patients is unknown."

This is still the case for the most recently released compound, Tysabri (natalizumab), which was approved in November 2004 [20]. Even though MRI is considered to be a surrogate endpoint for MS, there is no formal validation of the MRI metrics in comparison to clinical disability in clinical trials. While there is considerable information as to the technical requirements for using MRI in MS clinical trials, there is a paucity of the necessary clinical validation. This is in part due to the continually evolving perception of the role of MRI as a clinical endpoint and/or diagnostic. In one recent study by Sormani and colleagues, representing the European Study Group on Interferon-β-1b in Secondary Progressive MS, they claim that "the cMRI (conventional MRI) metrics should not be used as a stand-alone measure of outcome in phase III trials of IFNB in secondary progressive MS" [21].

This is further complicated by the nature of the therapeutic agents that are not considered to be "cures" for the disease, but rather having significant efficacious impact on the short-term outcome of the disease. With the development of disease-modifying therapies, we are defining and/or redefining the disease. The imaging technology is having a significant impact on this process. The problem remains that the methodological approaches for determining drug efficacy will not be the most "cutting edge" technology or application of the technology being employed. It is naïve to expect otherwise as by the time the necessary clinical and technical validation are completed to satisfy regulatory agencies such that an imaging technology may be considered "validated", the technology will be out of date in the eyes of the technologists. Perhaps we have unrealistic expectations?

2.3   Osteoarthritis

Due to the increased aging population, osteoarthritis (OA) will continue to develop into a major health problem. Most people over 60 will have some form of OA, while at least half will exhibit the symptoms [22]. At present, all therapies associated with OA treat the symptoms, i.e. pain, and not the disease itself. There are increased efforts to develop therapies that are specific for modifying the disease, known as disease-modifying osteoarthritis drugs

(DMOADs). Both European and US regulatory guidelines [23–25] specify that to gain a DMOAD indication, clinical studies need to demonstrate that a new therapeutic can slow down disease structural progression as measured by joint space narrowing (JSN) on plain X-rays, and that this delayed JSN translates into a clinical benefit for the patients. The limitation is that JSN is not sensitive to small changes and there is significant high precision error [26]. MRI is now being investigated as an approach to measure the cartilage itself. Both structural and chemical changes in the cartilage can be measured over time using MRI procedures [27, 28]. This is recognized as a more sensitive method than JSN and measures the targeted tissue response directly. Thus, shorter clinical trials may be possible. There are accumulated data available on these methods, and it is generally agreed that the technology is ready for phase II studies, but further work is need for phase III. Regulatory agencies recognize the advances and potential of such technologies as MRI. For example, in the FDA draft guidance for industry for the clinical development programs for regulated products related to OA, it is stated: "In the future, measurement of cartilage volume using MRI may be able to replace the X-ray measurement of JSN, but currently technical problems remain, and adequate studies correlating MRI with X-rays are not yet available."

In relation to the use of JSN as a method for measuring DMOAD efficacy, it is stated in the same guidance: "Determining what change in JSN of the knee or hip is clinically relevant to the patient with OA is fundamental, but currently unknown" [23].

The Committee for Proprietary Medical Products (CPMP) of the European Agency for the Evaluation of Medicinal Products (EMEA) in their 1998 document on clinical investigation of OA products only referred to the JSN as a measure of structural progression [24].

2.3.1 Regulatory considerations

The FDA shows a willingness to discuss new methodologies for measuring efficacy in the DMOAD class of compounds that are presently under considerable development. This is shown by their participation in the National Institutes of Health Osteoarthritis Initiative. However, it is clear that significant or at least appropriate validation needs to be done of all new approaches, both imaging and biochemical, before acceptance. A combined pharmaceutical industry/academia/government initiative is trying to develop standards for new endpoints [29]. The degree of change that will have to be measured using such techniques as MRI is not yet known, and will only be determined upon a measured response in the rate of change of the measured parameter upon therapeutic treatment, e.g., cartilage volume. The regulators are indicating that there must be clinical symptoms, i.e., pain measurements, associated, as there must be a measurable "clinical benefit". Using technologies such as MRI and specific biochemical markers, we are defining the disease-modifying measurement parameters of the OA process. An extensive OA initiative is presently in progress to evaluate the various potential biomarkers for OA, including imaging. Participants are from academia, government and industry (for an excellent review see http://www.niams.nih.gov/ne/oi/oabio-marwhipap.htm). A possible scenario is that a technology will measure significant changes in the rate of cartilage degradation but not demonstrate a significant change in the clinical symptoms. Such a compound would not be approved. However, in combination with an established agent for treating clinical symptoms, the regulatory decision process will be challenged. As for the case of MS discussed above, the science and subsequent understanding of the disease process/mechanism will usually be significantly ahead of the state of therapy and the clinical endpoints used to determine clinical efficacy. This type of challenge to the regulators and the pharmaceutical industry is prevalent in the development of new therapies in most therapeutic areas.

2.4 Alzheimer's disease

The increased prevalence of Alzheimer's disease (AD) continues to be synonymous with the increase in aging populations. The problem with dementia patients is that they often lack the ability to give informed consent due to cognitive impairment. Subsequently, it is often required that a surrogate decision maker serve as the guardian of the individual's rights [30]. This distinguishes AD from other diseases and highlights the need for a surrogate endpoint that is capable of replacing the clinical endpoint. The limitations of the present AD clinical endpoints in terms of clinical trials for evaluating new therapies are recognized. While there are a limited number of compounds that have been successfully approved for treatment of signs and symptoms, much of the emphasis of the pharmaceutical industry most recently has been on the development of compounds for purposes of prevention. Subsequently, there has been a need to evaluate new compounds in terms of modification of disease progression. The clinical signs and symptoms alone are not appropriate for evaluations of action of such compounds. This has resulted in significant efforts in academia and industry to develop biomarkers for evaluating disease progression with the ultimate goal of providing surrogate endpoints for AD disease progression. In terms of regulatory activities, the FDA, Division of Neuropharmacological Products, has shown great interest in such developments by participating in conferences and symposia and even publishing documents presenting their perspectives [31, 32]. Imaging has received significant attention due to its non-invasive nature with volumetric MRI (vMRI) being the most published approach [33]. Considerable studies have been made on the performance characteristics of vMRI in terms of monitoring disease progression [34], potential risk factor/diagnostic [35], and therapeutic studies [36]. FDG-PET will also play a significant role and has recently been approved for reimbursement for certain AD diagnoses [37, 38]. The use of FDG-PET as an imaging endpoint for AD clinical trials has also been investigated; however, it is limited due to the availability of sites and the exposure to the radioactive tracer. Other imaging approaches include MR spectroscopy [36], diffusion-weighted imaging [39] and perfusion MRI [40] as other possible approaches. Another PET methodology that has gained considerable attention is the amyloid plaque tracers that have been developed [41]. Upon validation, these could be very promising tools for evaluating plaque-modifying agents, or possibly as subject inclusion/exclusion criteria, or even as a diagnostic associated with prescribing the therapy(ies). An extensive government/academia/industry effort is underway to investigate and evaluate imaging procedures for AD. A consortium has been established for this purpose with financial support from industry and NIH (see http://www.nia.nih.gov/NewsAndEvents/Press-Releases/ADNIQandA.htm).

There have not yet been any AD drugs approved based on imaging surrogate markers. At present, FDA submission of an AD compound requires at least two separate randomized, double-blind, placebo-controlled trials of at least 3–6 months duration. Such trials will not be appropriate to obtain a disease-modifying approval indication. The FDA has participated and provided considerable discussion and direction in terms of the requirements for an AD imaging surrogate. In November 2002, the Peripheral and Central Nervous System Drugs Advisory Committee of the FDA, held a meeting to discuss the role of brain imaging as an outcome measure in phase III drug trials in AD [41]. There were many of the leading experts in imaging methodologies making presentations on the state of the art of imaging modalities for AD. Dr. Katz, the Director of the Division of Neuropharmacological Drug Products, opened the proceedings with a discussion on surrogate markers. He indicated support for the development of a surrogate marker for AD disease progression, but indicated that it was the job of the industry or the health sciences community to provide it. The general conclusion of the Advisory Committee was that none of the imaging modalities were validated. One would need a demonstrable effect by a therapeutic treatment before a decision could be made regarding the validity of the imaging surrogate. However, it was clear that clinical symptoms would be needed to accompany any submission. An interesting point that was raised by Dr. Katz "if you had a drug that effected a surrogate but had never had an effect on cognition, I'm not sure what you'd have." He followed this statement with "I think it would suggest that the surrogate's a failed surrogate." [41]. This statement was not disputed by any of the Committee. At the American Society for Experimental Neurotherapeutics, in March 2004, Dr. Katz provided an overview of this meeting with some additional comments [42]. However, it was clear that there was little if any progress in terms of the perception and use of imaging surrogates for AD from the Advisory Committee meeting 2 years earlier. Dr. Katz has published an article on an FDA perspective on biomarkers and surrogates in April 2004 [31]. In addition, there was a well-written document on a regulatory perspective on the evaluation of disease-modifying drugs for AD, by Dr. Mani, from Dr. Katz's division [31]. The FDA should not define the requirements for such an imaging surrogate. This can only be determined upon a successful clinical trial showing an effect of a therapeutic on an imaging surrogate that correlates with clinical signs and symptoms. To "validate" (and refine) the definition, subsequent therapeutic studies with other agents using these imaging criteria would be needed. As can be seen, there is a general willingness to recognize surrogate endpoints by the FDA in a number of different diseases; however, the issues vary from one disease to another. It will be difficult to establish a standard protocol for surrogate marker validation. Perhaps some consensus general guiding principles could be developed by the community to help the various stakeholders in their efforts to pursue new surrogates.

3   Confusion and unclear terminologies

The major debate regarding the use of imaging as a clinical endpoint generally focuses on their use as surrogate endpoints in clinical trials. There have been considerable publications, meetings, etc. on distinguishing between biomarkers and surrogate endpoints. At a recent FDA Pharmaceutical Sciences Advisory Committee Meeting on Biomarkers and Surrogate Endpoints, Dr. Lawrence Lesko, Director of the Office of Clinical Pharmacology and Biopharmeceutics, Center for Drug Evaluation and Research (CDER), FDA, began the proceedings by defining and distinguishing biomarkers from surrogates. He used the following definitions which were a product of the joint NIH/FDA Biomarkers meeting held in 1999. They are: "Biomarker (biological marker) – characteristic that is measured and evaluated as an indicator of normal biologic processes, pathogenic processes, or pharmacologic responses to a therapeutic intervention. Surrogate endpoint – A biomarker intended to substitute for a clinical endpoint." As can be seen, a surrogate endpoint belongs to the biomarker class. This is a widely accepted definition of the surrogate.

So, what distinguishes the surrogate from the general biomarker category? The answer is in the necessary standards to reach the surrogate status. A surrogate is considered to be a potential replacement for an existing clinical endpoint. Thus, the surrogate endpoint is expected to satisfy the rigorous and demanding requirements for registration of new therapeutics. The difficulty is that there are no written standards regarding requirements. In addition, can it be expected that the requirements for a surrogate marker for OA will be the same as one for cardiovascular (CV) disease or AD? Is it feasible to establish universal standards for development of surrogates?

The innovative document published by the FDA Office of the Commissioner, commonly referred to as the "Critical Path" document states: "Additional biomarkers (quantitative measures of biological effects that provide informative links between mechanism of action and clinical effectiveness) and additional surrogate markers (quantitative measures that can predict effectiveness) are needed to guide product development" [43].

There are a number of examples of accepted surrogate endpoints, including, pain measures, blood pressure, cholesterol, intraocular pressure (glaucoma), and tumor shrinkage. All of these endpoints measure the effect of the disease or some associated correlate, not the disease progress. Imaging endpoints could potentially determine changes in disease progression. What is it going to take to develop new surrogate endpoints?

At the same Advisory Committee in November 2004, Dr. Janet Woodcock, Acting Deputy Commissioner of the FDA, made the following points in her presentation regarding regulatory acceptance of surrogate endpoints: "re-assessment of the idea of validation; perhaps adoption of new nomenclature" and "replace idea of "validation" with understanding of degree of uncertainty in various dimensions". This demonstrated the awareness of the FDA in relation to a major hurdle for achieving surrogate status, the problem of validation.

The terms surrogate endpoint and validation are widely used in the same sentence. The problem is that the perceived definition of these terms alone and/or together is not aligned in terms of efforts in academia, industry and the regulatory agencies. I would like to propose what I consider to be general principles appropriate for validation of a technology to reach the surrogate status. I emphasize that the ultimate acceptance by the regulators MUST be done on a case-by-case basis.

4   Validation

As was indicated above, the term 'validation' has caused much misunderstanding and lack of agreement. There are no formal definitions of how a method should be validated. The US Federal Government has an Interagency Committee for Validation of Alternative Methods, but this has primarily focused on toxicity screens for environmental-related issues (see http://icc-vam.niehs.nih.gov/). There have been numerous articles and reviews all dealing or demonstrating 'validation' to various degrees, at least in the perspective of the author(s) [44–48]. The following distinction is proposed, technical validation vs. clinical validation.

4.1   Technical validation

This relates to the performance characteristic of the methodology, whether it is an imaging modality or a simple biochemical assay. In terms of the use of imaging as a surrogate endpoint, the major issues that need to be dealt with regarding technical validation are as follows, and in should be dealt with in the following sequential order:

1) Instrument standardization – Either similar imaging instruments or information collected regarding test/retest for instrument (inter- and intra-patient variability), scanning protocols, image inclusion/exclusion criteria, accuracy of instrument (phantoms), upgrades, compliance details, different manufacturers.

2) Subject issues – The majority of "noise" that contributes to many imaging methods is due to the subject variability. This should be minimized by standardizing location of images, number of sections, specific coils, inclusion and exclusion criteria for subjects.

3) Site standardization – The major issue for using an imaging method for diagnostic purposes versus clinical trials, is that in clinical trials multiple imaging sites are employed. This requires that there be some form of standardization process. There are a number of imaging Contract Research Organizations (CRO) which focus on this issue. The imaging centers must have manuals (imaging protocols), training and pre-training of technicians, monitoring of technicians and monitoring of instruments. There is also a core reading lab (or imaging CRO) analyzing the images. They must have manuals (SOPs for image analysis), training and re-training of readers, monitoring of readers (intra- and inter-reader variability), monitoring measurement hardware at the various sites through the acquired image quality.

4) Data acquisition – There must be a standardized format that is compatible for instruments at all sites. Instrument manufacturers may have to be involved or the core reading lab may need to prepare a standardized format.

5) Data storage – The core lab must have sufficient and appropriate storage capabilities that are compliant with regulatory requirements. Data protection in terms of back up/redundancy and security must be constantly maintained. It must be clear what the sponsor's role is in this, i.e., are they accountable or responsible for the data storage. This may depend on the sponsor's resources.

6) Data analysis – The software for analysis must be evaluated and validated. Reader variability should be determined. Semi-automation where possible may reduce variability. It should be compliant with regulatory standards (21CFR part 11 for the US).

All of the above factors contribute to the variability or "noise" in the measurement. It is desirable to minimize them where possible. However, the reality is that the majority of the noise comes from the subject. Looking at rate changes over time, i.e., more than one time point is collected for each subject, can reduce this by normalizing the intra-subject variability. If the other factors are controlled, then direct comparisons can be made over time within a subject. The remaining contributors to the variability can be reasonably controlled if the above factors are dealt with.

4.2   Clinical validation

Clinical validation is a much more controversial issue [45–48]. What comprises clinical validation has not ever been openly addressed. This relates to whether the methodology being validated has the potential of replacing a clinical endpoint. Below are listed a number of parameters that if addressed will supply supporting evidence for a clinical validation program for an imaging methodology.

1) Correlation with pathology – Non-invasive imaging data correlates with "gold standard" pathology.
2) Endpoint correlation with risk factors – Does the imaging data predict disease progression in a manner similar to known risk factors?
3) Imaging outcomes correlate with clinical endpoints – Progression studies correlate with clinical outcomes. Epidemiological studies.
4) A treatment effect can be measured by the imaging modality that correlates with standard signs and/or symptoms.

If all four of these factors are addressed, then a clinically meaningful change as determined in terms of the imaging methodology needs to be defined. This definition should be considered acceptable by the various stakeholders, including academia, advocacy groups, reimbursement agencies and to be considered representative by a majority of the pharmaceutical industries. This still does not provide any guarantee that the regulatory agencies will accept the final definition.

5   The impact of imaging on atherosclerosis

Treatment of CV diseases is the most advanced of all therapeutic areas. This is in large part due to technology development. Technologies such as electrocardiograms and sphygnamometers have allowed measurement of clinical endpoints, which has lead to the development of many therapeutic approaches. More recently, simple clinical laboratory assays of cholesterol and low-density lipoproteins have had tremendous impacts, as can be witnessed by the introduction of statin therapy. These simple tests have raised the awareness of the public for the disease and its associated characteristics [49]. An additional impact of these and other technologies is to provide an enhanced understanding of CV diseases by the scientific community, leading to continued refinement of the disease definition. The imaging technologies have been rapidly developed and applied to help us better understand the disease, and is leading to definition of specific risk factors. A front-page article of the prestigious Wall Street Journal indicated that inclusion of a rapid ultrasound procedure could significantly reduce the occurrence of stroke [50].

For atherosclerosis, the development of technologies and their application has occurred initially as a basic research tool, but further experimentation has resulted in their translation as clinical trial tools. The initial imaging modality that impacted atherosclerosis was quantitative coronary angiography (QCA) [51]. This methodology measures the lumen of the artery, which was considered to correlate to the disease. With the development and acceptance of Glagov's model in the 1980s it was clear that QCA was not the most accurate procedure for measuring atherosclerosis progression. This model demonstrated that there could be significant increase in plaque formation without any measurable change in the lumen [52]. This leads to increased efforts to measure the plaque known as the intima-medial thickness (IMT). The first and most accepted method developed for this purpose was carotid ultrasound, often referred to as carotid IMT (cIMT) [53, 54]. This method provides one or more 2D image(s) or slice(s) of the carotid artery. More recently, a modified ultrasound approach, intravascular ultrasound (IVUS) was developed to measure plaque volume in coronary arteries [55]. The development of the vulnerable plaque concept led to the desire of the research community to measure changes in the chemical composition of the plaque, as it was the chemistry of the plaque that was considered most important to its state of vulnerability [56]. Electron beam CT scanning provides high resolution images of plaque calcification, which, depending on the results and interpretation of the investigator, represents plaque vulnerability [57] or stability [58]. The controversy in the method would suggest the method requires considerable investigation before use in clinical trial. More promising is MRI of the carotid. The technique is being applied by an increasing number of laboratories and methods are being standardized [59]. The *in situ* plaque composition as visualized using MRI has been shown to correlate with that found by histological analysis of the same excised plaque [60]. This method has been shown to be able to predict statin-induced reduction in the lipid pool of plaque in a single study [61]. Multi-slice CT, PET and infrared approaches are also being developed to provide functional and chemical information of the plaque [62–64]. In addition, there are some novel molecular imaging approaches being investigated [64]. The development of the methodologies provides additional information on the biology of plaque. A summary is provided in Table 1.

The use of the imaging technologies in plaque research has provided important information that may lead to development of specific therapies. To evaluate these new therapies directed at specific targets related to the disease state, it may well require the associated technologies (e.g., MRI for plaque composition) to be included in the clinical evaluation of the therapeutics. They could be a provisional primary endpoint or a secondary endpoint that could affect the labeling.

Regulatory agencies have been engaged in discussions on the use of imaging for CV endpoints by participating in a number of scientific meetings. In the published proceedings of one such meeting, the FDA representative, Dr. David Orloff stated that "the burden to validate the method(s) chosen is on the sponsor" [65].

As an example, I will focus on cIMT. If we are to examine the issues raised in the previous section on technical and clinical validation, then cIMT is probably the best example of a validated imaging method. All of the technical issues described above in terms of technical validation have been dealt with by a number of cautious and fastidious laboratories, such that a number of facilities can now run multi-site therapeutic studies [53, 54]. Considerable effort has gone into understanding the source of the "noise" in such measurements to limit the variability.

In terms of clinical validation, I quote Dr. Orloff from the published proceedings: "For changes in vascular anatomy as assessed by a particular method of imaging to be acceptable as a surrogate for a reduction in risk for atherosclerotic events, mechanistic plausibility must be demonstrated as well as adequate evidence that the imaging method accurately reflects the disease

Table 1. Use of different imaging modalities in clinical evaluation of atherosclerosis progression and characterization

Imaging modality	Characteristic	Stage of development	Use in clinical trials	Invasive (I) or noninvasive (NI)	Refs
Quantitative coronary angiography (MRI)	Lumen volume	Routine diagnosis and clinical use	Yes	NI (contrast reagent)	
Carotid intima-media thickness (B-mode ultrasound)	2D carotid plaque thickness	Validated for diagnostic and clinical use	Yes	NI	[53, 54]
Intravascular ultrasound (IVUS)	3D coronary plaque volume	Used in clinical setting	Yes	I	[55]
Electron beam computed tomography (EBCT)	Coronary artery calcification	Used in clinical setting	Yes	NI	[57, 58]
Fluorodeoxyglucose positron emission tomography (FDG-PET) and FDG-PET/CT	Macrophage-related inflammation in coronary plaque	Experimental clinical	No	NI (radiotracer)	[63]
Carotid magnetic resonance imaging (MRI)	Carotid plaque composition (lipid core and fibrous cap)	Experimental clinical	No	NI	[59, 60, 61]
Infrared spectroscopy	Coronary plaque composition (lipid core)	Early experimental clinical	No	I	[64]

process. This is a tall order and must be supported by epidemiologic, pathologic, and clinical evidence linking changes in the "picture" of the vessel, by whatever method used, to changes in clinical course of the atherosclerotic disease."

cIMT has satisfied many of the requirements outlined by Dr. Orloff such that it fulfills the surrogate endpoint requirements for clinical validation. Much of the clinically relevant cIMT data can be summarized as follows:

1) In three major epidemiology studies, the linkage between baseline IMT and CV disease events involving a total of 26 684 subjects over 2.5–7 years have been demonstrated.

2) In nine clinical trials, the link of IMT progression to events was examined and demonstrated using a total of 6352 subjects over a 2- to 4-year period. Studies were performed in USA, Europe (Finland, The Netherlands) and Japan.

Dr. Orloff goes on to expand by suggesting that two different imaging modalities measuring two different vascular beds in active control studies will be necessary. For example, cIMT can be used for the carotids, and IVUS for the coronary arteries. While there is not the quantity of information on IVUS that there is on cIMT, we can take advantage of what has been learned from cIMT and develop the validation in a more focused manner. In reality, in some ways IVUS is a "refined" IMT application.

The difficulty with both of these methods as pointed out by Dr. Orloff at a number of recent presentations is that there are no data addressing the minimum change in vascular anatomy by these methods that denotes a clinical benefit (coronary heart disease risk).

In contrast, the Europeans have indicated in their Note for guidance on Clinical Investigation of Medicinal Products in the Treatment of Lipid Disorders [66]: "Atherosclerosis progression can be measured by validated and reliable techniques ... its validity should be justified properly. As stated in section 2.3, today these parameters are not considered as surrogates for hard clinical endpoints, but they may constitute appropriate secondary endpoints to support information on progression or regression of atherosclerosis." At a recent CV Biomarkers meeting, the European regulatory representative presented an uncompromising position compared to that of the FDA representatives.

However, while these imaging techniques may help in terms of evaluating efficacy, it must be emphasized as stated by Dr. Orloff "that there is still a need for large, long-term safety exposures before approval because these surrogate imaging endpoints may not ... be sufficient to define the safety profile of the drug."

As clearly stated by Dr. Robert Temple, Director, Center of Drug Evaluation and Research (CDER), FDA: "even if coronary ultrasound predicted event rate, would you really want to treat tens of millions of people without reasonable outcome data". (PhrMA 2004 Scientific Regulatory Meeting, May 4, 2004).

In conclusion, it should be noted that even if all of the criteria I have suggested have been fulfilled from the sponsor's perspective, it will always be at the discretion of the regulators to decide whether the data is suitable as a surrogate endpoint.

6   Tracer technologies – Molecular imaging

PET has been a major issue of attention over the last decade in terms of the FDA. A section was included in the FDA Modernization Act of 1997 [67]. This provides definition of a PET agent that is regulated.

The term "compounded positron-emission tomography drug" (1) means a drug that:

(A) exhibits spontaneous disintegration of unstable nuclei by the emission of positrons and is used for the purpose of providing dual photon positron-emission tomographic diagnostic images; and

(B) has been compounded by or on the order of a practitioner who is licensed by a State to compound or order compounding for a drug described in subparagraph (A), and is compounded in accordance with that State's law, for a patient or for research, teaching, or quality control;

and (2) includes any nonradioactive reagent, reagent kit, ingredient, nuclide generator, accelerator, target material, electronic synthesizer, or other apparatus or computer program to be used in the preparation of such a drug.

This was followed by the preliminary draft for the Current Good Manufacturing Practice for Positron Emission Tomography Drug Products published in Federal Register in April 2002 [68]. The final product was the detailed "Guidances for Industry on Medical Imaging Drug and Biological Products" released in June 2004. Three different sections were published: (1) Conducting Safety Assessments [69], (2) Clinical Indications [70], and (3) Design, Analysis and Interpretation of Clinical Studies [71]. There is a detailed analysis for the development of such agents not limited to PET agents exclusively but other contrast reagents for additional imaging modalities including MRI, ultrasound, CT, etc. These agents were historically regulated by the Center for Device and Radiological Health as they regulate the performance of the imaging instruments. The standards for development of such agents are as rigorous and demanding as the compounds are treated as "drugs". This is not the most favorable situation for development of PET ligands for clinical use as many of the sites producing ligands, e.g., hospital facilities, do not have the GMP capabilities. If the PET ligand is to be used as an internal decision making tool, the requirements are not as rigorous and do not necessarily demand the GMP requirements listed in the Guidance. However, if the data are to be included in the submission package to the Agency, they should be consulted for verification.

The use of PET has had considerable activity over the years. If a successful tracer can be developed, it can impact dosing, both concentrations and regimens [72–74]. Such data could be requested for review by the regulatory agencies. The FDA has shown some interest in the use of PET in microdosing, but it presently has had limited application in the pharmaceutical industry [75]. There is considerable caution in introducing new technologies.

Molecular imaging technologies are extremely popular and a number of agents are being developed for application as tools for clinical trials and studies [76, 77]. They will be developed according the regulatory guidance document that was released last year. This provides a positive environment for development of such agents, even if the requirements are stringent. It is expected that such agents will be readily used as tools for clinical efficacy and safety measures in pre-submission or phase IV clinical studies where the regulatory requirements will focus on the therapeutic compounds rather than the imaging agents.

7   Safety approaches

In Dr. Woodcock's presentation to the Pharmaceutical Sciences Advisory Committee meeting in November 2004, she mentioned the potential for imaging for development of new safety endpoints. There have been very few examples of safety impacts. There have been limited examples where imaging has had an impact on the safety evaluation of therapeutic agents except in the field of oncology where PET is used routinely in clinical studies and has significant impact on management of patients. It is used for toxicity-based decisions for dose setting and tumor size, simultaneously [72, 78].

Imaging modalities have been used in preclinical studies for safety evaluation. For example, PET and MR spectroscopy have been used to evaluate long-term toxicity of 3-nitropropionic acid in rat brain [79]. High-field MRI has been used to evaluate lesions due to toxins in numerous animal tissues [80]; however, they have not been translated to clinical studies.

An interesting example is the evaluation of vigabatrin, a compound that was approved for refractory epilepsy. In 2-week treatments in rats a variety of lesions were identified in rat brains including microvacuolation using MRI and histology [81]. However, an MRI study in humans found no significant effects [82]. These controversial animal data resulted in a "black box" on the label indicating toxicity to animals. More recently, vigabatrin has been removed from the US market for other safety reasons, ocular toxicity, but is still being used in Europe.

A number of probes have been developed for monitoring apoptosis. One in particular, a PET/SPECT probe, is commercially available and has been shown to be of use in oncology and CV applications [83, 84]. These probes are not routinely used in clinical trials, but there still continues to be considerable interest, particularly in the field of oncology.

There are many publications on the use of imaging for monitoring safety in animals; however, few of these have translated over to clinical studies [73, 74, 85], except in the therapeutic area of oncology [72, 84]. It would seem that, as there is greater emphasis on pediatric therapeutic evaluation, non-invasive approaches such as imaging could prove important. The identification of potential imaging applications in clinical safety should be driven by necessity, as is the case for all innovative technologies.

8   Conclusion

While there continues to be a tremendous interest in the use of imaging in drug development, the impact has not been as great as was originally expected. This is not that surprising when it is considered that the clinical evaluation of new drugs tends to be driven by the regulations, and the flexibility of the regulations are limited as they must focus on safety. Thus, therapeutic approval based on a new technology or clinical endpoint may be perceived by regulators as increasing the risk.

In addition, the challenges from the global regulatory community make the acceptance of imaging technologies an even riskier investment. As shown above, the FDA has shown a general willingness to consider imaging technologies. The problem in Europe is that, while the EMEA is viewed as an overseeing regulatory body, it really serves as an advisory group for all of the associated countries. The reality is that the imaging data needs to be evaluated by a number of European countries, many of which have different standards. Add to this the complexity of the situation in Japan and the challenge gets greater. It would be ideal if there were global standards for the regulatory requirement for acceptance of imaging endpoints as surrogates, but this may be naïve considering we cannot get a consensus amongst the investigators using and developing them.

In spite of this complex environment, the continued development and application of imaging methods in clinical trials must continue to advance, the one feature that has consensus agreement by all stakeholders in new therapeutic development and approval.

References

1   1Federation of American Societies for Experimental Biology (FASEB): MRI: From atomic physics to visualization, understanding and treatment of brain disorders. Breakthroughs in BioScience. *FASEB*: http://www.faseb.org/opa/mri/ (accessed June 2005)

2   Dohrmann CE (2004) Target discovery in metabolic syndrome. *Drug Discov Today* 9: 785–794

3   Desany B, Zhang Z (2004) Bioinformatics and cancer target discovery. *Drug Discov Today* 9: 795–802

4   Youdim MB, Buccafusco JJ (2005) Multi-functional drugs for various CNS targets in the treatment of neurodegenerative disorders. *Trends Pharmacol Sci* 26: 27–35

5   Zubrod CG, Schneiderman SM, Frei III BC, Gold GL, Schnider B et al (1960) Appraisal of methods for the study of chemotherapy of cancer in man: comparative therapeutic trial of mustard and other thiophosphoamide. *J Chronic Dis* 11: 7–33

6   Tharesse P, Arbuck SG, Eisenhauer EA, Wanders J, Kaplan RS, Rubinstein L, Verweij J, Van Glabbeke M, van Oosterom AT, Christian MC, Gwyther SG (2000) *J Natl Canc Inst* 92: 205–216

7   Padhani AR, Ollivier L (2001) The RECIST criteria: implications for diagnostic radiologists. *Brit J Radiol* 74: 983–986

8   Mazumdar M, Smith A, Schwartz LH (2004) A statistical simulation study finds discordance between WHO criteria and RECIST guideline. *J Clin Epidemiol* 57: 358–365

9   Prasad SR, Saini S, Sumner JE, Hahn PF, Sahani D, Boland GW (2003) Radiological measurement of breast cancer metastases to lung and liver: comparison between WHO (bidimensional) and RECIST (unidimensional) guidelines. *J Comput Assist Tomogr* 27: 380–384

10   Kimura M, Tominaga T (2002) Outstanding problems with response evaluation criteria in solid tumors (RECIST) in breast cancer. *Breast Cancer* 9: 153–159

11   James K, Eisenhauer E, Christian M, Terenziani M, Vena D, Mudal A et al (1999) Measuring response in solid tumors: unidimensional vs. bidimensional measurement. *J Nat Cancer Inst* 91: 5223–5528 ((A: 10 authors!))

12   Husband JE, Schwartz LH, Spencer J, Ollivier L, King DM, Johnson R, Reznek R (2004) Evaluation of the response to treatment of solid tumors – a consensus statement of the International Cancer Imaging Society. *Brit J Cancer* 90: 2256–2260

13   Poser CM, Brinar VV (2004) Diagnostic criteria for Multiple Sclerosis: an historical review. *Clin Neurol Neurosurgery* 106: 147–158

14   Pretorius PM, Quaghebeur G (2003) The role of MRI in the diagnosis of MS. *Clin Radiol* 58: 434–448

15   Mathews PM (2004) An update of neuroimaging of multiple sclerosis. *Curr Opin Neurol* 17: 453–458

16   McDonald WI, Compston A, Edan G, Goodkin D, Hartung HP, Lublin FD, McFarland HF, Paty DW, Polman CH, Reingold SC et al (2001) Recommended diagnostic criteria for multiple sclerosis: guidelines from the international panel on the diagnosis of multiple sclerosis. *Ann Neurol* 50: 121–127

17   Sormani MP, Bruzzi P, Beckmann K, Wagner K, Miller DH, Kappos L, Filippi M (2003) MRI metrics as surrogate endpoints for EDSS progression in SPMS patients treated with IFN β-1b. *Neurology* 60: 1462–1466

18   Barkhof F, Rocca M, Francis G, van Waesberghe J-HTM, Uitdehaag BMJ, Hommes OR, Hartung H-P et al (2003) Validation of diagnostic Magnetic Resonance Imaging criteria for multiple sclerosis and response to interferon β1a. *Ann Neurol* 53: 718–724

19   Miller JR (2004) The importance of early diagnosis of multiple sclerosis. *J Manage Care Pharm* 10: S4–S11

20   Biogen Idec Inc. (2004) Tysabri Description Label: http://www.fda.gov/cder/foi/label/ 2004/125104lbl.pdf. Cambridge, MA, p. 2

21   Freedman MS, Patry DG, Grand'Maison F, Myles ML, Paty DW, Selchen DH (2004) Treatment optimization in multiple sclerosis. *Can J Neurol Sci* 31: 157–168

22   Abadie E, Ethgen D, Avouac B, Buovenot G, Branco J, Bruyere O, Calvo G, Devogelear J-P et al (2004)Recommendations for the use of new methods to assess the efficacy of disease-modifying drugs in the treatment of osteoarthritis. *Osteoarthritis and Cartilage* 12: 263–268

23   US Department of Health and Human Services, Food and Drug Administration, Center for Drug Evaluation and Research (1999) Guidance for the industry. Clinical development programs for drugs, devices and biological products used in the treatment of osteoarthritis. July 1999: http://www.fda.gov/cder/guidance/2199fdt.htm (accessed May 2005)

24   European Agency for the Evaluation of Medicinal Products. Committee for Proprietary Medicinal Products (1998) Points to consider on clinical investigation of medicinal products used in the treatment of osteoarthritis. July 1998: http://www.emea.eu.int/ pdfs/human/ewp/078497en.pdf (accessed May 2005)

25   Group for the Respect of Ethics and Excellence in Sciences (GREES) (1996) Recommendations for the registration of drugs used in the treatment of osteoarthritis. *Ann Rheum Dis* 55: 552–557

26   Peterfy CG (2002) Imaging the disease process. *Curr Opin Rheum* 14: 590–596

27   Garnero P (2002) Osteoarthritis: biological markers for the future. *Joint Bone Spine* 69: 525–530

28   King KB, Lindsey CT, Dunn TC, Ries MD, Steinbach LS, Majumdar S (2004) A study of the relationship between molecular biomarkers of joint degeneration and the magnetic-resonance measured characteristics of cartilage in 16 symptomatic knees. *Mag Res Imag* 22: 1117–1123

29   The NIH Osteoarthritis initiative (2004) http://www.niams.nih.gov/ne/oi/index.htm (accessed May 2005)

30   Beck C, Shue V (2003) Surrogate decision-making and related issues. *Alz Dis Assoc Disorders* 17: S12–S16

31   Katz R (2004) Biomarker and surrogate markers: An FDA perspective. *NeuroRx* 1: 189–195

32   Mani RJ (2004) The evaluation of disease modifying therapies in Alzheimer's disease:a regulatory viewpoint. *Statistics Med* 23: 305–314

33   Lee BCP, Mintun M, Buckner RL, Morris JC (2003) Imaging of Alzheimer's disease. *J Neuroimaging* 13: 199–214

34   Barnes J, Scahill RI, Boyes RG, Frost C, Lewis EB, Rossor MN, Fox NC (2004) *Neuroimage* 23: 574–581

35   Zamrini E, De Santi S, Tolar M (2004) Imaging is superior to cognitive testing for early diagnosis of Alzheimer's disease. *Neurobiol Aging* 25: 685–691

36   Krishnan KR, Charles HC, Doraiswamy PM, Mintzer J, Weisler R, Yu X, Perdomo C, Ieni JR, Rogers S (2003) Randomized, placebo-controlled trial of the effects of donepezil on neuronal markers and hippocampal volumes in Alzheimer's disease. *Am J Psychiatr* 160: 2003–2011

37   Gill SS, Rochon PA, Guttman M, Laupacis A (2003) The value of positron emission tomography in the clinical evaluation of dementia. *J Am Geriatr Soc* 51: 251–264

38   Centers for Medicare and Medicare Services (2004) Decision Memo for Positron Emission Tomography (FDG) and Other Neuroimaging Devices for Suspected Dementia (CAG-00088R): http://www.cms.hhs.gov/mcd/viewdecisionmemo.asp?id=104 (accessed May 2005)

39   Horsfield MA, Jones DK (2002) Applications of diffusion-weighted and diffusion tensor MRI to white matter diseases – a review. *NMR Biomed* 15: 570–577

40   Giesel FL, Hempel A, Schonknecht P, Wustenberg T, Weber MA, Schroder J, Essig M (2003) Functional magnetic resonance imaging and dementia. *Radiologe* 43: 558–561

41   Peripheral and Central Nervous System Advisory Committee, US Department of Health and Human Services, Food and Drug Administration, Center for Drug Evaluation and Research (2002) Meeting of the Advisory Committee, November 18, 2002 Gaithersburg, Maryland: www.fda.gov/ohrms/dockets/ac/02/transcripts/3907T1.htm (accessed May 2005)

42   Schachter G (2004) NeuroTherapeutics: Trials and Tribulations. http://www.drugandmarket.com/default.asp?section=feature&article=041604 (accessed May 2005)

43   Department of Health and Human Services, Food and Drug Administration (2004) Innovation/Stagnation – Challenge and Opportunity on the Critical Path to New Medical Products: http://www.fda.gov/oc/initiatives/criticalpath/whitepaper.html, p. 23. (accessed May 2005)

44   Molenberghs G, Burzykowski T, Alonso A, Buyse M (2004) A perspective on surrogate endpoints in controlled clinical trials. *Stat Methods Med Res* 13: 177–206

45   Berger VW (2004) Does the Prentice criterion validate surrogate endpoints? *Stat Med* 23: 1571–1578

46   Baker SG, Kramer BS (2003) A perfect correlate does not a surrogate make. *BMC Med Res Methodol* 3: 16–21

47   Colburn WA, Lee JW (2003) Biomarkers, validation and pharmacokinetic-pharmacodynamic modelling. *Clin Pharmacokinet* 42: 997–1022

48   Buyse M, Molenberghs G, Burzykowski T, Renard D, Geys H (2000) The validation of surrogate endpoints in meta-analyses of randomized experiments. *Biostatistics* 1: 49–67

49   Stockbridge H, Hardy RI, Glueck CJ (1989) Public cholesterol screening: motivation for

participation, follow-up outcome, self-knowledge, and coronary heart disease risk factor intervention. *J Lab Clin Med* 114: 142–151

50   Burton TM (2004) Two simple tests can prevent stroke, but few get them. *Wall St. Journal* 244(60): A1

51   Blankenhorn DH, Hodis HN (1994) George Lyman Duff Memorial Lecture. Arterial imaging and atherosclerosis reversal. *Arterioscler Thromb* 14: 177–192

52   Glagov S, Bassiouny HS, Giddens DP, Zarins CK (1995) Pathobiology of plaque modeling and complication. *Surg Clin North Am* 75: 545–556

53   Kastelein JP, de Groot E, and Sankatsing R (2004) Atherosclerosis measured by B-Mode ultrasonography: effect of statin therapy on disease progression. *Am J Med* 116, S1: 31–36

54   O'Leary DH, Polak JF (2002) Intima-media thickness: a tool for atherosclerosis imaging and event prediction. *Am J Cardiol* 90: 18L–21L

55   Guedes A, Tardif JC (2004) Intravascular ultrasound assessment of atherosclerosis. *Curr Atheroscler Rep* 6: 219–224

56   Plutzky J (1999) Atherosclerotic plaque rupture: emerging insights and opportunities. *Am J Cardiol* 84: 15J–20J

57   Raggi P, James G (2004) Coronary calcium screening and coronary risk stratification. *Curr Atheroscler Rep* 6: 107–111

58   James G, Raggi P (2004) Electron beam tomography as a non invasive method to monitor effectiveness of antiatherosclerotic therapy. *Curr Drug Targets Cardiovasc Haematol Disord* 4: 177–181

59   Yuan C, Kerwin WS (2004) MRI of atherosclerosis. Magn Reson Imaging 19: 710–719

60   Yuan C, Miller ZE, Cai J, Hatsukami T (2002) Carotid atherosclerotic wall imaging by MRI. *Neuroimaging Clin N Am* 12: 391–401, vi

61   Fuster V (2001) Advances in the diagnosis of arterial disease by magnetic resonance imaging. *Rev Esp Cardiol* 54, Suppl 1: 2–7

62   Achenbach S, Daniel WG (2004) Imaging of coronary atherosclerosis using computed tomography: current status and future directions. *Curr Atheroscler Rep* 6: 213–218

63   Davies JR, Rudd JH, Weissberg PL (2004) Molecular and metabolic imaging of atherosclerosis. *J Nucl Med* 45: 1898–1907

64   Moreno PR, Muller JE (2003) Detection of high-risk atherosclerotic coronary plaques by intravascular spectroscopy. *J Interv Cardiol* 16: 243–252

65   Isaacsohn JL, Troendle AJ, Orloff DG (2004) Regulatory Issues in the Approval of new drugs for diabetes mellitus, dyslipidemia, and the metabolic syndrome. *Am J Cardiol* 93: 49C–52C

66   Committee for Medicinal Products for Human Use (2003) Note for guidance on clinical investigation of medicinal products in the treatment of lipid disorders. http://www.emea.eu.int/pdfs/human/ewp/302003en.pdf#search='CPMP/EWP/3020/03' (accessed May 2005)

67   Food & Drug Administration (1997) Food and Drug Administration Modernization Act. Section 121 and 122. http://www.fda.gov/cder/fdama/ (accessed May 2005)

68   Food & Drug Administration, Center for Drug Evaluation and Research (2002) Current Good Manufacturing Practice for Positron Emission Tomography Drugs. http://www.fda.gov/cder/fdama/cgmpdpr.pdf (accessed May 2005)

69   Food & Drug Administration, Center for Drug Evaluation and Research (2004) Guidance for Industry. Developing Medical Imaging Drugs and Biological Products. Part 1: Con-

ducting Safety Assessments. http://www.fda.gov/cder/guidance/5742prt1.pdf (accessed May 2005)

70   Food & Drug Administration, Center for Drug Evaluation and Research (2004) Guidance for Industry. Developing Medical Imaging Drugs and Biological Products. Part 2: Clinical Indications. http://www.fda.gov/cder/guidance/5742prt2.pdf (accessed May 2005)

71   Food & Drug Administration, Center for Drug Evaluation and Research (2004) Guidance for Industry. Developing Medical Imaging Drugs and Biological Products. Part 3: Design, Analysis and Interpretation of Clinical Studies. http://www.fda.gov/cder/guidance/5742prt3.pdf (accessed May 2005)

72   Seddon BM, Workman P (2003) The role of functional and molecular imaging in cancer drug discovery and development. *Br J Radiol* 76, Spec No 2: S128–138

73   Roselt P, Meikle S, Kassiou M (2004) The role of positron emission tomography in the discovery and development of new drugs; as studied in laboratory animals. *Eur J Drug Metab Pharmacokinet* 29: 1–6

74   Cherry SR (2001) Fundamentals of positron emission tomography and applications in preclinical drug development. *J Clin Pharmacol* 41: 482–491

75   Bergstrom M, Grahnen A, Langstrom B (2003) Positron emission tomography microdosing: a new concept with application in tracer and early clinical drug development. *Eur J Clin Pharmacol* 59 :357–366

76   Mandl SJ, Mari C, Edinger M, Negrin RS, Tait JF, Contag CH, Blankenberg FG (2004) Multi-modality imaging identifies key times for annexin V imaging as an early predictor of therapeutic outcome. *Mol Imaging* 3: 1–8

77   Blasberg RG, Gelovani J (2002) Molecular-genetic imaging: a nuclear medicine-based perspective. Mol Imaging 1: 280–300

78   Macapinlac HA (2004) FDG PET and PET/CT imaging in lymphoma and melanoma. *Cancer J* 10: 262–270

79   Brownell AL, Chen YI, Yu M, Wang X, Dedeoglu A, Cicchetti F, Jenkins BG, Beal MF (2004) 3-Nitropropionic acid-induced neurotoxicity--assessed by ultra high resolution positron emission tomography with comparison to magnetic resonance spectroscopy. *J Neurochem* 89: 1206–1214

80   Lester DS, Lyon RC, McGregor GN, Engelhardt RT, Schmued LC, Johnson GA, Johannessen JN (1999) 3-Dimensional visualization of lesions in rat brain using magnetic resonance imaging microscopy. *Neuroreport* 10: 737–741

81   Qiao M, Malisza KL, Del Bigio MR, Kozlowski P, Seshia SS, Tuor UI (2000) Effect of long-term vigabatrin administration on the immature rat brain. *Epilepsia* 41: 655–665

82   Guberman A, Bruni J (2000) Long-term open multicentre, add-on trial of vigabatrin in adult resistant partial epilepsy. The Canadian Vigabatrin Study Group. *Seizure* 9: 112–118

83   Kartachova M, Haas RL, Olmos RA, Hoebers FJ, van Zandwijk N, Verheij M (2004) *In vivo* imaging of apoptosis by 99mTc-Annexin V scintigraphy: visual analysis in relation to treatment response. *Radiother Oncol* 72: 333–339

84   Cook GJ (2003) Oncological molecular imaging: nuclear medicine techniques. *Br J Radiol* 76, Spec No 2: S152–158

85   Pogge A, Slikker W Jr (2004) Neuroimaging: new approaches for neurotoxicology. *Neurotoxicology* 25: 525–531

Index

The PDR-Series
Progress in Drug Research

Progress in Drug Research is a prestigious book series which provides extensive expert-written reviews on highly topical areas in current pharmaceutical and pharmacological research.

Founded in 1959 by Ernst Jucker, the series moved from its initial focus on medicinal chemistry to a much wider scope. Today it encompasses all fields concerned with the development of new therapeutic drugs and the elucidation of their mechanisms of action, reflecting the increasingly complex nature of modern drug research. Invited authors present their biological, chemical, biochemical, physiological, immunological, pharmaceutical, toxicological, pharmacological and clinical expertise in carefully written reviews and provide the newcomer and the specialist alike with an up-to-date list of prime references.

Starting with volume 61, *Progress in Drug Research* is continued as a series of monographs.

Forthcoming titles:

Unbiased Approaches to Drug Target Finding and Validation (PDR 64), D. Jeffery (Editor), 2006
Systems Biological Approaches in Infectious Diseases (PDR 65), H.I. Boshoff (Editor), 2006

Available volumes:

Advances in Targeted Cancer Therapy (PDR 63), R. M. Schultz (Editor), 2005
Peptide Transport and Delivery into the Central Nervous System (PDR 61), L. Prokai,
    K. Prokai-Tatrai (Editors), 2003
Progress in Drug Research, volumes 1–60, E. Jucker (Editor), 1959–2003